Modern Methods for Epidemiology

Yu-Kang Tu · Darren C. Greenwood
Editors

Modern Methods for Epidemiology

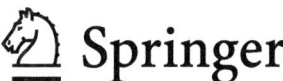

Editors
Yu-Kang Tu
Division of Biostatistics
Leeds Institute of Genetics
Health and Therapeutics
University of Leeds
Leeds, UK

Darren C. Greenwood
Division of Biostatistics
Leeds Institute of Genetics
Health and Therapeutics
University of Leeds
Leeds, UK

ISBN 978-94-007-3023-6   ISBN 978-94-007-3024-3 (eBook)
DOI 10.1007/978-94-007-3024-3
Springer Dordrecht Heidelberg New York London

Library of Congress Control Number: 2012934174

© Springer Science+Business Media Dordrecht 2012
This work is subject to copyright. All rights are reserved by the Publisher, whether the whole or part of the material is concerned, specifically the rights of translation, reprinting, reuse of illustrations, recitation, broadcasting, reproduction on microfilms or in any other physical way, and transmission or information storage and retrieval, electronic adaptation, computer software, or by similar or dissimilar methodology now known or hereafter developed. Exempted from this legal reservation are brief excerpts in connection with reviews or scholarly analysis or material supplied specifically for the purpose of being entered and executed on a computer system, for exclusive use by the purchaser of the work. Duplication of this publication or parts thereof is permitted only under the provisions of the Copyright Law of the Publisher's location, in its current version, and permission for use must always be obtained from Springer. Permissions for use may be obtained through RightsLink at the Copyright Clearance Center. Violations are liable to prosecution under the respective Copyright Law.
The use of general descriptive names, registered names, trademarks, service marks, etc. in this publication does not imply, even in the absence of a specific statement, that such names are exempt from the relevant protective laws and regulations and therefore free for general use.
While the advice and information in this book are believed to be true and accurate at the date of publication, neither the authors nor the editors nor the publisher can accept any legal responsibility for any errors or omissions that may be made. The publisher makes no warranty, express or implied, with respect to the material contained herein.

Printed on acid-free paper

Springer is part of Springer Science+Business Media (www.springer.com)

Preface

Statistical methods are important tools for scientific research to extract information from data. Some statistical methods are simple whilst others are more complex, but without such methods our data are just numbers and useless to our understanding of the world we are living in. In epidemiology, researchers use more advanced and complex statistical methods than colleagues who work with experimental data, often under more controlled conditions than can be achieved with the larger datasets and more "real-life" conditions required by observational data. The issues of observational data are not just about the amount of data but also the quality of data. Epidemiological data usually contains missing values in some variables for some patients, and the instruments used for data collection may be less accurate or precise than those used for experimental data. Therefore, textbooks of epidemiology often contain much discussion of statistical methods for dealing with those problems in analysis and interpretation of data, and very often they also contain some discussion of the philosophy of science. This is because elaborating causes and their consequences from observational data usually requires certain epistemological theories about what constitutes "causes" and "effects".

Routine applications of advanced statistical methods on real data have become possible in the last 10 years because desktop computers have become much more powerful and cheaper. However, proper understanding of the challenging statistical theory behind those methods remains essential for correct application and interpretation, and rarely seen in the medical literature. This textbook contains a general introduction to those modern statistical methods that are becoming more important in epidemiological research, to provide a starting point for those who are new to epidemiology, and for those looking for guidance in more modern statistical approaches. For those who wish to pursue these methods in greater depth, we provide annotated lists of further reading material, which we hope are useful for epidemiological researchers who wish to overcome the mathematical barrier of applying those methods to their research.

The Centre for Epidemiology and Biostatistics at the University of Leeds, United Kingdom, where we have been working for many years, has a masters degree programme in the field of Statistical Epidemiology, aiming to provide a unique opportunity for researchers to obtain further training in both epidemiology and statistics. Several modules in the programme teach statistical methods that are not discussed in standard textbooks of epidemiology or biostatistics. For example, very few textbooks of epidemiology discuss multilevel modelling, whilst very few textbooks of biostatistics discuss confounding using Directed Acyclic Graphs (DAGs). Here we bring these two important topics in modern epidemiology together in the same book. For topics such as G-estimation, latent class analysis, regression trees, or generalised additive modelling, students have previously had to dig into monographs or journal articles for those methods, which are usually aimed at more advanced readers. We feel that there is a need for a textbook that can be used for teaching modern, advanced statistical methods to postgraduate students studying epidemiology and biostatistics and also a good source of self-learning for researchers in epidemiology and medicine. We therefore invited colleagues from Leeds, Bristol, Cambridge and London in the United Kingdom, and colleagues in Denmark and South Africa, all leading experts in their respective fields, to contribute to writing this book.

This volume contains 17 chapters dedicated to modern statistical methods for epidemiology. The opening chapter starts with the most important, but also the most controversial concept in epidemiology: confounding. Before the introduction of DAGs into epidemiology, the definition of confounding was sometimes confusing and deficient. Graham Law and his co-authors provide an overview of DAGs and show why DAGs are so useful in statistical reasoning surrounding the potentially causal relationships in observational research. Chapter 2 discusses another troubling issue in observational research: incomplete data or missing data. James Carpenter and his colleagues provide an overview of incomplete data problems in biomedical research and various strategies for imputing missing values. At the heart of all epidemiology is an appropriate assessment of exposure. Chapter 3 discusses this problem of measurement error in epidemiological exposures. Darren Greenwood provides a concise introduction to the problems caused by measurement error and outlines some potential solutions that have been suggested. Chapter 4 discusses the issue of selection bias in epidemiology, a particular problem in the context of case-control studies. Graham Law and his co-authors use DAGs as a tool to explain how this problem affects the results of observational studies and how it may be resolved.

Chapter 5 discusses multilevel modelling for clustered data, a methodology also widely used in social sciences research. Andrew Blance provides an overview of the basic principles of multilevel models where random effects are assumed to follow a normal distribution. In Chap. 6, Mark Gilthorpe and his co-authors discuss the issues of outcomes formed from a mixture of distributions and use zero-inflated models as an example. Chapter 7 can be seen as an extension of Chaps. 5 and 6. Wendy Harrison and her co-authors discuss scenarios where the assumption that random effects follow a normal distribution is not appropriate, instead assuming a discrete distribution, describing discrete components that can be viewed as latent classes. Chapters 8 and 9 both discuss Bayesian approach for sparse data, where observations of events are scattered in space or time, Chap. 8 discussing bivariate disease mapping and Chap. 9 discussing multivariate survival mapping models. Samuel Manda and Richard Feltbower use data from the Yorkshire region in the United Kingdom and from the South Africa to illustrate these approaches. In Chap. 10, Darren Greenwood discusses meta-analysis of observational data. This is more complex than meta-analysis of randomised controlled trials because of greater heterogeneity in design, analysis, and reporting of outcome and exposure variables. Methods and software packages available to deal with those issues are discussed.

Chapter 11 returns to the concepts introduced in the opening chapters, focusing on the resemblance between DAGs and path diagrams. Yu-Kang Tu explains how to translate regression models into both DAGs and path diagrams and how those graphical presentations can inform us the causal relations in the data. Chapter 12 discusses latent growth curve modelling, which is equivalent to multilevel modelling for longitudinal data analysis. Yu-Kang Tu and Francesco D'Auito use a dataset from Periodontology to illustrate the flexibility of latent growth curve modelling in accommodating nonlinear growth trajectories. These ideas are extended in Chap. 13 by allowing random effects to follow a discrete distribution. Darren Dahly shows how growth mixture modelling can be used to uncover distinctive early growth trajectories, which may be associated with increased disease risk in later life. Chapter 14 focuses on the problem of time-varying confounding, and Kate Tilling and her colleagues explain how G-estimation may be used to overcome it.

Chapter 15 discusses generalised additive modelling for exploring non-linear associations between variables. Robert West gives a concise introduction to this complex method and shows how it can be extended to multivariable models. He then continues to explain regression trees and other advanced methods for classification of variables in Chap. 16. These methods have become popular in biomedical research for modelling decision-making. In the final chapter, Mark Gilthorpe and David Clayton discuss the intricate issues surrounding statistical and biological interaction. They use the example of gene-environment interaction to show that statistical interactions and biological interactions are different concepts and much confusion arises where the former is used to describe the latter.

Editing this book has been an exciting experience, and we would like to thank all the authors for their excellent contributions. We also want to thank Dr Brian Cattle for his help with the preparation of the book and our editors in Springer for their patience with this project.

Leeds, UK   Yu-Kang Tu
                                                   Darren C. Greenwood

Contents

1. **Confounding and Causal Path Diagrams**..................... 1
   Graham R. Law, Rosie Green, and George T.H. Ellison

2. **Statistical Modelling of Partially Observed Data Using Multiple Imputation: Principles and Practice** 15
   James R. Carpenter, Harvey Goldstein, and Michael G. Kenward

3. **Measurement Errors in Epidemiology**............................. 33
   Darren C. Greenwood

4. **Selection Bias in Epidemiologic Studies** 57
   Graham R. Law, Paul D. Baxter, and Mark S. Gilthorpe

5. **Multilevel Modelling** 73
   Andrew Blance

6. **Modelling Data That Exhibit an Excess Number of Zeros: Zero-Inflated Models and Generic Mixture Models**................ 93
   Mark S. Gilthorpe, Morten Frydenberg, Yaping Cheng, and Vibeke Baelum

7. **Multilevel Latent Class Modelling** 117
   Wendy Harrison, Robert M. West, Amy Downing, and Mark S. Gilthorpe

8. **Bayesian Bivariate Disease Mapping** 141
   Richard G. Feltbower and Samuel O.M. Manda

9. **A Multivariate Random Frailty Effects Model for Multiple Spatially Dependent Survival Data**..................... 157
   Samuel O.M. Manda, Richard G. Feltbower, and Mark S. Gilthorpe

10. **Meta-analysis of Observational Studies** 173
    Darren C. Greenwood

11	Directed Acyclic Graphs and Structural Equation Modelling......	191
	Yu-Kang Tu	
12	Latent Growth Curve Models...	205
	Yu-Kang Tu and Francesco D'Auito	
13	Growth Mixture Modelling for Life Course Epidemiology.........	223
	Darren L. Dahly	
14	G-estimation for Accelerated Failure Time Models..................	243
	Kate Tilling, Jonathan A.C. Sterne, and Vanessa Didelez	
15	Generalised Additive Models...	261
	Robert M. West	
16	Regression and Classification Trees..	279
	Robert M. West	
17	Statistical Interactions and Gene-Environment Joint Effects.......	291
	Mark S. Gilthorpe and David G. Clayton	
Index..		313

Contributors

Vibeke Baelum School of Dentistry, Faculty of Health Sciences, University of Aarhus, Aarhus, Denmark

Paul D. Baxter Division of Biostatistics, Centre for Epidemiology and Biostatistics, Leeds Institute of Genetics, Health & Therapeutics, University of Leeds, Leeds, UK

Andrew Blance Division of Biostatistics, Centre for Epidemiology and Biostatistics, Leeds Institute of Genetics, Health & Therapeutics, University of Leeds, Leeds, UK

James R. Carpenter Department of Medical Statistics Unit, London School of Hygiene and Tropical Medicine, London, UK

Yaping Cheng Division of Biostatistics, Centre for Epidemiology and Biostatistics, Leeds Institute of Genetics, Health & Therapeutics, University of Leeds, Leeds, UK

David G. Clayton Juvenile Diabetes Research Foundation/Wellcome Trust Diabetes and Inflammation Laboratory, Cambridge University, Cambridge, UK

Francesco D'Auito Department of Periodontology, Eastman Dental Institute, University College London, London, UK

Darren L. Dahly Division of Biostatistics, Centre for Epidemiology and Biostatistics, Leeds Institute of Genetics, Health & Therapeutics, University of Leeds, Leeds, UK

Vanessa Didelez School of Mathematics, University of Bristol, Bristol, UK

Amy Downing Cancer Epidemiology Group, Centre for Epidemiology and Biostatistics, University of Leeds, Leeds, UK

George T.H. Ellison Division of Biostatistics, Centre for Epidemiology and Biostatistics, Leeds Institute of Genetics, Health & Therapeutics, University of Leeds, Leeds, UK

Richard G. Feltbower Division of Epidemiology, Centre for Epidemiology and Biostatistics, Leeds Institute of Genetics, Health & Therapeutics, University of Leeds, Leeds, UK

Morten Frydenberg Department of Biostatistics, Faculty of Health Sciences, Institute of Public Health, University of Aarhus, Aarhus, Denmark

Mark S. Gilthorpe Division of Biostatistics, Centre for Epidemiology and Biostatistics, Leeds Institute of Genetics, Health & Therapeutics, University of Leeds, Leeds, UK

Harvey Goldstein Medical Statistics Unit, London School of Hygiene and Tropical Medicine, London, UK

Graduate School of Education, University of Bristol, Bristol, UK

Rosie Green Department of Nutrition and Public Health Intervention Research, London School of Hygiene and Tropical Medicine, London, UK

Darren C. Greenwood Division of Biostatistics, Centre for Epidemiology and Biostatistics, Leeds Institute of Genetics, Health & Therapeutics, University of Leeds, Leeds, UK

Wendy Harrison Division of Biostatistics, Centre for Epidemiology and Biostatistics, Leeds Institute of Genetics, Health & Therapeutics, University of Leeds, Leeds, UK

Michael G. Kenward Department of Medical Statistics Unit, London School of Hygiene and Tropical Medicine, London, UK

Graham R. Law Division of Biostatistics, Centre for Epidemiology and Biostatistics, Leeds Institute of Genetics, Health & Therapeutics, University of Leeds, Leeds, UK

Samuel O.M. Manda Biostatistics Unit, South Africa Medical Research Council, Pretoria, South Africa

Jonathan A.C. Sterne School of Social and Community Medicine, University of Bristol, Bristol, UK

Kate Tilling School of Social and Community Medicine, University of Bristol, Bristol, UK

Yu-Kang Tu Division of Biostatistics, Centre for Epidemiology and Biostatistics, Faculty of Medicine and Health, Leeds Institute of Genetics, Health & Therapeutics, University of Leeds, Leeds, UK

Robert M. West Division of Biostatistics, Centre for Epidemiology and Biostatistics, Leeds Institute of Genetics, Health & Therapeutics, University of Leeds, Leeds, UK

Chapter 1
Confounding and Causal Path Diagrams

Graham R. Law, Rosie Green, and George T.H. Ellison

1.1 Causal Models

The issue of causation is a challenging one for epidemiologists. Politicians and the public want to know whether something of concern causes a disease or influences the effectiveness of healthcare services. However, the training provided to statisticians, and to scientists more generally, tends to stress that non-experimental research will only ever offer evidence for association and that suitably designed experimental studies are required to offer robust evidence of causation. In the real world, where experimental data are rare, difficult or impossible to produce, the extent to which associations between variables can and should be interpreted as evidence of causality is less a technical question than a philosophical, moral, cultural or political one. These issues have been discussed at some length elsewhere (see for example Susser 1973; and Pearl 1998, 2000), and although these influence the extent to which associational evidence from non-experimental studies is (and should be) used in real-world settings, the following Chapter will focus on the more technical issue of strengthening the causal inferences drawn from non-experimental data by using causal path diagrams when designing and describing the analysis of data from non-experimental studies. In this chapter we will introduce causal path diagrams (specifically Directed Acyclic Graphs; DAGs) and explore the issue of confounding.

G.R. Law (✉) • G.T.H. Ellison
Division of Biostatistics, Centre for Epidemiology and Biostatistics, Leeds Institute of Genetics, Health & Therapeutics, University of Leeds, Room 8.01, Worsley Building, LS2 9LN Leeds, UK
e-mail: g.r.law@leeds.ac.uk

R. Green
Department of Nutrition and Public Health Intervention Research, London School of Hygiene and Tropical Medicine, London, UK

1.1.1 Directed Acyclic Diagrams (DAGs), Nomenclature and Notation

A causal path diagram is a visual summary of the likely (and, where relevant, the speculative) causal links between variables. Constructing these diagrams is based on *a priori* knowledge and, in the case of speculative and hypothesised relationships being explored in the analysis, on conjecture. Causal path diagrams have been used informally for many years in causal analysis and in recent years have been formally developed for use in expert-systems research (Greenland et al. 1999). Although such diagrams are beginning to be adopted by the epidemiological community (Hoggart et al. 2003; Hernandez-Dìaz et al. 2006; Shrier and Platt 2008; Head et al. 2008, 2009; Geneletti et al. 2011; Tu and Gilthorpe 2012), a causal diagram is still a novel epidemiological tool which can be used in a variety of ways: to think clearly about how exposure, disease and potential confounder variables, relevant to the research hypothesis, are related to each other; to communicate these inter-relationships to academic and professional audiences; to indicate which variables were important to measure; and to inform the statistical modelling process – particularly the identification of confounding, confounders and competing exposures.

In this Chapter we discuss the use of causal path diagrams (Pearl 2000), specifically Directed Acyclic Graphs (DAGs), to develop models that can inform the analysis of one variable (the 'exposure') as a potential cause of another (the 'outcome'). Within epidemiology, such analyses include exploring: the potential role of risk factors (as 'exposures') in the aetiology of disease (where the 'outcome' is the prevalence, incidence or severity of disease); and the role of specific characteristics of healthcare systems (where these characteristics are the 'exposures') in the effective and efficient delivery of health services (where this constitutes the 'outcome').

1.1.1.1 Nomenclature and the Construction of DAGs

The nomenclature of DAGs is still evolving, and can be off-putting to the uninitiated, particularly when accompanied by statistical notation (such as that developed by Geneletti et al. (2009)). However, the terminology that is developing helps to specify each of the components of DAGs in a way that facilitates their consistent application and further utility. And, with this in mind, we have provided a comprehensive glossary of terms in Table 1.1, and a more detailed explanation of these below.

Nodes, Arcs and Directed Arcs

In statistical parlance, each variable in a DAG is represented by a *node* (also known as a *vertex*), and relationships between two variables are depicted by a line connecting the nodes, called an *arc* (or alternatively an *edge* or a *line*). A *directed arc* indicates

1 Confounding and Causal Path Diagrams

Table 1.1 Glossary of terms for causal diagrams

Term	Description
Ancestor	A variable that causes another variable in a *causal path* in which there are intermediary variables situated along the *causal/direct path* between them
Arc	A line with one arrow that connects two *nodes* (synonymous with *edge* and *line*)
Backdoor path	A path that goes against the direction of the *arc* on the path, but can then follow or oppose the direction of any subsequent *arc*
Blocked path	A path that contains at least one *collider*
Causal path	A path that follows the direction of the *arcs* (synonymous with *direct path*)
Child	A variable that is directly affected by another variable, with no intermediary variables situated along the *causal path* between them
Collider	A variable that a *path* both enters and exits via *arcs*
Descendant	A variable that is caused by one or more preceding variables in a direct *causal path* in which there is one or more intermediary variables situated along the *causal path* between them
Direct path	A path that follows the direction of the *arcs* (synonymous with *causal path*)
Directed arc	An arrow between two variables that indicates a known, likely or speculative causal relationship between them
Edge	A line with one arrow that connects two *nodes* (synonymous with *arc* and *line*)
Line	A line with one arrow that connects two *nodes* (synonymous with *arc* and *edge*)
Node	A point within the diagram which denotes a variable, such as the (key) exposure variable of interest, the (key) outcome (of interest), and another covariates (synonymous with *vertex*)
Parent	A variable that directly affects another variable, with no intermediary variables situated along the *causal path* between them
Path	An unbroken route between two variables, in either direction (synonymous with *route*)
Route	An unbroken route between two variables, in either direction (synonymous with *path*)
Unblocked path	A *path* that does not contain a *collider*
Vertex	A point within the diagram which denotes a variable, such as the (key) exposure variable of interest, the (key) outcome (of interest), and another covariates (synonymous with *vertex*)

known (i.e. from a firm grasp of established functional biological, social or clinical relationships between variables); *likely* (i.e. from previous robust empirical studies); or *speculative* (i.e. hypothesised) relationships between any two variables, with an arrow representing causality – the direction of causality following in the direction of the arrow. For example, 'X causes Y' would be represented as $X \rightarrow Y$, where X and Y are nodes (or vertices) and the arrow between them is an arc (or edge or line).

Parents, Children, Ancestors and Descendants

DAGs are usually depicted with the nodes arranged in a temporal and thus causal sequence, with the preceding variables to the left of the diagram and subsequent variables to the right. This is not mandatory, but can help when deciding which of two closely related variables precedes the other and acts as its cause. A node immediately preceding another node to which it is connected (i.e. a node at the non-arrow end of an arc) is known as a *parent* of the node at the arrow end of the arc, which is in turn known as a *child*. Thus, in the example $X \rightarrow Y$, X is the parent node and Y is the child. Similarly, a node 'preceding' another node but connected to another node via at least one other node is known as an *ancestor,* whereas the preceding node from which it is separated is known as a *descendent*. Therefore, in the example $X \rightarrow Y \rightarrow Z$, X is the ancestor of Z, and Z is the descendent of X; while Y (which is a child of X and a parent of Z) lies on the causal pathway between X and Z.

Directed Paths, Backdoor Paths, Colliders and Blocked Paths

A *path* is the sequence of arcs connecting two or more nodes, thus $X \rightarrow Y \rightarrow Z$ is the path (or route) connecting the nodes X and Z. A *direct* (or *causal*) *path* is one where the arcs all follow in the direction of causality. In contrast, a *backdoor path* is where one exits a node along an arc pointing into it, against the causal direction, to another node across any number of arcs pointing in either direction. For example, when $X \leftarrow Z \rightarrow Y$ backdoor path exists between X and Y via Z. A node becomes a *collider* where both arcs of the path entering and leaving the node have arrows pointing into it. For example, Y is a collider when $X \rightarrow Y \leftarrow Z$ and a path is *blocked* if it contains at least one collider. A *directed acyclic graph* occurs if no directed path forms a closed loop, reflecting the assumption that that no variable can cause itself (an assumption that may limit the utility of DAGs for modelling functional processes containing positive or negative feedback loops).

Identification of Arcs

All arcs in a DAG reflect *a priori* presumptions about cause and effect in a specific context. Some of these presumptions will be based on *known* causal relationships between variables (drawing on established functional biological, social and clinical processes); others on *likely* causal relationships (drawing, for example, on the statistical findings of previous robust empirical studies); as well as speculative relationships (drawing on unsubstantiated hypotheses – including the specific hypotheses being tested in the analyses). These arc-related presumptions cannot (and should not) be inferred empirically from data on which the analyses will be conducted, but must be drawn from established mechanisms or strong research evidence, both of which are crucial for developing an accurate DAG as the basis on which suitable statistical analyses can then be designed (Tu et al. 2004; Weinberg 2005; Tu and Githorpe 2012).

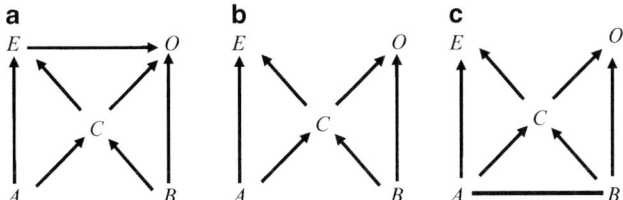

Fig. 1.1 An example of Directed Acyclic Graphs. Key to variables: E exposure, O outcome, A, B, C additional

1.1.1.2 Notation

An additional technical approach to represent the statistical relationships between variables (as nodes) in causal path diagrams is to use the notation developed by Geneletti et al. (2009). For example, the notation $A \perp\!\!\!\perp B | C$ signifies A as being independent of B given C, where A, B and C are known variables. For example the DAG represented in Fig. 1.1 consists of 5 variables: E the exposure of interest, O the outcome of interest and 3 other additional variables A, B, and C.

In Fig. 1.1a the exposure, E, causes the outcome, O. This can be represented as

$$O \not\!\perp\!\!\!\perp E$$

1.1.2 The Speculative Nature of DAGs and Their Limitations

In most research studies the causal pathways described and summarised within causal path diagrams are not established (i.e. 'proven') causal relationships, but are in the main based on evidence from whatever previous studies are available. Proof in this context is essentially more of a philosophical than a scientific concept, and can be subject to intense debate. The pathways included in the diagrams are therefore often based on: (i) incomplete or predominantly theoretical understanding (rather than established knowledge) of the functional relationships between the variables involved; (ii) the statistical findings of empirical research which may not themselves be definitive; and (iii) hypotheses based on putative, tentative or speculative beliefs about the sorts of relationships that exist – not least the one between the exposure(s) and the outcomes that the study set out to address. These three very different ingredients involved in the conceptualisation of causal pathways are important to recognise as they influence both: the extent to which different causal path diagrams can be drawn for the same variables (reflecting different views of what is *known*, *likely* or *speculative*) and the extent to which these different diagrams might be more (or less) useful for generating robust evidence of causality between two or more specific variables. Despite this DAGs are useful because they force researchers to make explicit their presumptions about the relationships between pairs of variables, whether or not these presumptions prove to be correct. Other analysts are then able to critique, (re)interpret and (where necessary) repeat and improve on the analyses conducted, based on different presumptions or firmer knowledge of the causal relationships involved.

However, alongside their assumption that no variable can be its own cause (which, as mentioned earlier, reduces the utility of DAGs for modelling systems containing feedback loops), a key limitation of DAGs is that they will only ever be able to include variables (as nodes) that are (as Donald Rumsfeld would have it) 'knowns' (i.e. are recognised as conceptual entities within the epistemological context concerned). Likewise, analyses based on DAGs will only ever be able to include those variables for which data are available (i.e. that have been measured – in Donald Rumsfeld's parlance, 'known knowns'). This is a fundamental limitation of all analyses of data from non-randomised non-experimental studies, not least because unknown or unmeasured confounders cannot be taken into account when modelling or analysing potential causal relationships. Nonetheless, using DAGs to identify the most appropriate statistical analyses for any given set of measured variables will reduce the likelihood that these are subject to confounding (from known and measured confounders) and help others to critique, (re)interpret and (where necessary and possible) repeat and improve on the analyses conducted. These then are the core strengths of using DAGs to design the analysis of data from non-experimental studies – strengths we explore in greater detail in Sect. 1.2.4, below.

Meanwhile, another potential limitation of DAGs is that, despite the potential for visual complexity (particularly for those DAGs with more than a handful of nodes), they are essentially an oversimplification of the causal relationships between variables. For example, a causal diagram does not indicate whether an effect is harmful or protective or whether effect modification is actually occurring (Hernan et al. 2004 – although Weinberg 2007 recently suggested how DAGs might be modified to include this), nor does a causal diagram identify whether a cause is sufficient or necessary to elicit the outcome(s) involved (Rothman 1976). Nonetheless, it bears restating that one of the key strengths of such diagrams is that they enable researchers to think clearly and logically about the research question at hand, and to make explicit any presumptions that are being made about the (presumed) relationships between the pairs of variables involved. This visual summary can then be used as an aid to communicate these inter-relationships to academic and professional audiences and to explicitly identify, for example, if important variables or relationships are missing from or misrepresented in the diagram or, indeed, whether any of the presumed relationships are contentious.

1.1.3 Notation

One way to represent the statistical relationships between variables (as nodes) in causal diagrams is to use the notation developed by Geneletti and colleagues (2009). For example, the notation $A \perp\!\!\!\perp B|C$ signifies A is independent of B given C, where A, B and C are known variables. For example the DAG represented in Fig. 1.1 consists of 5 variables: E the exposure of interest, O the outcome of interest and 3 other additional variables A, B, and C.

In Fig. 1.1a the exposure, E, causes the outcome, O. This can be represented as

$$O \not\!\perp\!\!\!\perp E$$

A common practice in epidemiology is to consider other covariates at the same time as the exposure. For example, these might include a measure of socio-economic status, age or sex.

1.2 Confounding and Confounders

Confounding is a central concept in epidemiological research. It is a process that can generate biased results when examining the association between exposure and outcome. Historically there have been many definitions of confounding, but they may be divided broadly into two main types: "comparability-based" and "collapsibility-based" (Greenland and Robins 1986):

- In terms of the "comparability-based" definition, confounding is said to occur when there are differences in outcome in the unexposed and exposed populations that are not due to the exposure, but are due to other variables that may be referred to as 'confounders'. This results in bias in the estimate of the effect of a particular exposure on a particular outcome (McNamee 2003).
- In terms of the "collapsibility-based" definition, confounding may be: (i) reduced by adjusting the data by the potential confounder; or (ii) eliminated by stratifying the data by the potential confounder (McNamee 2003). This second definition is therefore based solely on statistical considerations and confounding is said to occur if there is a difference between unadjusted or "collapsed" estimates of the effect of exposure on outcome and estimates that have been adjusted or stratified by the potential confounder.

Although these two definitions of confounding have often been considered indistinguishable, focusing on confounding as a causal rather than a statistical issue leads one to adopt the "comparability-based" definition over the "collapsibility-based" definition (Greenland and Morgenstern 2001). The "comparability-based" definition of confounding can then be used to establish which epidemiological criteria can and should be used to establish whether a variable should be classified as a confounder or not. First, the variable concerned must be a cause of the outcome (or a proxy for a cause) in unexposed subjects (i.e. a 'risk factor'). Second, the variable concerned must be correlated with the exposure variable within the study population concerned. Finally, the variable concerned must not be situated on any causal pathway between exposure and outcome (Hennekens and Buring 1987). More recently, the last of these three conditions has been replaced with an even stricter one: the variable concerned must not be an effect of the exposure (McNamee 2003).

Confounding can exist at the level of the population, or as a consequence of a biased sample. This is an important point; the consideration of confounding should not be solely based on a study sample, indeed it may be the case that apparent confounding in a study is due to sampling and is not true confounding in the population as a whole. Many studies are often able to identify more than one relevant confounder in their analyses, and we will discuss later how one might establish whether the analyses have accounted for a sufficient set of confounders (or whether too few/too many have been included in the analyses: see Sect. 1.2.3, below).

We may have a situation where $E \rightarrow O$ and $A \rightarrow O$, but there is no association between E and A. This happens in a successfully randomised controlled trial (RCT) where baseline variables (A) are balanced between groups – so A is independent of E (due to the success of randomisation for treatments). Nonetheless, because A is a competing exposure for O, the precision with which the relationship between E and O is characterised improves after adjusting for A.

1.2.1 Confounding and DAGs

The use of causal path diagrams to identify confounding and confounders in epidemiological research was introduced by Greenland et al. (1999). The use of DAGs represents a rigorous approach to assessing confounding and identifying confounders, and DAGs are particularly useful given the absence of any objective criteria or test for establishing the presence (or absence) of confounding. Compared with the use of traditional epidemiological criteria to identify confounders, the key additional insight that DAGs provide is the extent to which adjustment for a confounding variable may create further confounding which in turn requires adjustment (Greenland et al. 1999). DAGs also allow analysts to select a subset of potential confounders (i.e. a subset selected from all identified potential confounders) that is sufficient to adjust for potential confounding. Indeed, DAGs can be used to identify the full range of such subsets and thereby test and select the most appropriate one to use (Greenland et al. 1999).

1.2.2 Identifying Confounding

In order to explain how DAGs can be used to determine whether there is potential for confounding in the apparent relationship between an exposure and an outcome let us first use a simple DAG as an example (see Fig. 1.1a). To determine if confounding is present the following algorithm is applied to the DAG (Greenland et al. 1999):

(i) delete all single headed arrows that exit from the exposure variable (i.e. remove all exposure effects); and
(ii) check if there are any unblocked backdoor paths from exposure to outcome (i.e. examine whether exposure and outcome have a common cause).

If there are no unblocked backdoor paths the relationship between exposure and outcome should not be subject to potential confounding (albeit from those variables that have been measured precisely and are available for inclusion in the model and its related statistical analyses). For example, in order to check if the relationship of E on O in Fig. 1.1a is subject to potential confounding:

(i) the arrow between E and O is deleted; and
check if there are any unblocked backdoor paths from E to O (there are three: $E \leftarrow C \rightarrow O$; $E \leftarrow A \rightarrow C \rightarrow O$; and $E \leftarrow C \leftarrow B \rightarrow O$)

Because there are three unblocked backdoor paths from E to O, there is the potential for confounding of the effect of E on O, because we can identify three potential confounders – A and B, and C (which lies on the pathway between A and O, and between B and E). When confounding is present an additional algorithm can be applied to identify where adjustment is required and of which variables (see Sect. 1.2.3 below).

However, before we address this it is important to point out that two variables that are not associated with each other, and that share a child (or descendent) that is a confounder, may also become associated within at least one stratum of the confounder. This is a well-established observation in epidemiological research (Weinberg 1993). Adjusting for one confounder may also alter the associations between other variables. In a DAG, this is equivalent to creating a non-directed arc between the two variables and therefore a new backdoor path that has to be dealt with when adjusting for confounding. This can be illustrated using the example in Fig. 1.1a, where controlling only for C in the relationship between E and O may create an association between A and B, because both A and B are parents of C. If this is the case, then A and B must also be included as confounders, otherwise additional confounding will have been introduced by adjustment for C alone.

1.2.3 Sufficient Set of Confounders

Where confounding is present it is usually possible and desirable to identify a subset of variables (S) using a DAG that is sufficient to address confounding through adjustment. In other words, S constitutes the subset of variables with which it is possible to address <u>all</u> confounding through adjustment. In order to assesswhether S removes all confounding another algorithm is applied to the DAG (Pearl 1993):

(i) delete all single headed arrows that exit from the exposure variable;
(ii) draw non-directed arcs that connect each pair of variables that share a child that is either in S or has a descendant in S (i.e. account for any associations between variables that are generated by controlling for S); and
(iii) check if there are any unblocked backdoor paths from exposure to outcome that do not pass through S – if there is no unblocked backdoor path then S is sufficient for control of confounding.

If we apply this algorithm to the five-variable DAG described earlier in Fig. 1.1a to check whether a tentative set of variables (S') that contains A, B and C would be sufficient for controlling for any potential confounding control would involve:

(i) deleting the arrow between E and O;
(ii) drawing a nondirected arc between A and B (since C is a child of A and B; see Fig. 1.1c); and
(iii) assessing whether there are no unblocked backdoor paths from E to O that do not pass through A, B and C (there are none).

Using this approach in this example would therefore lead us to conclude that adjusting for A, B and C would be sufficient to address potential for confounding in the relationship between E and O.

However, in order to check whether there might be an even smaller *sub*set of the tentative subset of confounders (S'; A, B, and C) it is worth exploring the consequences of deleting each of these variables in turn:

Deleting A would still mean that:

- the backdoor path $E \leftarrow A - B \rightarrow O$ in Fig. 1.1c would be blocked at B;
- $E \leftarrow A - B \rightarrow C \rightarrow O$ would be blocked at B;
- $E \leftarrow A \rightarrow C \rightarrow O$ would be blocked at C; and
- $E \leftarrow C \rightarrow O$ would be blocked at C.

Therefore B and C are minimally sufficient. In other words, it is not necessary to adjust for A in addition to B and C.

Deleting B would mean that:

- the backdoor path $E \leftarrow A - B \rightarrow O$ in Fig. 1.1c would be blocked at A;
- $E \leftarrow A - B \rightarrow C \rightarrow O$ would be blocked at A;
- $E \leftarrow A \rightarrow C \rightarrow O$ would be blocked at A; and
- $E \leftarrow C \rightarrow O$ would be blocked at C.

Therefore A and C (like B and C, above) would also be minimally sufficient. *Deleting C* would mean that:

- the backdoor path $E \leftarrow A \rightarrow C \rightarrow O$ in Fig. 1.1c would be blocked at A;
- $E \leftarrow C \rightarrow B \rightarrow O$ would be blocked at B; and
- $E \leftarrow C \rightarrow O$ would be blocked

Therefore A and B would not be minimally sufficient.

As this example shows, there can be more than one minimally sufficient set (*S*). However, these sets may also vary in size and may not necessarily overlap (Greenland et al. 1999). It can therefore be helpful to identify *all* minimally sufficient sets so that the best one can be chosen for dealing with confounding through adjustment. For example, some sets may need to be rejected if they contain variables that were not measured in the study. Others may be rejected due to concerns about measurement error, or because they contain many more variables than other sets and would thereby generate less precise estimates from multivariable statistical analyses on the sample sizes available. As such an important advantage of using DAGs over traditional approaches to identifying potential confounding is that the latter are usually unable to identify any of the potential sufficient subsets of potential confounders, and all potential confounders would therefore need to be included in the analysis (at cost to the precision of the estimates produced).

1.2.4 Strengths and Weaknesses of Causal Path Diagrams

As we have shown in this chapter, DAGs can be used to identify confounding and confounders in a systematic way, and by helping researchers to identify these objectively and explicitly, DAGs can help to reduce bias and advance debate. Moreover, despite the various limitation mentioned earlier in this Chapter (see Sect. 1.1.2, above), one of the main strengths of using causal path diagrams in epidemiological analyses of data from non-experimental studies is that it enables researchers to think clearly and logically about the *known*, *likely* and *speculative* causal relationships between variables that are relevant to the research hypothesis and related analytical questions. Causal path diagrams thereby facilitate the communication of any causal presumptions that have been made during data analysis to academic and professional audiences using a structured approach that is explicit and easy to critique or re-model.

DAGs also enable the identification of variables that are important to measure in a prospective research study, and thereby improve the efficiency of both data collection and statistical analyses by avoiding the unnecessary measurement or inclusion of variables that are irrelevant to the study and its analysis.

Nonetheless, a somewhat surprising feature of tackling confounding using DAGs is that incorrect specification of the model itself can itself create more problems than it solves. For example, bias may be introduced by including variables that are consequences of the exposure, while additional confounding may be created by including variables that are common descendents of other confounders. Likewise, as we saw earlier, stratification may lead to key changes to some of the paths within the DAG, and these changes may lead to previously blocked paths becoming unblocked and causing further confounding. However, both of these potential flaws can be put to good use in identifying whether adjustment for specific confounders might create new associations between variables that may generate further confounding that will also need to be addressed. As such, these features are arguably an additional strength of using DAGs in analytical design.

One important weakness of DAGs is that with increasing numbers of highly inter-related variables they can rapidly become visually complex to read. DAGs also represent an inherent oversimplification of causal relationships between variables as they do not indicate whether: any relationships are positive or negative (e.g. harmful or protective); effect modification might occur; each causal relationship is weak or strong; and some of the variables might only be able to cause an effect in combination with other variables.

Moreover, as with all causal models, DAGs are only as good as the functional and empirical knowledge and speculative hypotheses on which they are based. In particular, DAGs may be based on a set of presumptions that are wrong (either as a result of incorrect knowledge, weak empirical evidence or fallacious hypotheses). However, because DAGs ensure that these presumptions are explicitly stated, the key benefit of DAGs is that they facilitate criticism, (re) interpretation and (where necessary) modification of the model to assess whether different conclusions would be reached about: which variables are true confounders (see Chap. 11 on structural equation modelling); and which subset of variables are best to adjust for in order to address confounding while taking into account the availability and quality of data on each of the variables involved.

1.3 Conclusions

Directed acyclic graphs (DAGs) have great potential utility in epidemiological analyses of data from non-experimental studies; not least because they encourage researchers to formally structure presumed and predicted causal pathways. These causal path diagrams are essentially intuitive to construct but nonetheless require considered thought. As with all models, careful interpretation remains imperative. Following established algorithms, they can nonetheless be used to identify sufficient sets of confounders which will greatly advance analytical modelling strategies and their subsequent interpretation, critique, testing and re-modelling by other researchers.

References

Geneletti, S., Richardson, S., & Best, N. (2009). Adjusting for selection bias in retrospective, case-control studies. *Biostatistics, 10*, 17–31.
Geneletti, S., Gallo, V., Porta, M., Khoury, M. J., & Vineis, P. (2011). Assessing causal relationships in genomics: From Bradford-Hill criteria to complex gene-environment interactions and directed acyclic graphs. *Emerging Themes in Epidemiology, 8*, 5.
Greenland, S., & Morgenstern, H. (2001). Confounding in health research. *Annual Review of Public Health, 22*, 189–212.

Greenland, S., & Robins, J. M. (1986). Identifiability, exchangeability, and epidemiological confounding. *International Journal of Epidemiology, 15*, 413–419.

Greenland, S., Pearl, J., & Robins, J. M. (1999). Causal diagrams for epidemiologic research. *Epidemiology, 10*, 37–48.

Head, R. F., Gilthorpe, M. S., Byrom, A., & Ellison, G. T. H. (2008). Cardiovascular disease in a cohort exposed to the 1940–45 Channel Islands occupation. *BMC Public Health, 8*, 303.

Head, R. F., Gilthorpe, M. S., & Ellison, G. T. H. (2009). Cholesterol levels in later life amongst UK Channel Islanders exposed to the 1940–45 German occupation as children, adolescents and young adults. *Nutrition and Health, 20*, 91–105.

Hennekens, C. H., & Buring, J. E. (1987). *Epidemiology in medicine* (1st ed.). Boston/Toronto: Little Brown and Company.

Hernan, M. A., Hernandez-Dìaz, S., & Robins, J. M. (2004). A structural approach to selection bias. *Epidemiology, 15*, 615–625.

Hernandez-Dìaz, S., Schisterman, E. F., & Hernan, M. A. (2006). The birth weight "paradox" uncovered? *American Journal of Epidemiology, 146*, 1115–1120.

Hoggart, C. J., Parra, E. J., Shriver, M. D., Bonilla, C., Kittles, R. A., Clayton, D. G., & McKeigue, P. M. (2003). Control of confounding of genetic associations in stratified populations. *American Journal of Human Genetics, 72*, 1492–1504.

McNamee, R. (2003). Confounding and confounders. *Occupational and Environmental Medicine, 60*, 227–234.

Pearl, J. (1993). Comment: Graphical models, causality and intervention. *Statistical Science, 8*, 266–269.

Pearl, J. (1998). Graphs, causality, and structural equation models. *Sociological Methods and Research, 27*, 226–284.

Pearl, J. (2000). *Causality: Models, reasoning and inference*. Cambridge: University Press.

Rothman, K. J. (1976). Causes. *American Journal of Epidemiology, 104*, 587–592.

Shrier, I., & Platt, R. W. (2008). Reducing bias through directed acyclic graphs. *BMC Medical Research Methodology, 8*, 70.

Susser, M. (1973). *Causal thinking in the health sciences*. New York: Oxford University Press.

Tu, Y.-K., & Gilthorpe, M. S. (2012). *Statistical thinking in epidemiology*. Boca Raton: CRC Press.

Tu, Y.-K., West, R. W., Ellison, G. T. H., & Gilthorpe, M. S. (2004). Why evidence for the fetal origins of adult disease can be statistical artifact: The reversal paradox examined for hypertension. *American Journal of Epidemiology, 161*, 27–32.

Weinberg, C. R. (1993). Toward a clearer definition of confounding. *American Journal of Epidemiology, 137*, 1–8.

Weinberg, C. R. (2005). Barker meets Simpson. *American Journal of Epidemiology, 161*, 33–35.

Weinberg, C. R. (2007). Can DAGs clarify effect modification? *Epidemiology, 18*, 569–572.

Chapter 2
Statistical Modelling of Partially Observed Data Using Multiple Imputation: Principles and Practice

James R. Carpenter, Harvey Goldstein, and Michael G. Kenward

2.1 Introduction

Missing data are inevitably ubiquitous in experimental and observational epidemiological research. Nevertheless, despite a steady flow of theoretical work in this area, from the mid-1970s onwards, recent studies have shown that the way partially observed data are reported and analysed in experimental research falls far short of best practice (Wood et al. 2004; Chan and Altman 2005; Sterne et al. 2009). The aim of this Chapter is thus to present an accessible review of the issues raised by missing data, together with the advantages and disadvantages of different approaches to the analysis.

Section 2.2 gives an overview of the issues raised by missing data, and Sect. 2.3 explores those situations in which a 'complete case' analysis, using those units with no missing data, will be appropriate. Section 2.4 describes the advantages and disadvantages of various methods for the analysis of partially observed data and argues that multiple imputation is the most practical approach currently available to applied researchers. Section 2.5 reviews some key issues that arise when using multiple imputation in practice. We conclude with a worked example in Sect. 2.6 and discussion in Sect. 2.7.

J.R. Carpenter (✉) • M.G. Kenward
Department of Medical Statistics, London School of Hygiene and Tropical Medicine, Keppel Street, London WC1E 7HT, UK
e-mail: James.Carpenter@lshtm.ac.uk

H. Goldstein
Graduate School of Education, University of Bristol, 35 Berkeley Square, BS8 1JA, Bristol

2.2 Issues Raised by Missing Data

We illustrate the issues raised by missing data using Fig. 2.1, which shows the frontage of a high-level mandarin's house in the New Territories, Hong Kong.

First, we notice missing data can either take the form of completely missing figurines, or damaged— i.e. partially observed—figurines. The former is analogous to what is usually termed unit non-response, while the latter is analogous to item non-response. However, the statistical issues raised are the same in both cases. For simplicity, we therefore assume there are no completely missing figurines.

Next, we see that the effect of missing data on any inference depends crucially on the question at hand. For instance, if interest lies in the position of the figurines in the tableau shown in Fig. 2.1, then missing data are not a problem. If, instead, interest is in the height, or facial characteristics of the figurines, then missing data raises issues that have to be addressed. Thus, when assessing the impact of missing data it is not the number, or proportion of missing observations per se that is the key, rather the extent of the missing information about the question at hand. Changing the example, if we are interested in the prevalence of a rare disease, missing the disease status of two individuals—potentially non-randomly—out of 1,000 means we have lost a substantial amount of information.

Now suppose we are interested in estimating a facial characteristic—say average hair length—of the four figurines shown. Two are missing their heads, and we cannot be sure why. In order to estimate the average hair length we need to make an assumption about why the two heads are missing, and/or how their mean hair length relates to those whose heads are present. Our assumptions must take one of the following three forms:

1. the reason for the missing heads is random, or at any rate unconnected to any characteristics of the figurines;
2. the reason for the missing heads is not random; but within groups of 'similar' figurines (e.g. with similar neckties) heads are missing randomly, or
3. the reason for the missing heads is not random, and—even within groups of apparently similar figurines—depends on hair length (i.e. depends directly on what we want to measure).

In case 1, the 'data' (hair length) are said to be Missing Completely At Random (MCAR). What is usually termed the missingness mechanism may depend on the position of the figurines relative to missing tiles in the roof above, but is independent of information relevant to the question at hand. Under this assumption there is no difference in the distribution of hair-length between the figurines, so we can get a valid estimate using the complete cases (i.e. figurines with heads). In case 2, the data are said to be Missing At Random (MAR). The reason for the missing data (hair length) depends on the unseen value (hair length) but we can form groups based on observed data (e.g. necktie) within which the reason for the missing data does not depend on the unseen value (missing hair length). If we assume hair length is MAR given necktie, we can estimate hair length among figurines with straight

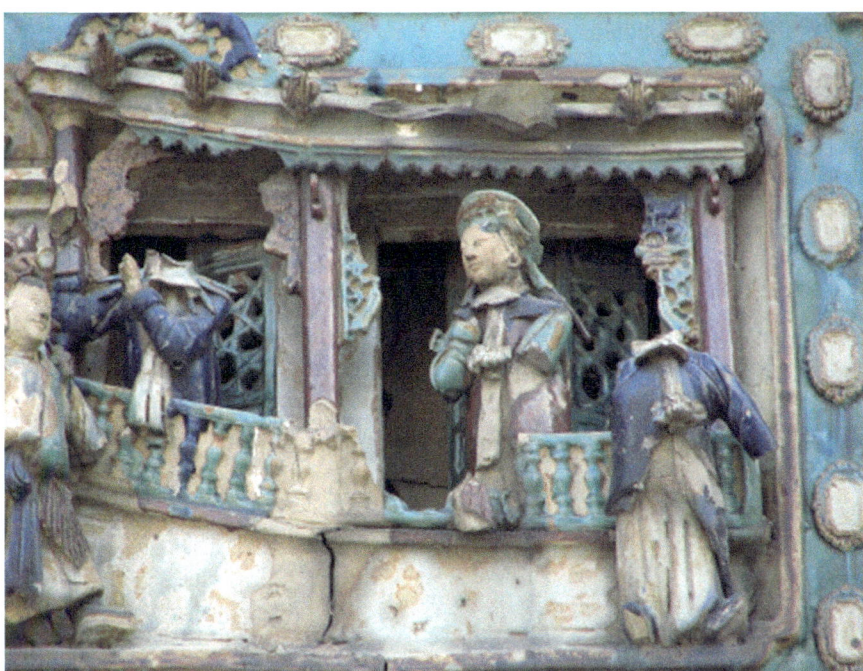

Fig. 2.1 Mandarin's house, New Territories, Hong Kong (Photo H. Goldstein)

neckties, and among those that end in a bobble. We can then calculate a weighted average of these—weighting by the number with each kind of necktie—to estimate mean hair length across the 'population' of figurines.

In case 3, the data are said to be Missing Not At Random (MNAR). In this case, we cannot estimate average hair length across the figurines without knowing either (i) the relationship between the chance of a headless figurine and hair length or (ii) the difference in mean hair length between figurines with, and without, heads.

This terminology was first proposed by Rubin (1976), and despite the slightly counter-intuitive meaning of 'Missing At Random' it is now almost universally used. We now highlight two things, implicit in the above discussion, which are universal in the analysis of partially observed data:

2.2.1 Ambiguity Caused by Missing Data

Given Fig. 2.1, we do not know which of the assumptions 1–3 above is correct; furthermore each has different implications for how we set about validly estimating mean hair length. Therefore, the best we can do is state our assumptions clearly, arrive at valid inference under those assumptions, and finally report how inference varies with the assumptions. The latter is referred to as sensitivity analysis, and is fundamental to inference from partially observed data. We hope that our inference is pretty robust to different assumptions about the missing data, so that we can be fairly confident about our conclusions. However, as we cannot verify our assumptions using the data at hand, our readers can reasonably be expected to be informed if this is indeed the case.

2.2.2 Duality of Missingness Mechanism and Distribution of Missing Data Given Observed Data

Each of the assumptions 1–3 above makes a statement both about the probabilistic mechanism causing the missing data (which we refer to as the missingness mechanism) and the difference between the distribution of the missing data given the observed data. To see this, suppose that Y is hair length, X is characteristics of the body (observed on all figurines) and $R = 1$ if the head is present and 0 if absent.

Under MCAR, the chance of $R = 1$ given X, Y —for which we use the notation [R|X, Y]—does not depend on X or Y, that is [R|X, Y] = [R]. This means that the distribution of Y given X does not depend on R. More formally, using the definition of conditional probability,

$$[Y|X,R] = \frac{[Y,X,R]}{[X,R]} = \frac{[R|X,Y][X,Y]}{[R|X][X]}$$
$$= \frac{[R][Y,X]}{[R][X]} \quad \text{(because of MCAR assumption)}$$
$$= [Y|X] \qquad (2.1)$$

Thus the missingness mechanism tells us about the distribution of the missing data given the observed, and vice versa.

A similar argument gives (2.1) if data are MAR, for then the chance of $R = 1$ does not depend on Y once we take X into account, so that [R |Y, X] = [R|X]. Thus, if data are MCAR or MAR, the distribution of the partially observed variables (hair length) given the fully observed ones (body characteristics) is the same across individuals, regardless of whether—for a particular individual—the partially observed variable (hair length) is seen or not.

However, this relationship does not hold if data are MNAR. In that case the chance of $R = 1$ depends on both X and Y, and this means that the distribution of [Y |X] is different depending on whether Y is observed or not (i.e. whether $R = 1$ or not). This makes MNAR analyses more difficult, as we either have to say (i) exactly how [R] depends on Y, X or (ii) exactly how [Y |X] differs according to R—i.e. whether Y is observed or not.

The aim of this Section was to use a pictorial example to sketch out the intuition behind the standard jargon in the missing data literature. This is a key step in understanding its relevance to the analysis of any partially observed dataset. It is also important to bear in mind the question the analysis is addressing, and how the answers might be affected by plausible missing data mechanisms.

The next Section elaborates this further.

2.3 When Will Complete Cases Do?

Analyses of a partially observed data set which include only individuals with no missing data (or at least no missing data on the variables in the current model) are often called 'Complete Case' analyses.

The question in the section heading is often posed, but given the discussion above is not appropriate as it stands. Instead, the question is whether a complete case estimator is appropriate given the inferential question at hand and assumptions about the missing data mechanism. An important secondary question concerns the efficiency of a complete case estimator, relative to other estimators such as those obtained using multiple imputation. We now discuss this further, taking a simple setting as an example.

Suppose we have four variables, W, X, Y, Z. In a more general setting, these could be groups of covariates. Let our model of interest be the regression of Y on X and Z. We consider two situations: first that the response Y is partially observed but the other variables are complete, and second that the covariate X is partially observed.

2.3.1 Response Y Partially Observed, Other Variables Complete

Given the results in the previous Section we know that, if Y values are MCAR, then the complete case analysis is unbiased. Now suppose Y is MAR given X and Z. In this situation, the complete case analysis is also unbiased. To see this, we note that the contribution to the likelihood for an individual with missing data is simply the likelihood with the missing data integrated out. With a missing response it is thus

$$\int [Y|X,Z]dY = 1 \tag{2.2}$$

This also means that in this setting a complete case analysis is efficient.

Next, we suppose that W is predictive of the response Y being missing, so that Y is MAR given W and possibly the X, Z, but values of W are independent of Y (this also means W is not a confounder). This situation may occur, for example, when W describes how the data collection process has changed over time, but this administrative change is unrelated to the actual values of Y. Once again, the complete case analysis is unbiased, as W contains no information on the parameters in the regression of interest.

Now suppose that W is both not independent of Y and predictive of Y being missing, so that Y is MAR given W and possibly X, Z. Here a complete case analysis is inconsistent. Consistent estimation requires that we take account of the information in W. We could include W as an additional covariate; however this changes the model of interest. This may not be desirable, because it changes the goal of the analysis. In this setting, we need to use one of the more sophisticated methods described below.

The last possibility is that the response Y is MNAR. From the discussion in the previous Section it should be clear that a complete case analysis will be inconsistent here. We need to make an assumption about the difference between $[Y \mid X, Z, R = 1]$ (i.e. the complete case estimate) and $[Y \mid X, Z, R = 0]$ (i.e. the regression relationship in individuals where Y is missing). Only given such an assumption can we estimate the regression parameters relating Y to X and Z.

2.3.2 Covariate X Partially Observed

We again consider the regression of Y on X, Z but now suppose that Y, Z are fully observed and X is partially observed. If X is MCAR, then the complete case analysis will be unbiased, as above. However, in this setting (in contrast to that of a missing response, equation (2.2) we can recover information about the regression coefficients from individuals with Y and Z observed. The key to this is the introduction of an assumed distribution for X in terms of Y and Z. This distribution buys information about the missing data, though it cannot be definitively validated from the observed data. This information can be incorporated using for example multiple imputation or EM-type algorithms, as described in Sect. 2.4.

Next suppose X is MAR given Z, but given Z the mechanism does not depend on Y. In this case, analysis using complete cases will again be unbiased, but—as with X MCAR—more information on the regression coefficients can be obtained from individuals with Y and Z observed. If the covariate X is MAR and the mechanism depends on the response Y and covariate Z, then analysis based on complete cases will be biased, as well as potentially inefficient. In such settings a more sophisticated analysis is needed, taking account of the information in the partially observed cases. As usual, this relies on an assumed distribution of the missing data given the observed data, which cannot be definitively validated from the observed data. Again, this information can be incorporated using for example multiple imputation or EM-type algorithms.

Similarly, if X is MAR but the mechanism depends on another variable W which is not in our model of interest, but which is associated with Y, then the complete case analysis will be biased, and an analysis valid under MAR is required. However, if—as above—W is associated with the chance of seeing X, but not with the distribution of X, then there is no gain in including W in the analysis.

Next, if the covariate X is MNAR, depending on X and possibly Z but given these not on the response Y, then the complete case analysis is unbiased. A more efficient analysis is possible, but only if we correctly specify the MNAR missingness mechanism. In practice, we are unlikely to be able to do this. Further, an analysis under the MAR assumption is not valid here—as the true missingness mechanism is MNAR. Since for this particular MNAR mechanism the complete case analysis is unbiased, an analysis under MAR could introduce bias.

Finally, if X is MNAR, depending on X, Y and possibly Z then the complete case analysis is biased, as is an analysis under the MAR mechanism. Quite often the MAR analysis will be less biased than the complete case analysis but this is not guaranteed. Only if we can correctly specify the MNAR mechanism—i.e. the difference in the conditional distribution of X when X is observed and unobserved—will our analysis be unbiased in general.

Taken together, the above underlines the importance of exploring the data carefully, and understanding plausible missingness mechanisms, before using a more sophisticated—and potentially time consuming—analysis. This can yield important insights about whether a more sophisticated analysis is required, how to formulate it, and how plausible the results are likely to be. Nevertheless, the uncomfortable fact remains that all analysis with partially observed data rest on inherently untestable assumptions. Thus sensitivity analyses—where we explore the robustness of our inference to different assumptions about the missing data—have a key role to play.

2.4 Methods for Analysis of Partially Observed Data

Here we briefly review the advantages and disadvantages of different methods for analysing partially observed data. All the methods have an extensive literature, to which we give some pointers.

2.4.1 Inverse Probability Weighting

Under this approach, we calculate the probability of cases being complete as a function of the observed data, usually using logistic regression. Then, we weight the complete case analysis, weighting each case (typically observations from an individual) by the inverse of the probability of observing their data. Thus, those complete cases which represent individuals who are likely to have missing data are up-weighted relative to individuals whose data are more likely to be observed. See, for example, Carpenter and Plewis (2011).

This approach only re-weights those with no missing data, whereas other approaches (discussed later in this section) assume a distribution for the missing data given the observed. Thus we can view inverse probability weighting as trading efficiency for robustness. If our weight model is correctly specified, our parameter estimates are consistent. However, if we are prepared to specify a distribution of the missing data given the observed we can obtain consistent and more efficient estimates. Note that neither approach avoids the need to make untestable assumptions. Specifically with regard to inverse probability weighting, the data we need to check the assumptions made in estimating the weights are missing.

This point has triggered extensive methodological work, and the emergence of *augmented inverse probability weighting* and *doubly robust estimation*. These approaches both make some additional assumptions in order to buy information relative to inverse probability weighting. Thus doubly robust methods incorporate a term which is a function of the mean of the missing data given the observed data. Assuming that the (as usual inherently untestable) assumption under which this mean is estimated is correct, and that the model for the weights is correct, the resulting estimates are consistent and comparably precise to those obtained using the methods described in the rest of this section. They also have the desirable property that if either the weights are wrong, or the mean of the missing data given the observed data is wrong, consistent parameter estimates result. For a relatively accessible introduction see Carpenter et al. (2006) or Vansteelandt et al. (2010). The principal drawback of these approaches remain the difficulty of dealing with the non-monotone missing data patterns (which arise naturally in most observational data and some experimental data) under a general MAR mechanism, concern about instability in the weights (now an active research area, see Cao et al. (2009)), and the lack of software. For a lively discussion see Kang and Schafer (2007).

2.4.2 EM-Algorithm and Related Methods

The second widely used approach to parameter estimation with missing data is the Expectation-Maximisation (EM) algorithm and its derivatives, which was developed in the early 1970s (Orchard and Woodbury 1972; Dempster et al. 1977). This is an iterative method for obtaining maximum likelihood estimates with missing data, based on iteratively calculating the expectation of the likelihood over the distribution of the missing data given the observed data, and then maximising this expected likelihood with respect to the parameters of interest. Although it can work well, convergence is often slow, estimating the standard errors of parameters can be tricky (Louis 1982) and calculating the expectations involved can be tricky. This has led to the development of various approaches which use Monte-Carlo methods to estimate the expectations involved; see for example Little and Rubin (2002) and Clayton et al. (1998), who also discuss other algorithms for maximising incomplete data likelihoods. Once Monte-Carlo methods are used in the estimation, a key attraction of the EM algorithm relative to multiple imputation is removed. This, convergence difficulties and difficulties in developing general software—in particular to take account of information in auxiliary variables such as W in the discussion in the previous Section, has limited its use.

2.4.3 Repeated Measures Modelling

If missing data are primarily in an outcome measured repeatedly over time, it may often be possible to embed the simpler model of interest in a more complex repeated measures model. If there are no missing data, the two give the same inference for the parameters of interest, but if data are missing, the latter gives inference under a broader class of MAR mechanisms. This approach requires care, but is most suitable for clinical trials with continuous repeatedly measured outcome data subject to patient withdrawal. This approach is reviewed and applied in this context in Chap. 3 of Carpenter and Kenward (2008), and also compared to multiple imputation. It is limited by the difficulty of setting up such model in general, particularly when covariates are missing.

2.4.4 Multiple Imputation

The fourth option we consider here, Multiple Imputation (MI), was conceived as a two-stage Bayesian approach for parameter estimation in the presence of missing data. However, if done properly, inferences have very good frequentist properties. Thus MI can be viewed as a method of maximising an incomplete data likelihood. Indeed, provided the underlying incomplete data likelihood is the same, asymptotically equivalent estimates will be obtained from the EM-type algorithms and repeated measures modelling. It follows that MI can also be viewed an approximation to a full Bayesian analysis in which the analyst's model of interest and the imputation model for the missing data given the observed are fitted concurrently.

MI was introduced by Rubin (Rubin 1987, 1996); for a recent review see Kenward and Carpenter (2007). A joint model is formed for the observed data, where partially observed variables are the response. This model is fitted, and then used to create a number of imputed datasets, by drawing the missing data from its conditional distribution given the observed data, taking care to fully accommodate the statistical uncertainty in this process. This results in a number of 'complete' datasets. Then the model of interest is fitted to each of these in turn, and the results combined for final inference using Rubin's rules. These rules are simple and general, and although naturally derived using a Bayesian argument, the resulting inferences have good frequentist properties.

The attraction of MI relative to the methods above include (i) it can be implemented in terms of regression models, so developing general robust software is more straightforward; (ii) convergence issues do not arise in the same way as with

Table 2.1 Some of the software packages available for multiple imputation

Imputation method	Software package	Name of imputation package	Available from
Full conditional specification	Stata	*ice*[a]	Install within Stata using the ssc command; packaged with Stata 12 onwards
	R	*mice*[a]	Install as additional package from http://cran.r-project.org/
		mi[a]	Install as additional package from http://cran.r-project.org/
	SAS	*IVEware*[a]	Download from http://www.isr.umich.edu/src/smp/ive/
Joint modelling	MLwiN	*mi* macros[b]	Download from http://www.missingdata.org.uk
	SAS	PROC MI (with the MCMC option)	Standard from SAS v9
	Stand alone	*norm, PAN*[b], *mix*[a]	Download from http://sites.stat.psu.edu/~jls/misoftwa.html
	Stata	*MI*	Standard with Stata version 11 and later
	Stand alone	*REALCOM*[a,b]	Download from http://www.bristol.ac.uk/cmm/
			Designed to work with MLwiN; interface to Stata and other packages from http://www.misssingdata.org.uk

All websites accessed 25 Jan 2012
[a] indicates software which does not treat discrete data as continuous
[b] indicates software allowing for multilevel structure

EM-type algorithms; (iii) information from auxiliary variables, not in the model of interest, can naturally be included, and (iv) it can readily be used for sensitivity analysis to the MAR assumption. Thus it is becoming increasingly established as the leading practical approach to analysing partially observed datasets (Sterne et al. 2009; Klebanoff and Cole 2008). Although there is an increasing range of statistical software packages available, they vary in their accessibility to data analysts. More fundamentally, some software uses the full conditional specification approach (also known as the chained equation approach; for an early example see van Buuren et al. (1999)), which does not explicitly model the joint distribution but forms univariate models for each incomplete variable in turn conditional on all the others. There is no guarantee in general that these correspond to a proper joint model. Other software is based on an explicit joint model, as described for example in Schafer (1997). Moreover, some software treats discrete data as continuous in the imputation model, and most packages do not allow for a multilevel structure (Kenward and Carpenter 2007). Table 2.1 gives some more details.

In the light of the above, we believe multiple imputation is currently the most general and accessible method for a wide range of analyses. In the next Section, we therefore review some key issues that arise in its application, before illustrating its use in a multilevel setting in Sect. 2.6.

2.5 Practical Application of MI: Issues to Consider

Assuming that the user knows the model of interest they wish to fit in the absence of missing data, the multiple imputation procedure follows a fixed set of standard steps once the user has specified the imputation model. This is because the computer fits the imputation model to the partially observed data, imputes the missing data from this to create the 'completed' data sets, fits the user's model of interest to each imputed dataset and then combines the results for final inference using Rubin's rules.

2.5.1 Formulating the Imputation Model

The implication is that care needs to be taken in formulating the imputation model—this is the make or break step. In particular this needs to be compatible/congenial with the model of interest—in the sense described below—and valid under a general missing at random mechanism.

By compatibility we mean that the imputation model should ideally allow the same richness of structure between the variables as the model of interest. Thus all the variables in the model of interest, including the response, need to go into the imputation model. This is important, for otherwise the imputed data will be independent of these variables. For most outcomes, this is straightforward; for survival data we need to remember to include the censoring indicator as well as a suitable measure of survival. Work by White and Royston (2009) suggests the cumulative hazard is preferable. Survival data with censoring—when we know the event occurred after censoring—can also be viewed as an example of situations where we have prior information about the range of values the missing data can take. Goldstein et al. (2009) discuss how such information can be incorporated.

2.5.2 Non-linear Relationships and Interactions

Problems are more likely to arise when the model of interest contains non-linearities and/or interactions. If these are functions of fully observed variables, then they should be included as covariates in the imputation model. However, if they include partially observed variables then more care needs to be taken, and in some settings it is challenging to handle this correctly. If this is not done correctly, estimates of interactions and non-linearities in the model of interest will tend to be biased towards the null. This is obviously of greatest concern where inference focuses on precisely these interactions/non-linearities. For a detailed discussion and worked example, see Carpenter and Plewis (2011).

2.5.3 Multilevel Data

A further issue of compatibility concerns the correlation structure of the data. If the data are multilevel, then this structure should be reflected in the imputation model. Failure to do this will generally result in the imputations being weighted towards those level two units with the most data, and the variance of the imputed data will be too small. Multilevel multiple imputation is more problematic with the full conditional specification approach (Royston 2007; van Buuren et al. 2006). However, it can be handled naturally within a joint modelling approach, as can missing values for level two variables. This approach is described in Goldstein et al. (2009) and can handle discrete and continuous variables at different levels of the multilevel data hierarchy. Experimental software implementing this is available at http://www.bristol.ac.uk/cmm/.

2.5.4 Auxiliary Variables

Validity under a general missing at random mechanism is most plausible if we include in the imputation model additional variables, associated with both the chance of data being missing and the actual unseen values, but not in the model of interest. Such auxiliary variables, for example may lie on the causal path between our exposure and response. However, the desire to include a number of such variables needs to be balanced against the risk of numerical problems in fitting the imputation model that may arise. Such problems are most likely when a number of the partially observed variables are binary. In practice, it seems best to include key auxiliary variables, rather than all auxiliary variables, and monitor the imputation model to check for evidence of overfitting (e.g. unduly large standard errors for some coefficients in the conditional regression imputation models).

2.5.5 Multiple Imputation Is Not Prediction

In conclusion, we note that multiple imputation does not have the same goal as prediction. To see this, consider a model with a number of covariates, such as the model for obtaining educational qualifications by age 23, fitted to the 1958 National Childhood Development Study data by Carpenter and Plewis (2011). For fitting the model of interest, there were only 10,279 complete cases, i.e. 65% of the target sample. The advantage of multiple imputation is that, even if our imputations are very imprecise, we can bring in the information from the observed data for the 35% of individuals with incomplete data. In most cases—especially with the judicious use of auxiliary variables (Spratt et al. 2010)—improved prediction will result in more accurate inference for the model of interest. However, multiple imputation can be useful when prediction is poor. For a full discussion of these points see Rubin (1996).

2.6 Example: Multilevel Multiple Imputation

In this Section we illustrate some of the key points above, using data from a study of the effect of class size on children's achievement in their first 2 years at school. We explore the importance of multilevel structure in the imputation model. The data come from a class size study kindly made available to us by Peter Blatchford at the Institute of Education, London. This study sought to understand the effect of class size on development of literacy and numeracy skills in the first 2 years of English children's full time education. The analysis below is illustrative; for a fuller analysis and more details of the study see Blatchford et al. (2002).

The version of the dataset we explore below was derived from the original; we restrict the analysis to a complete subset of 4,873 pupils in 172 schools. School sizes vary greatly in these data and this is reflected in the number of pupils each school contributes to the analysis, which ranges from 1 to 88. The dataset is thus multilevel, with children at level 1 belonging to classes at level 2. Our model of interest regresses literacy score at the end of the first year on class size, adjusting for literacy measured when the children started school, eligibility for free school meals and gender. The pre- and post- reception year (i.e. first school year) literacy scores were normalised as follows. For each test, the pupils' results were ranked. Then for observation in rank order i, where N pupils sat the test, the normalised result was calculated as the inverse normal of $i/(n+1)$.

We will explore the following:

1. fitting the multilevel model of interest to the 4,873 complete cases;
2. fitting the same model ignoring the multilevel structure;
3. making some values of pre-reception literacy score missing at random, and

   (a) analysing the remaining complete cases;
   (b) using multilevel multiple imputation to handle the missing data, and
   (c) using single level multiple imputation to handle the missing data.

Let j denote class and i denote pupil. Our illustrative model of interest is:

$$\begin{aligned} nlitpost_{ij} &= \beta_{0ij} + \beta_1 nlitpre_{ij} + \beta_2 gend_j + \beta_3 fsmn_j \\ \beta_{0ij} &= \beta_0 + u_j + e_{ij} \\ u_j &\sim N(0, \sigma_u^2) \\ e_{ij} &\sim N(0, \sigma_e^2) \end{aligned} \tag{2.3}$$

where the variable names are given in Table 2.2.

Parameter estimates from fitting this to the 4,873 cases are shown in column 2 of Table 2.3. Estimates from the single level model, where σ_u^2 is constrained to be 0, are shown in column 3. We see that there is a substantial component of variability between schools, and that when this is taken out of the analysis the gender coefficient in particular changes by more than one standard error, consistent with a stronger effect of gender in the larger schools.

Table 2.2 Description of variables in class size data used in this analysis

Variable name	Description
nlitpost	Normalised literacy score at the end of 1st school year
nlitpre	Normalised literacy score at the start of 1st school year
fsmn	Binary variable, 1 indicates pupil is eligible for free school meals
gend	Binary variable, 1 for boys and 0 for girls

Table 2.3 Parameter estimates from fitting model (2.3) to various datasets; full details in text

	Estimates (standard errors) from				
	Original data Multilevel model	Original data Single level model	Reduced data Complete cases	Multilevel MI on reduced data	Single level MI on reduced data
Parameter	(n = 4,873)	(n = 4,873)	(n = 3,313)	(n = 3,313)	(n = 3,313)
β_0	0.088 (0.040)	0.065 (0.017)	0.121 (0.041)	0.092 (0.041)	0.107 (0.037)
β_1	0.733 (0.010)	0.662 (0.012)	0.717 (0.012)	0.731 (0.011)	0.647 (0.012)
β_2	−0.058 (0.018)	−0.086 (0.022)	−0.020 (0.022)	−0.056 (0.020)	−0.070 (0.022)
β_3	−0.068 (0.027)	−0.095 (0.030)	−0.036 (0.037)	−0.101 (0.034)	−0.103 (0.034)
σ_u^2	0.237 (0.028)	–	0.231 (0.028)	0.243 (0.029)	0.182 (0.022)
σ_e^2	0.372 (0.008)	0.573 (0.012)	0.360 (0.009)	0.367 (0.009)	0.425 (0.011)

We now make the data missing according to the following mechanism:

$$\log\mathrm{it}\{\Pr(\text{observe nlitpre}_{ij})\} = 1.5 + 0.5 \times \text{nlitpost}_{ij} - \text{fsmn}_j - \text{gend}_j. \quad (2.4)$$

This mechanism says we are more likely to see *nlitpre* for girls with higher *nlitpost* who are not eligible for free school meals. Using these probabilities, we generate 4,873 random numbers from a uniform distribution on [0, 1] and make each individual's data missing if these are greater than their probability implied by (2.4). This results in 3,313 complete cases. Fitting the model of interest to these, we see that the gender effect, and to a lesser extent the eligibility for free school meals, are diluted so that they are no longer significant (column 4, Table 2.3).

We now perform multilevel multiple imputation, using *MLwiN* 2.15 and the multiple imputation macros available from www.missingdata.org.uk. We first fit our model of interest, (2.3). The software then analyses this and proposes the following imputation model, where j indexes school and i pupil:

$$\text{nlitpre}_{ij} = \beta_0 + \beta_1 \text{gend}_j + \beta_2 \text{nlitpost}_{ij} + u_{1j} + e_{1ij}$$
$$\text{fsmn}_{ij} = \beta_3 + \beta_4 \text{gend}_j + \beta_5 \text{nlitpost}_{ij} + u_{2j} + e_{2ij}$$
$$\begin{pmatrix} u_{1j} \\ u_{2j} \end{pmatrix} \sim N(0, \Omega_u)$$
$$\begin{pmatrix} e_{1ij} \\ e_{2ij} \end{pmatrix} \sim N(0, \Omega_e) \quad (2.5)$$

for 2 × 2 covariance matrices Ω_u, Ω_e. Note that the fully observed *fsmn* has been included as a response, since the software requires two or more responses in the imputation model in order to perform multiple imputation. Although this is not strictly compatible with (2.3), as the missing data is in *nlitpre*, the error induced by treating *fsmn* as continuous is negligible. This is because the properties of the bivariate normal distribution mean that we would get similar imputations if we instead had *fsmn* as a covariate in a univariate imputation model for *nlitpre*. The software fits this imputation model using Markov Chain Monte Carlo (MCMC), taking improper priors for the regression coefficients and Wishart priors for the covariance matrices. It then imputes the missing data as draws from the Bayesian posterior, fits the model of interest to each imputed dataset and combines the results for inference using Rubin's rules.

We used a 'burn in' of 500 MCMC updates and updated the sampler a further 200 times between drawing each of 50 imputed datasets. The results are shown in the rightmost two columns of Table 2.3. Column 5 shows the result of multilevel multiple imputation; in column 6 we create the imputations using (2.5), but with Ω_u set to zero. This is equivalent to single level imputation, as available in other packages. Looking at the results, we see that multilevel multiple imputation gives point estimates much closer to the original, fully observed, data but with slightly increased standard errors (reflecting the lost information in the partially observed data). Comparing with single level multiple imputation, we see the latter results in an overestimated gender coefficient. This is because the difference between boys and girls is greater in the larger schools; single level imputation carries this stronger effect to all schools and results in a greater gender coefficient. Further, the school level component of variance is substantially reduced after single level multiple imputation, compared with multilevel multiple imputation. The pupil level variance is correspondingly increased. This makes sense: single level imputation puts extra variability at the pupil level. Finally, each multiple imputation analysis took about 90s with a 2.4 GHz chip.

Although our model is quite simple, we can readily handle additional variables with missing data. These are included as additional responses on the left hand side. In general, as described in Goldstein et al. (2009) this can include appropriate models for discrete and unordered categorical variables. This example illustrates the potential of multiple imputation, and also illustrates the importance of allowing for the multilevel structure in the imputation, when it is present in the data.

2.7 Conclusions

In this Chapter we have argued that, when data are missing, analysis cannot proceed without inherently untestable assumptions about the missingness mechanism. We gave an intuitive illustration of missingness mechanisms and related this to common terminology in the literature. Armed with this, we described the likely effect of missing covariate and response data, under different mechanisms.

We then gave a brief review of the advantages and disadvantages of various statistical methods for handling missing data, concluding that MI currently has the edge in terms of the range of problems that can be tackled using available software. Another attraction is that it is possible to explore the sensitivity of the conclusions to departures from MAR to MNAR missing data mechanisms, see for example Carpenter et al. (2007, 2012). This is important in many applications. We illustrated the potential of multiple imputation using educational data. In common with much medical and social science data, this has a multilevel structure and the analysis indicated the importance of multilevel multiple imputation in this setting.

Acknowledgements James Carpenter is funded by ESRC research fellowship RES-063-27-0257. We are grateful to Peter Blatchford for permission to use the class size data.

References

Blatchford, P., Goldstein, H., Martin, C., & Browne, W. (2002). A study of class size effects in English school reception year classes. *British Educational Research Journal, 28*, 169–185.

Cao, W., Tsiatis, A. A., & Davidian, M. (2009). Improving efficiency and robustness of the doubly robust estimator for a population mean with incomplete data. *Biometrika, 96*, 723–734.

Carpenter, J. R., & Kenward, M. G. (2008). Missing data in clinical trials — A practical guide. *Birmingham: National Health Service Co-ordinating Centre for Research Methodology.* Freely downloadable from www.missingdata.org.uk. Accessed 25 Jan 2012.

Carpenter, J. R., & Plewis, I. (2011). Coming to terms with non-response in longitudinal studies. In M. Williams & P. Vogt (Eds.), *SAGE handbook of methodological innovation.* London: Sage.

Carpenter, J. R., Kenward, M. G., & Vansteelandt, S. (2006). A comparison of multiple imputation and inverse probability weighting for analyses with missing data. *Journal of the Royal Statistical Society: Series A (Statistics in Society), 169*, 571–584.

Carpenter, J. R., Kenward, M. G., & White, I. R. (2007). Sensitivity analysis after multiple imputation under missing at random — A weighting approach. *Statistical Methods in Medical Research, 16*, 259–275.

Carpenter, J. R., Roger, J. H., & Kenward, M. G. (2012). Analysis of longitudinal trials with missing data:—A framework for relevant, accessible assumptions, and inference via multiple imputation (Submitted).

Chan, A., & Altman, D. G. (2005). Epidemiology and reporting of randomised trials published in PubMed journals. *The Lancet, 365*, 1159–1162.

Clayton, D., Spiegelhalter, D., Dunn, G., & Pickles, A. (1998). Analysis of longitudinal binary data from multi-phase sampling (with discussion). *Journal of the Royal Statistical Society, Series B (statistical methodology), 60*, 71–87.

Dempster, A. P., Laird, N. M., & Rubin, D. B. (1977). Maximum likelihood from incomplete data via the EM algorithm (with discussion). *Journal of the Royal Statistical Society Series B (Statistical Methodology), 39*, 1–38.

Goldstein, H., Carpenter, J. R., Kenward, M. G., & Levin, K. (2009). Multilevel models with multivariate mixed response types. *Statistical Modelling, 9*, 173–197.

Kang, J. D. Y., & Schafer, J. L. (2007). Demystifying double robustness: A comparison of alternative strategies for estimating a population mean from incomplete data (with discussion). *Statistical Science, 22*, 523–539.

Kenward, M. G., & Carpenter, J. R. (2007). Multiple imputation: Current perspectives. *Statistical Methods in Medical Research, 16*, 199–218.

Klebanoff, M. A., & Cole, S. R. (2008). Use of multiple imputation in the epidemiologic literature. *American Journal of Epidemiology, 168*, 355–357.

Little, R. J. A., & Rubin, D. B. (2002). *Statistical analysis with missing data* (2nd ed.). Chichester: Wiley.

Louis, T. (1982). Finding the observed information matrix when using the EM algorithm. *Journal of the Royal Statistical Society, Series B, 44*, 226–233.

Orchard, T., & Woodbury, M. (1972). A missing information principle: theory and applications. In L. M. L. Cam, J. Neyman, & E. L. Scott (Eds.), *Proceedings of the Sixth Berkely Symposium on Mathematics, Statistics and Probability: Vol. 1* (pp. 697–715). Berkeley: University of California Press.

Royston, P. (2007). Multiple imputation of missing values: Further update of ice with emphasis on interval censoring. *The Stata Journal, 7*, 445–464.

Rubin, D. B. (1976). Inference and missing data. *Biometrika, 63*, 581–592.

Rubin, D. B. (1987). *Multiple imputation for nonresponse in surveys*. New York: Wiley.

Rubin, D. B. (1996). Multiple imputation after 18 years. *Journal of the American Statistical Association, 91*, 473–490.

Schafer, J. L. (1997). *Analysis of incomplete multivariate data*. London: Chapman and Hall.

Spratt, M., Sterne, J. A. C., Tilling, K., Carpenter, J. R., & Carlin, J. B. (2010). Strategies for multiple imputation in longitudinal studies. *American Journal of Epidemiology, 172*, 478–487.

Sterne, J. A. C., White, I. R., Carlin, J. B., Spratt, M., Royston, P., Kenward, M. G., Wood, A. M., & Carpenter, J. R. (2009). Multiple imputation for missing data in epidemiological and clinical research: Potential and pitfalls. *British Medical Journal, 339*, 157–160.

van Buuren, S., Boshuizen, H. C., & Knook, D. L. (1999). Multiple imputation of missing blood pressure covariates in survival analysis. *Statistics in Medicine, 18*, 681–694.

van Buuren, S., Brand, J. P. L., Groothuis-Oudshoorn, C. G. M., & Rubin, D. B. (2006). Fully conditional specification in multivariate imputation. *Journal of Statistical Computation and Simulation, 76*, 1049–1064.

Vansteelandt, S., Carpenter, J. R., & Kenward, M. G. (2010). Analysis of incomplete data using inverse probability weighting and doubly robust estimators. *Methodology, 6*, 37–48.

White, I. R., & Royston, P. (2009). Imputing missing covariate values for the Cox model. *Statistics in Medicine, 28*, 1982–1998.

Wood, A. M., White, I. R., & Thompson, S. G. (2004). Are missing outcome data adequately handled? A review of published randomized controlled trials in major medical journals. *Clinical Trials, 1*, 368–376.

Chapter 3
Measurement Errors in Epidemiology

Darren C. Greenwood

3.1 Background to the Problem of Measurement Error

3.1.1 General Context

The purpose of many epidemiological studies is to attempt an exploration of possible relationships between disease and an exposure of interest within a defined population. The exposure may be an environmental factor, an occupation, a lifestyle, another disease, or an individual's genotype or phenotype, for example. Generalised Least Squares models handle variation in the outcome measure but assume that predictor variables, e.g. exposures and potential confounders, are perfectly known. However, in epidemiological settings this is rarely the case. Many characteristics of human beings and our environment vary over time; long-term measurements may be impractical or the relevant time window may not be known. Some characteristics, like personality, may be impossible to measure perfectly. Aspects of long-term nutrition and diet are particularly difficult to measure. Exposures based on laboratory analysis are not immune: methods may give very precise results, but often only relate to short periods of time. For example, use of doubly labelled water as a recovery biomarker for total energy intake will give a precise measure of intake over 24 h, but not a lifetime. Thus laboratory measures are still subject to potentially large random error or variation when compared to long-term true exposure. These are all examples of what is referred to as "measurement error" or "errors-in-variables" and can lead to biased estimates and loss of power.

D.C. Greenwood (✉)
Division of Biostatistics, Centre for Epidemiology and Biostatistics,
Leeds Institute of Genetics, Health & Therapeutics, University of Leeds, Leeds, UK
e-mail: D.C.Greenwood@leeds.ac.uk

Measurement error relative to the true exposure is also introduced by categorisation of an exposure or confounder. It is common practice for epidemiologist to categorise variables to facilitate simple presentation and interpretation of results. However, it is not widely recognised that this is at the expense of information loss, which is simply another phrase for measurement error. Whether introduced in exposure assessment or analysis, measurement error is a cause of much bias in estimates from observational epidemiology.

3.1.2 Biased Estimates

There is a widespread view that such measurement error in an exposure can only dilute any association between exposure and outcome (Bashir and Duffy 1997; Fuller 1987; Gladen and Rogan 1979; Weinberg et al. 1994; Wong et al. 1999a). However, the belief that this is always the case is flawed for several reasons (Bjork and Stromberg 2002; Carroll et al. 1995; DelPizzo and Borghesi 1995; Dosemeci et al. 1990; Flegal 1999; Phillips and Smith 1991; Richardson and Ciampi 2003; Sorahan and Gilthorpe 1994; Weinberg et al. 1994; White et al. 2001; Wong et al. 1999b): First, even in simple situations where this is generally the case, this is only "on average", so situations will exist where by chance the bias is away from the null; second, this assumes a simple linear regression scenario with classical additive non-differential measurement error (see Sect. 3.2.2) (Carroll et al. 1995), and for logistic regression, for instance, the resulting bias may be in either direction (Stefanski and Carroll 1985). Even if the *exposure* is measured without error, biased estimates can be caused by measurement error in *confounding* variables (Brenner 1993; Greenland 1980; Wong et al. 1999b). Even with additive measurement error in linear regression, measurement error in a confounding variable often leads to under-adjustment for the confounder and this can readily lead to distortion of the estimated effect of the exposure in *either* direction, depending on the direction of the confounder's effect (Wong et al. 1999b). In addition, bias away from the null is possible under certain situations with other more complex error structures (Carroll et al. 1995; Fuller 1987). One implication of the effects of measurement error not always biasing estimates towards the null is that trends are not always preserved (Carroll et al. 1995; Weinberg et al. 1994), even under non-differential measurement error (Sect. 3.2.2.4). One situation where bias may not be relevant is in the context of prediction, e.g. a risk score based on measured exposures (Wikipedia contributors 2007). However, in aetiological epidemiology, such bias could substantially influence conclusions relating to the true level of exposure.

It can be argued that, for the purposes of prediction or public health advice, measurement error in an exposure is irrelevant, because the prediction is based on the measured exposure, not the true exposure. The problem with interpreting such models based on error-prone exposures is that few clinicians have a good appreciation for the amount of variation in such measures. Therefore, an analysis based on an error-prone exposure may lead to the erroneous conclusion that a particular exposure is unimportant or does not strongly (or significantly) predict the outcome. Many naïve analyses may lead to this variable being dropped from the model entirely, or the public health implications being under-estimated. If the measurement error is in a confounder, then this would lead to under-adjustment for the confounder, again potentially leading to incorrect interpretation of the model. Finally, if there is a nonlinear association between the outcome and an error-prone exposure, then this can lead to a shift in location as well as a bias in the regression slopes.

3.1.3 Loss of Power

In addition to potential bias in estimates, leading to incorrect conclusions surrounding the magnitude of an association, the observed variance structure is altered, so that for a given measured exposure, the outcome is generally more varied than if the true exposure were used. These distortions not only lead to the biases described above, but in addition, the altered variance structure and biased estimates can lead to a loss of power using the measured exposure compared to the true exposure (Aiken and West 1991; DelPizzo and Borghesi 1995; Elmstahl and Gullberg 1997; Freedman et al. 1990; Kaaks et al. 1995; Rippin 2001; Schatzkin et al. 2001a; White et al. 1994). Whilst methods to correct for the effects of measurement error will generally reduce bias, they have little effect on loss of power (Armstrong 1998).

3.2 The Structure of Measurement Error

3.2.1 Characterising Measurement Error

When considering the exposure-disease relationship it is helpful to consider the overall model as three submodels, based on terminology introduced by Clayton (1992):

1. the disease model (relating outcome Y to true exposure X and other error-free covariates Z);
2. the exposure model (describing the distribution of true exposure X);
3. the measurement model (relating measured exposure W to true exposure X).

3.2.2 Underlying Mechanisms for Measurement Error

There is a large literature on measurement error in linear regression, going back many years. This is comprehensively discussed by Fuller (1987). More recent work has focussed on nonlinear models such as logistic regression (Carroll et al. 1995) (nonlinear in the sense of using a link function other than the identity link). This more recent work is of far greater relevance to most branches of epidemiology because exposures are often being related to dichotomous disease outcomes using logistic regression or Poisson regression models, or through methods for survival analysis. The mechanisms underlying measurement error in covariates are common to both linear and nonlinear models, though their impact on estimates may differ.

One general distinction to be drawn between assumed underlying mechanisms is based on whether the measurement error model focuses on modelling the observed measure (W) conditional on the true exposure (X) and other covariates (Z), the classical model, or whether the focus is on modelling the true measure (X) conditional on the observed (W) and the other covariates (Z), the Berkson model.

3.2.2.1 Classical Measurement Error

In its simplest form the classical measurement error model is:

$$W = X + U, \text{ where } U \sim N(0, \sigma_u^2), E(U|X) = 0$$

Under this model there is random error around the true value and it is assumed that any measurement error is not associated with the *true* exposure. In more complicated forms, it is assumed that measurement error is only independent of true exposure conditional upon other covariates.

Classical measurement error can be described using the three submodels outlined above, where it is helpful to express the conditional independence assumptions of this model in terms of model conditional distributions:

Disease model:	$[Y|X, Z, \beta]$
Exposure model:	$[X|Z, \pi]$
Measurement model:	$[W|X, \lambda]$

Where β, π and λ are model parameters, which in the general case are vector quantities.

Disease status Y is only dependent on the true exposure X, the known covariates Z and the unknown parameters β. Therefore, conditional on the true exposure, X, being known, the imperfect observed measures W do not contribute any information to the outcome Y.

The aim of methods to control for measurement error is to discover the disease model free of any bias caused by measurement error. To achieve this, one needs to know the distribution of $X|W$, ignoring perfectly measured covariates and other parameters for the moment. Knowledge of the measurement model $W|X$ is not sufficient in itself to identify the true disease-exposure relationship. One also requires the exposure model, the distribution of X, as demonstrated by Bayes' theorem: prob($X|W$) $\propto$ prob($W|X$) prob(X).

This provides the Bayes estimate of X and is the basis for Bayesian approaches to handling classical measurement error, because we now have an estimate of the true exposure. This provides a justification for conceptually separating the mechanism into three sub-models.

3.2.2.2 Berkson Measurement Error

The basic form of the Berkson measurement error model is:

$$X = W + U, \text{where } U \sim N(0, \sigma_u^2), E(U|W) = 0$$

For the Berkson measurement error model, it is assumed that any measurement error is not associated with the *measured* exposure. In terms of the three submodels, where β and λ are model parameters:

Disease model:	$[Y|X, Z, \beta]$
Exposure model:	not required
Measurement model:	$[X|W, \lambda]$

This type of measurement error is also known as "control-knob" error because the knob operator of, say, a piece of machinery, turns the knob to a setting he/she believes to be the true exposure. However, what they see on the dial is a measure W that contains a component of error. That error is simply a random component in addition to the measured W and is independent of the measured exposure W. This is an example of Berkson error.

3.2.2.3 Random and Systematic Error

Both classical and Berkson error models assume random errors. Alternative mechanisms extend these fundamental approaches to encompass systematic errors (Thomas et al. 1993) where values that are measured are not randomly distributed around the truth (classical) or measured values (Berkson). For example, food frequency questionnaires are notorious for either over-estimating energy and nutrient intakes (Byers 2001; Cade et al. 2002; Calvert et al. 1997) or under-estimating them (Kipnis et al. 2001, 2003; Schatzkin et al. 2003; Subar et al. 2003). A situation where dietary intake is under-estimated for people (in absolute terms) for people with larger intakes, and over-estimated for people with lower intakes would be a systematic error that depended systematically on the true exposure. The underlying measurement error mechanism potentially may be more complicated if it systematically depends on unmeasurable person-specific characteristics. This is a particular problem in the field of nutrition epidemiology.

3.2.2.4 Differential and Non-differential Error

Both systematic and random measurement error structures can be sub-divided into differential or non-differential. This distinction depends on whether the errors in the exposure variable are conditionally independent of the outcome Y, given true exposure X and perfectly known covariates Z. If the misclassification of the measured exposure depends on the outcome, then this is a differential measurement error. If, on the other hand, the measured exposure W given true exposure X and known covariates Z contains no additional information about Y, then the measurement error is said to be non-differential, i.e. $p(Y/X,Z,W) = p(Y/X,Z)$. When this occurs, W can be said to be a surrogate for X, because W is conditionally independent of the outcome Y. Where measurement error can be assumed to be non-differential, then relatively straightforward methods can be used to correct for the measurement error bias.

3.2.2.5 Additive and Multiplicative Error Structures

Measurement error models have also traditionally been considered to fall into two separate categories: additive or multiplicative. Additive error structures are those that define the measurement error model in terms of adding a component of error, e.g. $W = X + U$ in the classical model, or $X = W + U$ in the Berkson model. Multiplicative error structures are those that define the measurement error model in terms of multiplying a component of error, e.g. $W = XU$ or $X = WU$. However this distinction is often a false one, when a multiplicative error structure is additive on the log scale, e.g. $W = XU$ implies $ln(W) = ln(XU) = ln(X) + ln(U)$.

3.2.2.6 Functional and Structural Modelling

Along with these basic mechanisms and distinctions between approaches, historically there has been a distinction in the approach to correcting for measurement error between functional modelling and structural modelling (Carroll et al. 2006). In the functional modelling approach the distribution of the true predictor is not modelled parametrically, but the values of the true exposure X are regarded as fixed. An example of this approach, introduced later in Sect. 3.3.5.1, is regression calibration. In contrast, the approach of structural modelling is to model the distribution of the true predictor, e.g. Bayesian modelling, introduced in Sect. 2.2.6. There is some controversy as to which approach is better, functional or structural (Carroll et al. 2006): for example, structural models make assumptions about the distribution of X that may not be appropriate.

3.2.3 A Simple Example

3.2.3.1 Biased Slope

Consider a straightforward non-differential additive measurement error model in the case of simple linear regression. In this situation the regression model is given by $Y = \beta_0 + \beta_x X + \varepsilon$ where Y is the outcome, the true exposure $X \sim N(\mu, \sigma_x^2)$, the error term ε is independent of X, and $\varepsilon \sim N(0, \sigma_\varepsilon^2)$. Consider also the observed exposure W where $W = X + U$, and U is the amount of measurement error, independent of X, such that $U \sim N(0, \sigma_u^2)$. If we regress Y on W then the standard least squares estimate of the slope β_W, denoted β_X^*, is:

$$\begin{aligned} \beta_X^* &= \frac{Cov(Y,W)}{Var(W)} = \frac{Cov(Y,X)}{Var(W)} \text{ if } U \text{ is independent of } X. \\ &= \frac{Cov(Y,X)}{Var(X) + Var(U)} \\ &= \frac{Var(X)}{Var(X) + Var(U)} \times \frac{Cov(Y,X)}{Var(X)} \\ &= \lambda \beta_X \end{aligned} \qquad (3.1)$$

Therefore, if we regress Y on W then we do not get a consistent estimate of β_x but a biased estimate β_x^* where $\beta_x^* = \lambda \beta_x$ and where the constant λ (often referred to as the reliability ratio or the attenuation ratio, with $0 \le \lambda \le 1$) is:

$$\lambda = \frac{Var(X)}{Var(X) + Var(U)} \qquad (3.2)$$

3.2.3.2 Biased Intercept

In this simple example of linear regression with additive error in the classical model, the intercept is also biased. If we regress Y on W, the standard least squares estimate of the intercept is:

$$\begin{aligned} \beta_0^* &= \mu_Y - \beta_X^* \mu_W \\ &= \mu_Y - \lambda \beta_X \mu_W \\ &= \beta_0 + \beta_X \mu_X - \lambda \beta_X \mu_X \\ &= \beta_0 + (1 - \lambda) \beta_X \mu_X \end{aligned}$$

So that the estimated intercept is biased by the constant $(1-\lambda)\beta_X \mu_X$

3.2.3.3 Inflated Residual Variance

Similarly, in a standard least squares regression of Y on W, the residual variance is estimated as:

$$Var(Y|W) = \frac{1}{n-2}\left(s_{YY}^2 - \beta_W s_{WY}\right)$$

using s_{YY}^2 to represent the observed sample variance of Y and s_{WY} to represent the observed sample covariance of W and Y. Since, from Eq. 3.1, $\beta_W = \lambda\beta_X$, this becomes:

$$= \frac{1}{n-2}\left(s_{YY}^2 - \lambda\beta_X s_{WY}\right)$$

and from the working given above demonstrating the biased estimate of the slope, $s_{WY} = s^2{}_W\beta_W = (s^2{}_X + s^2{}_U)\beta_W = (s^2{}_X + s^2{}_U)\lambda\beta_X = s^2{}_X\beta_X$, so the residual variance becomes

$$= \frac{1}{n-2}\left(s_{YY}^2 - \lambda\beta_X^2 s_X^2\right)$$
$$= \frac{1}{n-2}\left\{\left(s_{YY}^2 - \beta_X^2 s_X^2\right) + \left([1-\lambda]\beta_X^2 s_X^2\right)\right\}$$

Which is the true residual variance inflated by the factor $(1-\lambda)\beta_X^2\sigma^2{}_X$.

3.2.3.4 Reduced Power

The estimate of λ also affects power. In general sample size calculations, for a given required power, dividing the effect size one wishes to detect by a constant c increases the number of subjects required by c^2. Using this argument, if the estimated regression coefficient changes by multiplying by λ, then the number of study participants required will change by $1/\lambda^2$ (Carroll et al. 2006). When λ is <1, this leads to a substantial increase in the required sample size, or loss of power for the same sample size.

3.2.3.5 Summary of Simple Example

In this simple example, the constant λ tends to be less than 1 because of shrinkage. This is because classical measurement error in an exposure will, in the long run, tend to make the measured exposure appear more extreme than the true exposure. For this simple example it is relatively straightforward to demonstrate how the constant λ can be used to quantify, on average, the amount of attenuation of the association (flattening of the regression slope) caused by measurement error, bias in the intercept, and in the residual variance.

In many epidemiological settings, however, the simple classical model may not hold. For radiation exposures, the Berkson model is sometimes more appropriate. Multiplicative error structures may also hold for some exposures. In nutrition epidemiology, dietary exposures often have intercept and slope components to the measurement model, and in particular may well have correlated errors (Day et al. 2004; Kipnis et al. 2001). Adjustment for confounding, measured with or without error, adds further complexity. In these more complicated examples the algebra is more involved than that presented here and the potential for bias could easily be in either direction. Measurement error in gene-environment interactions also poses different problems (Greenwood et al. 2006a; Huang et al. 2005; Murad and Freedman 2007; Wong et al. 2003, 2004).

3.3 Reducing the Effects of Measurement Error

3.3.1 Design

The effects of measurement error can be reduced by using a more precise measure of exposure, and more precise measures of important confounders. In practice, this may mean that more lengthy or costly exposure measures are used, and that smaller samples are all that can be achieved. However, this is almost always offset by the reduction in the effects of measurement error outlined earlier. For example, in nutrition epidemiology, coding of weighed food diaries to derive nutrient intake is very expensive compared to simpler food frequency questionnaires, but will yield far more realistic results. Use of objective measures of dietary intake such as biomarkers or itemised till receipts will reduce bias further (Greenwood et al. 2006b; Kipnis et al. 1999).

The effect of measurement error can also be reduced by increasing the variance of the true exposure (Freedman et al. 2007; Schatzkin et al. 2001b). This is because increasing σ^2_X has the benefit of making λ closer to 1 and therefore reducing bias on average. The easiest way to do this is to ensure sampling a wide range of exposures.

Whilst the best approach to reducing the effects of measurement error are to avoid it in the first place through better exposure measure, the effects can be mitigated by statistical techniques using additional information from external or internal validation samples based on comparison with a measure of the true exposure (if one exists), or surrogate measures (including replicated measures).

3.3.2 Correction Using Aggregate-Level Surrogates

Use of aggregate-level surrogate measures of exposure is most prominent in occupational epidemiology where exposure information is not widely available for individuals, and must be derived from aggregate-level information on groups of individuals. For example, a nuclear power plant may have a precise and accurate measure of the radioactive emissions released from the facility. However, only a cheap error-prone measure of the radiation dose to an individual is available using a tag clipped to an individual's uniform. The more accurate measure is, however, the aggregate measure applying to everyone in the plant. Ideally, one would like to somehow calibrate the inaccurate and imprecise measures from the individuals by using the accurate and precise aggregate measure. This differs from designs with individual-level surrogates because imprecision in the exposure information applied to the individual has also to be accounted for. In nutrition epidemiology this may occur when diet is measured at the household level using household inventories or records of purchases, but inferences are required regarding the health of individuals. This second situation may become more common if databases of supermarket purchasing behaviour for households are linked to individuals' subsequent health (Greenwood et al. 2006b; Ransley et al. 2001, 2003).

3.3.3 Correction Using Individual-Level Surrogate Measures

Use of individual-level measures of diet, where dietary information (the measured exposure) is available on individuals, is far more common than aggregate-level measures (Richardson 1996). Designs can be further specified according to the source of the individual-level information required to estimate λ:

(a) *A validation sample* where the true X are known for a sub-sample of individuals. Wider use of the true measure of exposure on the entire sample is often limited by cost, time to complete, difficulty to implement or invasiveness, so the sub-sample is often small by comparison.
(b) *A replicate sample* where the measured exposure W is repeated at least once on a sample of individuals. This allows σ_u^2 to be estimated, and hence λ, assuming a simple classical measurement error model, i.e. the measure is unbiased and the error is purely random, with no systematic component. It is important for the sub-sample to be selected at random, rather than self-selected to avoid underestimating between-individual variation, with associated underestimation of measurement error (Wang et al. 1996).
(c) *An instrumental variable* where an instrument T exists on a sub-sample, and T is an unbiased measure of X, but contains random measurement error. T will be an imprecise surrogate of the true exposure X measured at the same time as W. T may be a second measure of the exposure obtained by a completely different method that may even be a biased measure providing it is an internal sub-sample. In a recent book, Dunn makes the point that T need not even be a measure of X, so long as it is correlated with it (Dunn 2004). To be an instrumental variable, T must be: (i) correlated with X, (ii) independent of $W - X$, i.e. errors independent from those in W. (e.g., the instrumental variable must not be prone to the same problem as the observed measure W), and (iii) a surrogate for X in that, given Z, it does not contribute anything more than X to the outcome Y.

Using an instrumental variable requires a weaker assumption than a replicate because it may be a biased measure. However, use of an instrumental variable is less desirable than using the original measure X for validation purposes because it introduces greater imprecision.

3.3.4 Using External Sources of Information

Sometimes, instead of a sub-sample from the same study, the repeat or validation sample is from an external source, a second study. However, even if the same exposure measure is used in the second study, it is unlikely that the distribution of X would be identical, and therefore unlikely that λ would be the same. Rather than try to apply the reliability ratio λ to the data, it is more sensible to extract the measurement error variance itself, σ_u^2, from the second study, and use this in conjunction with the distribution of X found in the study needing correction for the effects of measurement error (Carroll et al. 2006). The ability to use a parameter (such as the reliability ratio or measurement error variance) obtained from one study to inform another is known as "transportability". For the reasons I have outlined above, the measurement error variance is considered more transportable than the reliability ratio (Carroll et al. 2006).

The different combination of internal and external sources of information in the context of nutritional epidemiology has been summarised by Spiegelman et al. (2005). Whilst Lyles et al. explore the possibility of combining both internal and external validation (Lyles et al. 2007).

3.3.5 Statistical Methods

There are many statistical methods suggested for correcting for measurement error in a variety of situations. Many approaches for linear regression have been reviewed by Fuller et al. (Fuller 1987), and for nonlinear models (nonlinear link functions) by Carroll et al. (2006). I now introduce a few of the common or widely applicable methods that are available using standard statistical software.

3.3.5.1 Regression Calibration

Regression calibration is a widely applicable approach to measurement error in generalised linear models. The basis of it is replacing X (which we can't measure), with the regression of X on Z and W (which we can estimate) in the analysis model. This approximation on which regression calibration is based is exact for linear regression (apart from a change in the intercept parameter) where $Var(X|Z,W)$ is constant, and is an "almost exact" approximation for logistic regression (Carroll et al. 1995) and Cox's proportional hazards model (Hughes 1993).

In its simplest form, regression calibration follows the algorithm below:

1. Using replicates, a validation sample or instrumental data, estimate $\hat{X}$, the regression of X on Z and W.
2. Replace the unobserved X by its estimate $\hat{X}$ from step 1 and run the standard analysis to derive the parameter estimates.
3. Adjust the standard errors of these parameters to allow for the fact that X is only estimated in the calibration model, using either bootstrapping or sandwich estimates.

If we define $E(Y|X,Z) = f(Z,X,B)$, then the approximation made in the regression calibration model is to assume: $E(Y|W,Z) \approx f(Z,\hat{X},B)$. Since in this equation the X is replaced by $\hat{X}$, the expected values no longer depends on X, but on W. This assumes non-differential measurement error. With replicate data, the measurement error variance matrix Σ_{uu} can be estimated from a variance components model (Carroll et al. 2006). Estimation of the standard errors of the resulting parameters requires bootstrapping or sandwich estimates.

Where a validation sample exists, it is still preferable to use these true measures of X wherever they are known. To facilitate this, it is advisable to insert a dummy variable indicating the source of the X – whether exactly observed, or estimated from the first stage of the regression calibration.

Regression calibration is generally applicable to generalised linear models, though this depends to some extent on the linear approximation used in the calibration equation (Carroll et al. 2006). Some exploration of alternative "better" approximations have been made, but the linear approximation has been shown to be "adequate" providing the effects of X are "not too large" (Carroll et al. 1995; Kuha 1994; Rosner et al. 1989, 1990; Spiegelman et al. 1997; White et al. 2001; Whittemore 1989). Where imperfectly measured covariates are a mixture of continuous and binary, conventional regression calibration may lead to over-correction, because errors in the binary covariate are not independent of the true value. Extensions to the method are required in this situation (Bashir and Duffy 1997; Kuha 1997; Richardson and Gilks 1993b; White et al. 2001).

In the case of logistic regression, the conditions for regression calibration are satisfied if the disease is rare, the relative risk small, and measurement error small (Kuha 1994; Rosner et al. 1989). Carroll, in particular, has explored the application of regression calibration to logistic regression under what he calls four worst case scenarios covering additive and multiplicative error, normally distributed and skewed error distributions (Carroll et al. 2006). All four scenarios include very large measurement error. In each of these the regression calibration algorithm still works well and gives good estimates. In addition, in epidemiology, any effects of environmental exposures on outcomes such as cancer or death are generally either large and already known, or quite small and under investigation. This, then, also supports the use of the approximation in most future research.

Historically, the regression calibration method has been suggested as a general method by Carroll and Stefanski (1990), Gleser (1990), and Armstrong (1985), whilst Prentice, Clayton and Hughes have extended its use to the context of survival analysis and Cox proportional hazards regression (Clayton 1992; Hughes 1993; Prentice 1982), where it has been used in two large cohorts: the Nurses' Health Study (Spiegelman et al. 1997) and EPIC (Gonzalez et al. 2006a, b). The method was "popularised" amongst statisticians by Rosner et al. (Carroll et al. 1995; Rosner et al. 1989, 1990), though methods are still not widely used, even amongst statisticians or epidemiologists, and they are certainly not well recognised yet within clinical circles.

Caroll et al.'s version of regression calibration is available in Stata (StataCorp 2005) for a range of generalised linear models characterised by any sensible combination of link function and distribution families (Hardin et al. 2003a). Versions are also available in SAS (Rosner et al. 1992; Weller et al. 2007). It is also easy to implement the algorithms in R.

3.3.5.2 Simulation Extrapolation (SIMEX)

SIMEX and regression calibration are both functional approaches to adjusting for the effects of measurement error. Regression calibration uses a modelling-based solution to this, but in contrast SIMEX is simulation-based, using a particular resampling algorithm (Carroll et al. 1995; Cook and Stefanski 1994). This simple method is widely applicable to a broad range of models. Loosely speaking, the algorithm keeps adding a small known amount of error and re-estimates the parameters each time. A trend in the effect of the measurement error is then estimated, and extrapolation made to the case where there is no measurement error. The algorithm is as follows:

1. The model is fitted "as is" to obtain estimated coefficients $\hat{\beta}$ and an estimate of $\hat{\sigma}_u^2$ based on variance components analysis (Carroll et al. 2006) or deemed "known" from external validation data.
2. Additional error is added as follows:
    (a) Additional random error is generated at θ times the estimated $\hat{\sigma}_u^2$ and added to the original values of X, such that added error $\varepsilon_\theta \sim N(0, \theta\hat{\sigma}_u^2)$.
    (b) The model is then refitted to the new X and new coefficients $\hat{\beta}$ estimated.
3. This is repeated r times and the mean or median coefficient $\bar{\hat{\beta}}$ of these parameter estimates is then calculated. Step 2 is then repeated for different of values of θ, e.g. {.5, 1, 1.5, 2}. The original model fitted in step 1 is taken as an additional observation with $\theta = 0$.
4. For each coefficient in the model, the estimate is plotted against the value of θ used. The trend is then extrapolated back to $\theta = -1$. This then is the estimate without measurement error. Methods for extrapolation include linear or quadratic extrapolants. The most stable of these is the quadratic extrapolant (Carroll et al. 1995, 1996; Cook and Stefanski 1994; Hardin et al. 2003b; Wang et al. 1998).

The SIMEX method does allow for plots that can be informative in terms of the effects of measurement error, and the robustness of the results from taking this approach.

This approach does not have the elegance of a simple closed formula, and it may be sensitive to the choice of method used to extrapolate the curve over the values of θ. However, in practice it appears to work well. SIMEX is available in Stata for a range of generalised linear models characterised by any sensible combination of link function and distribution families (Hardin et al. 2003b). SIMEX is also available through R's `simex` package. It is also easy to implement the algorithm in SAS.

3.3.5.3 Multiple Imputation

The historical divergence of methods to handle missing data from those for mismeasured data is charted by Caroll (Carroll et al. 1995). Longford, however, has proposed multiple imputation (Rubin 1987; Schafer 1997) as a general approach to all forms of missingness in data, including variables measured with error, rounding error, coarse data, and completely missing data (Longford 2001). There is some conceptual advantage in using the same approach to handle these different types of "corrupted" observations, and it has been suggested that under some situations multiple imputation has greater power than other methods (Cole et al. 2006). As with multiple imputation of missing data, a number of imputed datasets would then be available for standard statistical analyses before simple pooling of estimates, making results corrected for measurement error more accessible to non-statisticians. However, one disadvantage is that multiple imputation requires validation data on a sub-sample (rather than replicates or instruments), and in many situations may have less power than other methods (White 2006). Multiple imputation is discussed at greater length in Chap. 2, and procedures are widely available in standard software such as Stata, R, and SAS.

3.3.5.4 Latent Variable and Multilevel Methods

Measurement error can profitably be viewed as a latent variable problem, with the latent true exposure estimated on the basis of replicates, surrogate measures or instrumental variables. The methods and software described elsewhere in this book for latent traits and latent classes are therefore directly relevant to correcting for errors in continuous and categorical exposure variables (see Chaps. 6 and 7). Two particularly flexible approaches to estimating disease associations with latent true exposures are Bayesian and quadrature-based methods.

3.3.5.5 Bayesian Approaches

Bayesian methods are ideally suited for modelling the conditional dependency models described by the disease, exposure and measurement models outlined in Sect. 3.2.2. The structural modelling approach has the advantage of naturally taking account of the hierarchical structure of data incorporating latent true exposures, repeated observed exposures and measurement error. In addition they allow the incorporation of prior information on the measurement error variance or the distribution of the true covariate. Through inclusion of prior information they may also provide a solution to non-identifiability of the measurement error model in some circumstances (White et al. 2001). This leads to very flexible models in that they can be applied to a wide range of measurement error problems.

Whilst regression calibration has two main steps (regressing X on W to estimate $\hat{X}$, then using $\hat{X}$ in place of X in the standard analysis), the Bayesian approach models all the estimates (nodes) simultaneously. This means that cyclical structural equation models cannot be fitted using some popular software (Spiegelhalter et al. 1996, 2004). In addition, Gustafson suggests that the need for an exposure model with the structural Bayesian approach, and the possibility of misspecifying this, makes it more susceptible to bias than regression calibration (Gustafson 2004).

Richardson has applied a range of Bayesian models in the context of both validation samples and replicate samples (Richardson and Gilks 1993a, b). She has extended these models to the situation where the prior distribution is a mixture of different distributions, to allow greater flexibility (Richardson et al. 2002), and has outlined how the approach may be used on aggregate level data (Gilks and Richardson 1992; Richardson 1996; Richardson and Best 2003). In addition, some discussion and development of these tools for use in epidemiology has been made by Bashir and Duffy (1997), by Mishra and Day (Day and Mishra 2003, 2004), by Gustafson (Gustafson et al. 2002; Gustafson 2004) and others (Bashir and Duffy 1997; Bennett and Wakefield 2001; Berry et al. 2002; Dunson 2001; Moala and Baba 2003; Raghunathan and Siscovick 1998; Schmid and Rosner 1993; Song et al. 2002; Whittaker et al. 2003).

Advantages of using MCMC within a Bayesian framework include the ability to model measurement error correlation structures, extension of simple classical measurement error models to include correlated person-specific biases and flattening of the regression of X on W. A range of exposure distributions can be modelled, or a mixture of distributions could be used if justified, e.g. for zero-inflated data (see Chap. 6). Disadvantages of Bayesian methods include possible subjectivity in specification of priors, potential lack of convergence to a stationary distribution, and length of time taken to achieve convergence, given the heavy computational requirement.

MCMC methods are implemented in the BUGS software family (Classic BUGS, WinBUGS, and OpenBUGS) (Spiegelhalter et al. 1996, 2007), JAGS (Plummer 2003), and for a limited range of models in MLwiN (Browne 2004; Rasbash et al. 2004). Bayesian models are often described using directed acyclic graphs (DAGs), and this graphical approach to modelling is described in detail in Chap. 9.

3.3.5.6 Quadrature-Based Methods

An alternative to using MCMC methods to perform numerical integration is Gauss-Hermite quadrature. This procedure evaluates the integral approximately by taking a weighted sum of the integrand evaluated at each of a set of values (known as quadrature points or masses) of the variable being integrated out (Skrondal and Rabe-Hesketh 2004). However, a large number of quadrature points may be required in many circumstances relating to correcting for measurement error (Crouch and Spiegelman 1990), so the procedure may take a considerable time to achieve accurate approximation. Adaptive quadrature allows the standard methods for quadrature to be fine-tuned, so that the quadrature points are placed in the most efficient places, e.g. under the peak of the integrand. These methods are implemented in Stata's `gllamm` (Rabe-Hesketh et al. 2001) and `cme` (Rabe-Hesketh et al. 2003), a Stata command based on `gllamm` with simplified syntax specific to measurement error problems. They are also implemented through R's `npmlreg` and SAS PROC NLMIXED.

This approach to maximum likelihood using adaptive quadrature is very flexible and can be extended to a variety of measurement error models that MCMC can handle (Rabe-Hesketh et al. 2001, 2002, 2003), including allowing for non-classical error structures and the use of instrumental variables (see Sect. 3.3.3). Criticisms of quadrature include its slow speed, particularly when implemented in Stata, but offset by its great flexibility.

3.4 Practical Example

The importance of correcting for the effects of measurement error are well demonstrated by research into the relationship between dietary fat and breast cancer (Bingham et al. 2003). Researchers in Cambridge investigated this association using both a food frequency questionnaire (FFQ) and a 7-day food diary. FFQs are known to lack precision, but are often used in large cohort studies because they are cheaper to administer and derive nutrient intakes from for large numbers of participants.

A nested case-control design was used, with four controls for every case, matched on age and date of entry to the study. Conditional logistic regression was then used to derive odds ratios (equivalent here to hazard ratios). After adjustment for potential confounders, including energy intake from non-fat sources, the FFQ measure of total fat yielded a hazard ratio of 1.06 (95% CI: 0.89–1.25) for each fifth of total fat intake. The same analysis based on the food diary gave a hazard ratio of 1.17 (95% CI: 1.00–1.36). For saturated fat, the contrast was just as clear, with 1.10 (0.94–1.29) using the FFQ and 1.22 (1.06–1.40) using the diary.

With the less precise measure, estimates of the size of the association were small and confidence intervals spanned the null, whilst using the more precise measure the association appeared stronger and confidence intervals further from the null. Yet food diaries themselves have been strongly criticised for containing a large component of error, and that error being correlated between repeat measures, and with other self-report tools such as FFQs (Day et al. 2004; Greenwood et al. 2006b; Kipnis et al. 1999, 2001). The implication is that even food diaries yield strongly biased estimates of diet-disease associations, possibly as much as halving the true association. Only the use of unbiased, objective measures such as recovery biomarkers, till receipts or household inventories can offer unbiased results.

3.5 Future Developments

Measurement error methods have only recently started to be used in major cohorts, e.g. the Nurses' Health Study (Spiegelman et al. 1997), EPIC (Ferrari et al. 2009; Gonzalez et al. 2006a, b), The UK Women's Cohort (Cade et al. 2007), and the Centre for Nutritional Epidemiology in Cancer Prevention and Survival (Dahm et al. 2010), but their use is not yet widespread. As their benefits are more widely recognised and they become accepted in the clinical community, we will begin to see less biased estimates of some difficult to measure environmental exposures. Recent incorporation into standard software packages should also facilitate their use. Areas of further development may be specific to particular exposures, such as development of a wider range of objective biomarkers of various exposures, including dietary exposures.

References

Aiken, L. S., & West, S. G. (1991). Reliability and statistical power. In *Multiple regression: Testing and interpreting interactions* (pp. 139–171). Newbury Park: Sage publications.
Armstrong, B. (1985). Measurement error in generalised linear models. *Communications in Statistics-Simulation and Computation, 14*, 529–544.
Armstrong, B. G. (1998). Effect of measurement error on epidemiological studies of environmental and occupational exposures. *Occupational and Environmental Medicine, 55*, 651–656.
Bashir, S. A., & Duffy, S. W. (1997). The correction of risk estimates for measurement error. *Annals of Epidemiology, 7*, 154–164.
Bennett, J., & Wakefield, J. (2001). Errors-in-variables in joint population pharmacokinetic/pharmacodynamic modeling. *Biometrics, 57*, 803–812.
Berry, S. M., Carroll, R. J., & Ruppert, D. (2002). Bayesian smoothing and regression splines for measurement error problems. *Journal of the American Statistical Association, 97*, 160–169.
Bingham, S. A., Luben, R., Welch, A., Wareham, N., Khaw, K. T., & Day, N. E. (2003). Are imprecise methods obscuring a relation between fat and breast cancer? *Lancet, 362*, 212–214.
Bjork, J., & Stromberg, U. (2002). Effects of systematic exposure assessment errors in partially ecologic case-control studies. *International Journal of Epidemiology, 31*, 154–160.
Brenner, H. (1993). Bias due to non-differential misclassification of polytomous confounders. *Journal of Clinical Epidemiology, 46*, 57–63.

Browne, W. (2004). *MCMC estimation in MLwiN*. London: Institute of Education/University of London.
Byers, T. (2001). Food frequency dietary assessment: How bad is good enough? *American Journal of Epidemiology, 154*, 1087–1088.
Cade, J., Thompson, R., Burley, V., & Warm, D. (2002). Development, validation and utilisation of food-frequency questionnaires – A review. *Public Health Nutrition, 5*, 567–587.
Cade, J. E., Burley, V. J., & Greenwood, D. C. (2007). Dietary fibre and risk of breast cancer in the UK Women's Cohort Study. *International Journal of Epidemiology, 36*, 431–438.
Calvert, C., Cade, J., Barrett, J. H., & Woodhouse, A. (1997). Using cross-check questions to address the problem of mis-reporting of specific food groups on food frequency questionnaires. *European Journal of Clinical Nutrition, 51*, 708–712.
Carroll, R. J., & Stefanski, L. A. (1990). Approximate quasi-likelihood estimation in models with surrogate predictors. *Journal of the American Statistical Association, 85*, 652–663.
Carroll, R. J., Ruppert, D., & Stefanski, L. A. (1995). *Measurement error in nonlinear models*. London: Chapman & Hall.
Carroll, R. J., Kuchenhoff, H., Lombard, F., & Stefanski, L. A. (1996). Asymptotics for the SIMEX estimator in nonlinear measurement error models. *Journal of the American Statistical Association, 91*, 242–250.
Carroll, R. J., Ruppert, D., Stefanski, L. A., & Crainiceanu, C. M. (2006). *Measurement error in nonlinear models* (2nd ed.). London: Chapman & Hall.
Clayton, D. G. (1992). Models for the longitudinal analysis of cohort and case-control studies with inaccurately measured exposures. In J. H. Dwyer et al. (Eds.), *Statistical models for longitudinal studies of health* (pp. 301–331). Oxford: Oxford University Press.
Cole, S. R., Chu, H., & Greenland, S. (2006). Multiple-imputation for measurement-error correction. *International Journal of Epidemiology, 35*, 1074–1081.
Cook, J. R., & Stefanski, L. A. (1994). Simulation-extrapolation estimation in parametric measurement error models. *Journal of the American Statistical Association, 89*, 1314–1328.
Crouch, E. A. C., & Spiegelman, D. (1990). The evaluation of integrals of the form integral-infinity + infinity F(T)Exp(-T2) Dt – Application to logistic normal-models. *Journal of the American Statistical Association, 85*, 464–469.
Dahm, C. C., Keogh, R. H., Spencer, E. A., Greenwood, D. C., Key, T. J., Fentiman, I., Shipley, M. J., Brunner, E. J., Cade, J. E., Burley, V. J., Mishra, G., Stephen, A. M., Kuh, D., White, I. R., Luben, R., Lentjes, M. A. H., Khaw, K. T., & Rodwell, S. A. (2010). Dietary fiber and colorectal cancer risk: A nested case–control study. *Journal of the National Cancer Institute, 102*(9), 614–626.
Day, J. G., Mishra, G. D. (2003). *Correcting for measurement error using data from two different measurement instruments*, Practical Bayesian Statistics 5 Conference, Milton Keynes.
Day, J. G., Mishra, G. D. (2004). *A Bayesian approach to correcting for measurement error where there is no calibration data*. 22nd International Biometrics Conference, Cairns, Australia.
Day, N. E., Wong, M. Y., Bingham, S., Khaw, K. T., Luben, R., Michels, K. B., Welch, A., & Wareham, N. J. (2004). Correlated measurement error–implications for nutritional epidemiology. *International Journal of Epidemiology, 33*, 1373–1381.
DelPizzo, V., & Borghesi, J. L. (1995). Exposure measurement errors, risk estimate and statistical power in case-control studies using dichotomous-analysis of a continuous exposure variable. *International Journal of Epidemiology, 24*, 851–862.
Dosemeci, M., Wacholder, S., & Lubin, J. H. (1990). Does nondifferential misclassification of exposure always bias a true effect toward the null value? *American Journal of Epidemiology, 132*, 746–748.
Dunn, G. (2004). *Statistical evaluation of measurement errors: Design and analysis of reliability studies* (2nd ed.). London: Arnold.
Dunson, D. B. (2001). Commentary: Practical advantages of Bayesian analysis of epidemiologic data. *American Journal of Epidemiology, 153*, 1222–1226.

Elmstahl, S., & Gullberg, B. (1997). Bias in diet assessment methods–consequences of collinearity and measurement errors on power and observed relative risks. *International Journal of Epidemiology, 26*, 1071–1079.

Ferrari, P., Roddam, A., Fahey, M. T., Jenab, M., Bamia, C., Ocke, M., Amiano, P., Hjartaker, A., Biessy, C., Rinaldi, S., Huybrechts, I., Tjonneland, A., Dethlefsen, C., Niravong, M., Clavel-Chapelon, F., Linseisen, J., Boeing, H., Oikonomou, E., Orfanos, P., Palli, D., de Santucci, M., Bueno-de-Mesquita, H. B., Peeters, P. H., Parr, C. L., Braaten, T., Dorronsoro, M., Berenguer, T., Gullberg, B., Johansson, I., Welch, A. A., Riboli, E., Bingham, S., & Slimani, N. (2009). A bivariate measurement error model for nitrogen and potassium intakes to evaluate the performance of regression calibration in the European Prospective Investigation into Cancer and Nutrition study. *European Journal of Clinical Nutrition, 63*, S179–S187.

Flegal, K. M. (1999). Evaluating epidemiologic evidence of the effects of food and nutrient exposures. *American Journal of Clinical Nutrition, 69*, 1339S–1344S.

Freedman, L. S., Schatzkin, A., & Wax, Y. (1990). The impact of dietary measurement error on planning sample size required in a cohort study. *American Journal of Epidemiology, 118*, 1185–1195.

Freedman, L. S., Schatzkin, A., Thiebaut, A. C. M., Potischman, N., Subar, A. F., Thompson, F. E., & Kipnis, V. (2007). Abandon neither the food frequency questionnaire nor the dietary fat-breast cancer hypothesis. *Cancer Epidemiology, Biomarkers & Prevention, 16*, 1321–1322.

Fuller, W. A. (1987). *Measurement error models*. New York: Wiley.

Gilks, W. R., & Richardson, S. (1992). Analysis of disease risks using ancillary risk factors, with application to job-exposure matrices. *Statistics in Medicine, 11*, 1443–1463.

Gladen, B., & Rogan, W. J. (1979). Misclassification and the design of environmental studies. *American Journal of Epidemiology, 109*, 607–616.

Gleser, L. J. (1990). Improvements of the naive approach to estimation in nonlinear errors-in-variables regression models. In P. J. Brown & W. A. Fuller (Eds.), *Statistical analysis of measurement error models and applications* (pp. 99–114). Providence: American Mathematical Society.

Gonzalez, C. A., Jakszyn, P., Pera, G., Agudo, A., Bingham, S., Palli, D., Ferrari, P., Boeing, H., Del Giudice, G., Plebani, M., Carneiro, F., Nesi, G., Berrino, F., Sacerdote, C., Tumino, R., Panico, S., Berglund, G., Siman, H., Nyren, O., Hallmans, G., Martinez, C., Dorronsoro, M., Barricarte, A., Navarro, C., Quiros, J. R., Allen, N., Key, T. J., Day, N. E., Linseisen, J., Nagel, G., Bergmann, M. M., Overvad, K., Jensen, M. K., Tjonneland, A., Olsen, A., Bueno-de-Mesquita, H. B., Ocke, M., Peeters, P. H., Numans, M. E., Clavel-Chapelon, F., Boutron-Ruault, M. C., Trichopoulou, A., Psaltopoulou, T., Roukos, D., Lund, E., Hemon, B., Kaaks, R., Norat, T., & Riboli, E. (2006a). Meat intake and risk of stomach and esophageal adenocarcinoma within the European Prospective Investigation into Cancer and Nutrition (EPIC). *Journal of the National Cancer Institute, 98*, 345–354.

Gonzalez, C. A., Pera, G., Agudo, A., Bueno-de-Mesquita, H. B., Ceroti, M., Boeing, H., Schulz, M., Del Giudice, G., Plebani, M., Carneiro, F., Berrino, F., Sacerdote, C., Tumino, R., Panico, S., Berglund, G., Siman, H., Hallmans, G., Stenling, R., Martinez, C., Dorronsoro, M., Barricarte, A., Navarro, C., Quiros, J. R., Allen, N., Key, T. J., Bingham, S., Day, N. E., Linseisen, J., Nagel, G., Overvad, K., Jensen, M. K., Olsen, A., Tjonneland, A., Buchner, F. L., Peeters, P. H., Numans, M. E., Clavel-Chapelon, F., Boutron-Ruault, M. C., Roukos, D., Trichopoulou, A., Psaltopoulou, T., Lund, E., Casagrande, C., Slimani, N., Jenab, M., & Riboli, E. (2006b). Fruit and vegetable intake and the risk of stomach and oesophagus adenocarcinoma in the European Prospective Investigation into Cancer and Nutrition (EPIC-EURGAST). *International Journal of Cancer, 118*, 2559–2566.

Greenland, S. (1980). The effect of misclassification in the presence of covariates. *American Journal of Epidemiology, 112*, 564–569.

Greenwood, D. C., Gilthorpe, M. S., & Cade, J. E. (2006a). The impact of imprecisely measured covariates on estimating gene-environment interactions. *BMC Medical Research Methodology, 6*, 21.

Greenwood, D. C., Ransley, J. K., Gilthorpe, M. S., & Cade, J. E. (2006b). Use of itemized till receipts to adjust for correlated dietary measurement error. *American Journal of Epidemiology, 164*, 1012–1018.

Gustafson, P. (2004). *Measurement error and misclassification in statistics and epidemiology: Impacts and Bayesian adjustments.* London: Chapman & Hall.

Gustafson, P., Le, N. D., & Vallee, M. (2002). A Bayesian approach to case-control studies with errors in covariables. *Biostatistics, 3*, 229–243.

Hardin, J. W., Schmiediche, H., & Carroll, R. J. (2003a). The regression-calibration method for fitting generalized linear models with additive measurement error. *The Stata Journal, 3*, 361–372.

Hardin, J. W., Schmiediche, H., & Carroll, R. J. (2003b). The simulation extrapolation method for fitting generalized linear models with additive measurement error. *The Stata Journal, 3*, 373–385.

Huang, L. S., Wang, H. K., & Cox, C. (2005). Assessing interaction effects in linear measurement error models. *Journal of the Royal Statistical Society Series C-Applied Statistics, 54*, 21–30.

Hughes, M. D. (1993). Regression dilution in the proportional hazards model. *Biometrics, 49*, 1056–1066.

Kaaks, R., Riboli, E., & van Staveren, W. A. (1995). Calibration of dietary-intake measurements in prospective cohort studies. *American Journal of Epidemiology, 142*, 548–556.

Kipnis, V., Carroll, R. J., Freedman, L. S., & Li, L. (1999). Implications of a new dietary measurement error model for estimation of relative risk: Application to four calibration studies. *American Journal of Epidemiology, 150*, 642–651.

Kipnis, V., Midthune, D., Freedman, L. S., Bingham, S., Schatzkin, A., Subar, A., & Carroll, R. J. (2001). Empirical evidence of correlated biases in dietary assessment instruments and its implications. *American Journal of Epidemiology, 153*, 394–403.

Kipnis, V., Subar, A. F., Midthune, D., Freedman, L. S., Ballard-Barbash, R., Troiano, R. P., Bingham, S., Schoeller, D. A., Schatzkin, A., & Carroll, R. J. (2003). Structure of dietary measurement error: Results of the OPEN Biomarker Study. *American Journal of Epidemiology, 158*, 14–21.

Kuha, J. (1994). Corrections for exposure measurement error in logistic-regression models with an application to nutritional data. *Statistics in Medicine, 13*, 1135–1148.

Kuha, J. (1997). Estimation by data augmentation in regression models with continuous and discrete covariates measured with error. *Statistics in Medicine, 16*, 189–201.

Longford, N. T. (2001). Multilevel analysis with messy data. *Statistical Methods in Medical Research, 10*, 429–444.

Lyles, R. H., Zhang, F., & Drews-Botsch, C. (2007). Combining internal and external validation data to correct for exposure misclassification: A case study. *Epidemiology, 18*, 321–328.

Moala, F. A., Baba, M. Y. (2003). *Bayesian analysis of the simple linear regression with measurement errors.* Practical Bayesian Statistics 5 Conference, Milton Keynes.

Murad, H., & Freedman, L. S. (2007). Estimating and testing interactions in linear regression models when explanatory variables are subject to classical measurement error. *Statistics in Medicine, 26*(23), 4293–4310.

Phillips, A. N., & Smith, G. D. (1991). How independent are independent effects – Relative risk-estimation when correlated exposures are measured imprecisely. *Journal of Clinical Epidemiology, 44*, 1223–1231.

Plummer, M. (2003). JAGS: A program for analysis of bayesian graphical models using gibbs sampling. *Proceedings of the 3rd International Workshop on Distributed Statistical Computing (DSC 2003)*, March 20–22, Vienna, Austria.

Prentice, R. L. (1982). Covariate measurement errors and parameter estimation in failure time regression models. *Biometrika, 69*, 331–342.

Rabe-Hesketh, S., Pickles, A., & Skrondal, A. (2001). *GLLAMM manual: Technical report 2001/01.* London: Department of Biostatistics and Computing, Institute of Psychiatry, King's College, University of London.

Rabe-Hesketh, S., Skrondal, A., & Pickles, A. (2002). Reliable estimation of generalised linear mixed models using adaptive quadrature. *The Stata Journal, 2*, 1–21.

Rabe-Hesketh, S., Skrondal, A., & Pickles, A. (2003). Maximum likelihood estimation of generalized linear models with covariate measurement error. *The Stata Journal, 3*, 386–411.

Raghunathan, T. E., & Siscovick, D. S. (1998). Combining exposure information from various sources in an analysis of a case-control study. *Journal of the Royal Statistical Society Series D-the Statistician, 47*, 333–347.

Ransley, J. K., Donnelly, J. K., Khara, T. N., Botham, H., Arnot, H., Greenwood, D. C., & Cade, J. E. (2001). The use of supermarket till receipts to determine the fat and energy intake in a UK population. *Public Health Nutrition, 4*, 1279–1286.

Ransley, J. K., Donnelly, J. K., Botham, H., Khara, T. N., Greenwood, D. C., & Cade, J. E. (2003). Use of supermarket receipts to estimate energy and fat content of food purchased by lean and overweight families. *Appetite, 41*, 141–148.

Rasbash, J., Steele, F., Browne, W., & Prosser, B. (2004). *A user's guide to MLwiN version 2.0*. London: Institute of Education/University of London.

Richardson, D. B., & Ciampi, A. (2003). Effects of exposure measurement error when an exposure variable is constrained by a lower limit. *American Journal of Epidemiology, 157*, 355–363.

Richardson, S. (1996). Measurement error. In W. R. Gilks, S. Richardson, & D. J. Spiegelhalter (Eds.), *Markov chain Monte Carlo in practice* (pp. 401–417). London: Chapman & Hall.

Richardson, S., & Best, N. (2003). Bayesian hierarchical models in ecological studies of health-environment effects. *Environmetrics, 14*, 129–147.

Richardson, S., & Gilks, W. R. (1993a). A Bayesian approach to measurement error problems in epidemiology using conditional independence models. *American Journal of Epidemiology, 138*, 430–442.

Richardson, S., & Gilks, W. R. (1993b). Conditional independence models for epidemiological studies with covariate measurement error. *Statistics in Medicine, 12*, 1703–1722.

Richardson, S., Leblond, L., Jaussent, I., & Green, P. J. (2002). Mixture models in measurement error problems, with reference to epidemiological studies. *Journal of the Royal Statistical Society: Series A (Statistics in Society), 165*, 549–566.

Rippin, G. (2001). Design issues and sample size when exposure measurement is inaccurate. *Methods of Information in Medicine, 40*, 137–140.

Rosner, B., Willett, W. C., & Spiegelman, D. (1989). Correction of logistic regression relative risk estimates and confidence intervals for systematic within-person measurement error. *Statistics in Medicine, 8*, 1051–1069.

Rosner, B., Spiegelman, D., & Willett, W. C. (1990). Correction of logistic-regression relative risk estimates and confidence-intervals for measurement error – The case of multiple covariates measured with error. *American Journal of Epidemiology, 132*, 734–745.

Rosner, B., Spiegelman, D., & Willett, W.C. (1992). Correction of logistic regression relative risk estimates and confidence intervals for random within person measurement error. *American Journal of Epidemiology, 136*, 1400–1413.

Rubin, D. B. (1987). *Multiple imputation for nonresponse in surveys*. New York: Wiley.

Schafer, J. L. (1997). *Analysis of incomplete multivariate data*. London: Chapman & Hall.

Schatzkin, A., Midthune, D., Subar, A., Thompson, F., & Kipnis, V. (2001a). The national institutes of health-American association of retired persons (NIH-AARP) diet and health study: Power to detect diet-cancer associations after adjusting for measurement error. *American Journal of Epidemiology, 153*, 966.

Schatzkin, A., Subar, A. F., Thompson, F. E., Harlan, L. C., Tangrea, J., Hollenbeck, A. R., Hurwitz, P. E., Coyle, L., Schussler, N., Michaud, D. S., Freedman, L. S., Brown, C. C., Midthune, D., & Kipnis, V. (2001b). Design and serendipity in establishing a large cohort with wide dietary intake distributions – The National Institutes of Health-American Association of Retired Persons Diet and Health Study. *American Journal of Epidemiology, 154*, 1119–1125.

Schatzkin, A., Kipnis, V., Carroll, R. J., Midthune, D., Subar, A. F., Bingham, S., Schoeller, D. A., Troiano, R. P., & Freedman, L. S. (2003). A comparison of a food frequency questionnaire with a 24-hour recall for use in an epidemiological cohort study: Results from the biomarker-based Observing Protein and Energy Nutrition (OPEN) study. *International Journal of Epidemiology, 32*, 1054–1062.

Schmid, C. H., & Rosner, B. (1993). A bayesian-approach to logistic-regression models having measurement error following a mixture distribution. *Statistics in Medicine, 12*, 1141–1153.

Skrondal, A., & Rabe-Hesketh, S. (2004). *Generalized latent variable modeling*. London: Chapman & Hall.

Song, X., Davidian, M., & Tsiatis, A. A. (2002). An estimator for the proportional hazards model with multiple longitudinal covariates measured with error. *Biostatistics, 3*, 511–528.

Sorahan, T., & Gilthorpe, M. S. (1994). Non-differential misclassification of exposure always leads to an underestimate of risk: An incorrect conclusion. *Occupational and Environmental Medicine, 51*, 839–840.

Spiegelhalter, D. J., Thomas, A., Best, N. G., & Gilks, W. (1996). *BUGS 0.5: Bayesian inference using Gibbs sampling manual*. Cambridge: MRC Biostatistics Unit.

Spiegelhalter, D. J., Thomas, A., Best, N. G., & Lunn, D. (2004). *WinBUGS user manual: Version 1.4.2*. Cambridge: MRC Biostatistics Unit.

Spiegelhalter, D. J., Thomas, A., Best, N. G., & Lunn, D. (2007). *WinBUGS user manual: Version 1.4.3*. Cambridge: MRC Biostatistics Unit.

Spiegelman, D., McDermott, A., & Rosner, B. (1997). Regression calibration method for correcting measurement-error bias in nutritional epidemiology. *American Journal of Clinical Nutrition, 65*, S1179–S1186.

Spiegelman, D., Zhao, B., & Kim, J. (2005). Correlated errors in biased surrogates: Study designs and methods for measurement error correction. *Statistics in Medicine, 24*, 1657–1682.

StataCorp. (2005). *Stata statistical software: Release 9.2*. College Station: Stata Corporation.

Stefanski, L. A., & Carroll, R. J. (1985). Covariate measurement error in logistic regression. *The Annals of Statistics, 13*, 1335–1351.

Subar, A. F., Kipnis, V., Troiano, R. P., Midthune, D., Schoeller, D. A., Bingham, S., Sharbaugh, C. O., Trabulsi, J., Runswick, S., Ballard-Barbash, R., Sunshine, J., & Schatzkin, A. (2003). Using intake biomarkers to evaluate the extent of dietary misreporting in a large sample of adults: The OPEN study. *American Journal of Epidemiology, 158*, 1–13.

Thomas, D., Stram, D. O., & Dwyer, J. H. (1993). Exposure measurement error: Influence on exposure-disease relationships and methods of correction. *Annual Review of Public Health, 14*, 69–93.

Wang, N., Carroll, R. J., & Liang, K. Y. (1996). Quasilikelihood estimation in measurement error models with correlated replicates. *Biometrics, 52*, 401–411.

Wang, N. Y., Lin, X. H., Gutierrez, R. G., & Carroll, R. J. (1998). Bias analysis and SIMEX approach in generalized linear mixed measurement error models. *Journal of the American Statistical Association, 93*, 249–261.

Weinberg, C. R., Umbach, D. M., & Greenland, S. (1994). When will nondifferential misclassification of an exposure preserve the direction of a trend? *American Journal of Epidemiology, 140*, 565–571.

Weller, E., Milton, D., Eisen, E., Spiegelman, D. (2007). Method in regression calibration for logistic regression with multiple surrogates for one exposure. *Journal of Statistical Planning and Inference, 137*, 449–461.

White, I. R. (2006). Commentary: Dealing with measurement error: multiple imputation or regression calibration? *International Journal of Epidemiology, 35*, 1081–1082.

White, E., Kushi, L. H., & Pepe, M. S. (1994). The effect of exposure variance and exposure measurement error on study sample-size – Implications for the design of epidemiologic studies. *Journal of Clinical Epidemiology, 47*, 873–880.

White, I., Frost, C., & Tokunaga, S. (2001). Correcting for measurement error in binary and continuous variables using replicates. *Statistics in Medicine, 20*, 3441–3457.

Whittaker, H., Best, N., & Nieuwenhuijsen, M. (2003). *Modelling exposure estimates for an epidemiological study of disinfection by-products in drinking water and adverse birth outcomes*. Practical Bayesian Statistics 5 Conference, Milton Keynes.

Whittemore, A. S. (1989). Errors in variables regression using Stein estimates. *The American Statistician, 43*, 226–228.
Wikipedia contributors. Regression dilution. http://en.wikipedia.org/w/index.php?title=Regression_dilution&oldid=159186428. 20-9-2007. Wikipedia, The Free Encyclopedia. 2-11-2007.
Wong, M. Y., Day, N. E., Bashir, S. A., & Duffy, S. W. (1999a). Measurement error in epidemiology: The design of validation studies – I: Univariate situation. *Statistics in Medicine, 18*, 2815–2829.
Wong, M. Y., Day, N. E., & Wareham, N. J. (1999b). Measurement error in epidemiology: The design of validation studies – II: Bivariate situation. *Statistics in Medicine, 18*, 2831–2845.
Wong, M. Y., Day, N. E., Luan, J. A., Chan, K. P., & Wareham, N. J. (2003). The detection of gene-environment interaction for continuous traits: Should we deal with measurement error by bigger studies or better measurement? *International Journal of Epidemiology, 32*, 51–57.
Wong, M. Y., Day, N. E., Luan, J. A., & Wareham, N. J. (2004). Estimation of magnitude in gene-environment interactions in the presence of measurement error. *Statistics in Medicine, 23*, 987–998.

Chapter 4
Selection Bias in Epidemiologic Studies

Graham R. Law, Paul D. Baxter, and Mark S. Gilthorpe

Bias is inherent in epidemiology, and researchers go to great lengths to avoid introducing bias into their studies. However, some bias is inevitable, and bias due to selection is particularly common. We discuss ways to identify bias and how authors have approached removing or adjusting for bias using statistical methods.

4.1 Introduction

Observational epidemiological studies are designed to elucidate the association between disease and risk factors through making observations on people, in contrast to randomised controlled trials and other designed experiments where exposures are assigned by the researcher. All epidemiological studies, whether randomised controlled trials or observational studies, are prone to various possible errors that can lead to bias. Bias is the distortion of truth that leads to inappropriate conclusions, and this needs to be minimised. The potential for incorrect conclusions needs to be minimised through robust study design and appropriate statistical analysis. The job of the epidemiologist is to minimise the potential for research to draw incorrect or distorted conclusions. With this aim, it is often helpful to consider the various sources of potential error.

G.R. Law (✉) • P.D. Baxter • M.S. Gilthorpe
Division of Biostatistics, Centre for Epidemiology and Biostatistics,
Leeds Institute of Genetics, Health & Therapeutics, University of Leeds,
Room 8.01, Worsley Building, LS2 9LN Leeds, UK
e-mail: g.r.law@leeds.ac.uk

4.2 Observational Epidemiology and Bias

There are three main types of error recognised in epidemiology: random error or chance, confounding, and systematic error. *Random error* is the most widely-understood form of error, and is introduced through the inevitable use of random samples from the population. Confidence intervals and statistical analysis have for a long time been used to address this form of error. The epidemiologist seeks also to address the other forms of error and associated potential bias. A substantive potential for bias can arise from what is characterised as *confounding*, when associations are inappropriately attributed as caused by an exposure of interest rather than to some other characteristic of the study participants. The identification and control of confounding was described in Chap. 1 and are further explored in Chap. 11.

The third source of error, bias due to *systematic error*, has traditionally been characterised by the cause of the bias. Bias due to errors in measuring the observed exposure or outcome, known as *information bias*, can have many causes. Chapter 2 discusses bias introduced through missing data, an extreme form of information bias. Chapter 3 discussed a subtler form of information bias, caused by errors in measuring the exposure or confounders. A more widely recognised source of information bias is differential recall, which arises where people with different outcomes remember information in different ways; this can be controlled and reduced through the design and implementation of a study.

4.2.1 Selection Bias

Selection bias is a form of systematic error in observational studies; though this is perhaps less well-understood by most biomedical researchers compared to other forms of bias (especially that due to random error). Part of the training for an epidemiologist is to consider carefully the design of a study to avoid initially selecting their subjects in an inappropriate way (random selection is always preferred where possible, though may not be achievable). Randomised selection from lists, for both people with a disease of interest, or for those without a disease, is usually implemented in research studies. However, despite the best designed selection process, active participation of human subjects is desirable, and indeed often essential, for investigating putative risk factors for disease. A sample of individuals, affected by participation, may not represent the population from which it was drawn. Unfortunately, participation rates in health-related studies have been decreasing over recent years (Galea and Tracy 2007). These studies are also looking for increasingly smaller and smaller effect sizes. Therefore, the problems arising from participation bias, which in turn stem from selection bias, are likely to be ever more important to the understanding of future epidemiological research.

4.2.2 Selection Bias and Study Design

Selection bias, particularly through differential participation, may arise in commonly-used study designs such as the case-control study. Frequently problems may arise when the design of the study is retrospective to the development of disease of interest. This leads to differing motivation amongst potential participants, and often different sampling frames to be used for capturing the various categories of participant. We focus here on the two most commonly implemented designs in observational epidemiology: case-control study and cohort study.

The case-control study has become embedded as a standard epidemiological tool, with application to a wide range of human disease research. The inherent strength of this design, that it uses individual rather than aggregated data, is also a potential weakness. Many case-control studies are unable to assess the characteristics of those individuals that did not participate, leading to an absence of information about the magnitude of participation bias and its potential impact. Reassurance has often come from the understanding that 'adjusting' for a variable related to selection employs the same process as adjusting for a confounder: i.e. selection bias is effectively 'removed' during the analysis phase of the study (Law et al. 2002). However, this is an oversimplification of an important issue, which we address in this chapter in more detail.

In contrast to the case-control study, the cohort study design has fewer problems with recruitment and participation being differential between groups. Historical cohorts may sometimes require participants to volunteer after the disease outcome is known, and so be more prone to the problem than traditional cohorts, but such historical or "retrospective", cohorts are less common than their traditional counterparts (Henderson and Page 2007).

In this chapter we focus on participation bias arising in a case-control study due to differential selection between cases and controls. We address the different ways in which bias may arise, identifying criteria under which there are possibilities for statistical adjustment. In particular, we demonstrate how one approach, extensively used in epidemiology, does not always provide the correct statistical adjustment – indeed, the bias may be increased. To proceed with this discussion, we first introduce the valuable tool of graphical models.

4.3 Graphical Models and Notation

We use graphical models (Pearl 2000), or Directed Acyclic Graphs (DAGs), to explore model specification for investigating the exposure as a cause of the outcome (see Chap. 1 for definitions) and the impact of selection bias (Greenland et al. 1999).

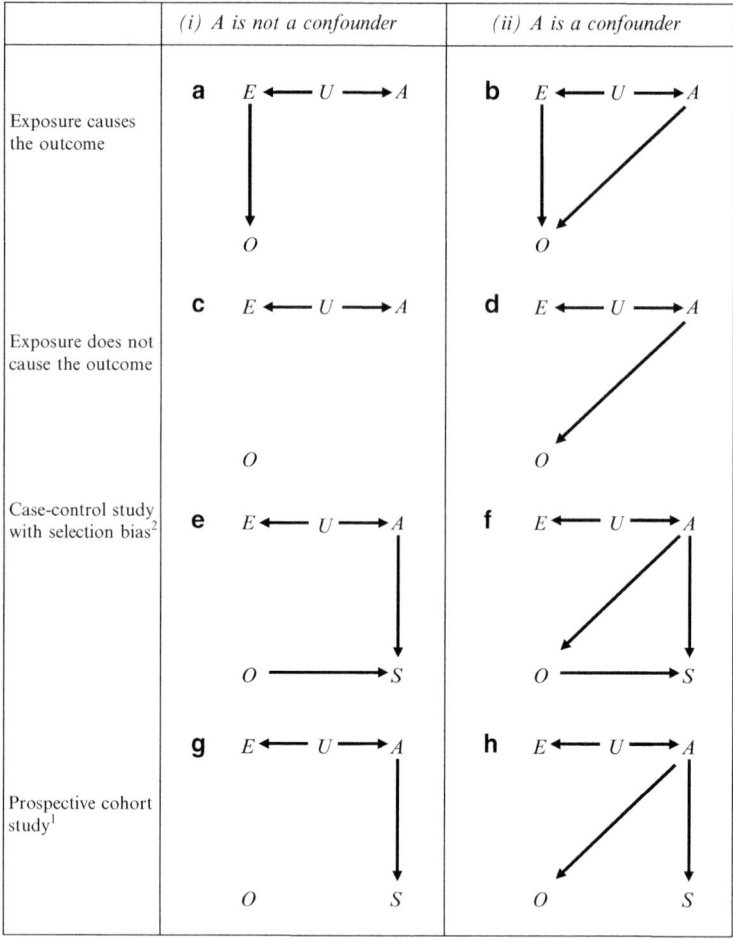

Fig. 4.1 Directed acyclic graphs representing two scenarios (**i**) one where an auxiliary factor (A) is not a confounder for the exposure (**ii**) and one where it is. Key to variables: E exposure, A auxiliary, O outcome, O_S sampled outcome, S selection, U-unmeasured; [1]balanced case and control sampling; [2]differential control sampling

4.3.1 An Epidemiological Illustration

Imagine an epidemiological investigation in a population is to be conducted into whether an exposure (E) causes an outcome (O). Figure 4.1 shows DAGs depicting causal relationships for this population, with an arrow between O and E representing the focus of a study to determine whether the exposure causes the outcome.

In notation for Fig. 4.1a

$$O \not\perp E \tag{4.1}$$

A common practice in epidemiology is to consider other covariates in parallel with an exposure. For example, these might include a measure of socio-economic or educational status, age, sex or ethnic group and we will refer to these as auxiliary variables (A). An auxiliary variable may have a cause in common (U) with the risk factor (E), such as depicted in Fig. 4.1a but not be a cause of the outcome.

$$E \not\perp A \tag{4.2}$$

A confounder may be present in any study, regardless of the study design. To consider a variable to be a confounder, it must be: (i) a cause, or a proxy of a cause, of the disease (ii) correlated with the exposure under study (iii) unaffected by the exposure, that is not on the causal pathway from exposure to the outcome (Tu et al. 2004). When these criteria are satisfied, a confounder is present, indicating that adjustment should be made within the analysis. DAGs are a particularly useful tool in identifying a confounder. If a backdoor path exists between the outcome and the exposure, via an auxiliary variable, then that variable should be considered a confounder (Greenland et al. 1999; McNamee 2003). Figure 4.1b shows such a situation, where the auxiliary variable is a cause of the outcome (O), thus leading to the conclusion that A is a confounder. Again, further to Eqs. 4.1 and 4.2:

$$O \not\perp A \tag{4.3}$$

It is important to be aware of variables that might impact upon the outcome of interest but not qualify as a confounder. These variables may be considered *competing exposures* as they qualify as an exposure were they of direct interest for their role on affecting outcome, yet they are not assigned this status in the study in question. Although not confounders, and therefore of little concern in the statistical adjustment for potential confounding, inclusion of these variables in the statistical analysis may prove beneficial by improving precision in the estimated impact of the exposure of interest. This is demonstrated for Fig. 4.1 where both E and A affect O, but A is independent of E; A may thus be considered an *independent* competing exposure.

By introducing A in the statistical analyses (e.g. in regression analysis), the variation in the O ~ E relationship is reduced – one might think of the varying O ~ E relationships as being coalesced when the variable A is introduced. The improved precision from introducing A into the analysis is offset by consuming a greater number of degrees of freedom. Therefore there may not always be an advantage in including independent competing exposures. In general, it is important not only to consider which variables are confounders (of the main exposure of interest), but also to identify which variables are independent competing exposures and to explore the value of including these in the analyses where parsimony is attained.

4.4 Representing Selection Bias

In order to consider selection bias, Geneletti and colleagues (2009) imagine that in the study population there is no causal link between the exposure and the outcome:

$$O \not\!\perp E \tag{4.4}$$

This is shown as a DAG in Fig. 4.1c, d depending on the absence or presence of a confounder respectively.

Selection for a study may be represented as a node, S, in the DAGs as summarized by Greenland and Brumback (Greenland and Brumback 2002) where S is either 0 or 1 for each individual, representing refusal or participation respectively. Figure 4.1e shows a causal diagram, from the study population represented in Fig. 4.1c where a variable A, such as socioeconomic status, is associated with the probability that someone will participate in a study. In this situation the selection and participation into a study is also associated with the disease outcome. This is the situation for a case-control study.

When the study conditions on S, all participants have S equal to unity, and an artefactual association between A and O will be found. This is a frequently observed result, for example see Smith and colleagues (Smith et al. 2004). Again using notation:

$$O \not\!\perp E | S = 1 \tag{4.5}$$

This is key to describing the results from many case-control studies where an association is shown but it can be explained through effects due to selection. In this situation some epidemiologists incorrectly believe that statistical adjustment for A will remove the bias due to selection. However this is a simplification of a more complex situation; this will be developed later.

Figure 4.1f shows a similar situation to Fig. 4.1e, though this time the A variable can be considered to be a true confounder. This is not due to conditioning on selection, but A is a separate and distinct cause of the outcome. In this situation making statistical adjustment for A would be appropriate for interpreting whether E causes the outcome O.

4.5 Study Design and Selection Bias

4.5.1 Case-Control Study

The case-control study is a popular design, particularly for rare diseases, to investigate putative risk factors in epidemiology. A "target-population" (Geneletti et al. 2009) is defined and the whole, or a random sample of the whole, population with a disease (cases) arising within that population are targeted for study: selection for a case-control study follows the diagnosis of disease in the cases. For two reasons selection bias is a particularly important issue for case-control studies: (i) the direct participation by the study subjects is usually required to obtain data on disease, risk factors, other auxiliary factors, and for ethical reasons, and (ii) cases are usually selected through a health system, such as clinic lists for the relevant disease, whilst controls are usually selected from a different sampling frame. When the researcher is aiming to recruit controls that represent the general population, a population register will be employed, such as birth registers.

If the case and control selection procedures produce a representative sample of the target-population, whereby selection bias is not present, the DAGs for the case-control study are an exact copy of those defined for the population, as shown in Fig. 4.1a, b. In practice, the probability that any individual, selected for inclusion in a study, will participate is usually higher for cases than for those without the disease (controls). It has been recognised that the effect of such differential or non-random sampling, and the bias it introduces, must be taken into account in the analysis of a case-control study. This is represented in Fig. 4.1e, f, dependent upon whether A is a true confounder or not.

4.5.2 Prospective Cohort Design

In a prospective cohort study, a sample from the target-population is made and the exposure measured, in advance of any diagnosis. After an appropriate length of follow-up time the proportion of cases of the disease could be compared in respect of their exposure. Every person in the target-population has equal probability of being approached at the outset: selection would not be conditioned on outcome (O). Figures 4.1g, h show the situation where selection is not associated with the outcome. This situation would be normal for prospective studies such as a cohort study. Within the cohort sample, conditioned on S, there would not be an arc between O and S. For this reason Eq. 4.4 holds.

4.6 Suggested Solutions to Selection Bias in a Case-Control Study

A large number of possible solutions to selection bias have been suggested, following the important step of recognising that selection bias may be a problem. When using most study designs, researchers are governed by practical and ethical constraints which require individuals to agree to participate. Of course, the best and most reliable option is to avoid the problem in the first place. When a case-control study can be conducted without requiring active participation from study subjects the design may allow a selection bias-free implementation. However, as most studies do require permission from study subjects, they are left open to error in selection and its effects. The aspect of the study most prone to error is control selection. This has long been recognised. Indeed, one of the first books detailing the conduct of case-control studies by Schlesselman (1982) explained that "The best-designed sampling scheme, assuring complete ascertainment of cases and a probability sample of control, can be vitiated by high rates of refusal."

4.6.1 Illustrative Example

The UK Childhood Cancer Study (UKCCS), amongst other research questions, sought to identify whether radon gas causes acute lymphoblastic leukaemia (ALL) in children (The UK Childhood Cancer Study Investigators 2002). The UKCCS aimed to enrol all cases of cancer, diagnosed in persons under the age of 15, in England, Scotland and Wales (The UK Childhood Cancer Study Investigators 2000). A comparison group was created: two children for each case were selected from all children living in the same National Health Service administration region (Family Health Services Authority for England and Wales and Health Board for Scotland) as the case.

It was argued that most of the cases arising in the target-population were recruited: multiple sources of case notification were interrogated (The UK Childhood Cancer Study Investigators 2000). The initial selection of control children has been shown to be reassuringly similar to the target-population for which it was designed to represent (Law et al. 2002). In contrast, it has been demonstrated that control participation was associated with a measure of socioeconomic status (Law et al. 2002), where it is thought that this acts as a proxy for closely related factors, such as educational status, which directly influences willingness to participate in the study as a control.

In our illustrative example, there is substantial evidence of an association between the socioeconomic status of the area in which a household resides (the auxiliary A) and the level of radon gas in their home (E) (Gunby et al. 1993; The UK Childhood Cancer Study Investigators 2002). This link is complex, but household income (U in Fig. 4.1) allows double glazing and draught proofing to be installed which can cause radon to increase in the home (Gunby et al. 1993). Household income also provides for greater material wealth and hence a higher measure of socioeconomic status (A). There was no evidence of any direct causal relationship between socioeconomic status and the probability of a child developing ALL (the outcome O) (Law et al. 2003). These variable inter-relationships suggest that Fig. 4.1a is the most appropriate representation of the population addressed by the UKCCS. Given this, the best model for estimating the association between radon and childhood leukaemia is not to adjust for the auxiliary variable, socioeconomic status. Hence, the population-level risk estimate in the UKCCS for the

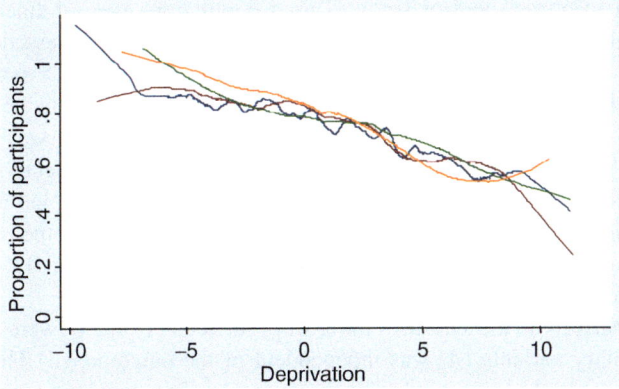

Fig. 4.2 Proportion of controls participating by deprivation categorised into control choice groups

sample, with selection bias, cannot be recovered by statistical adjustment for the auxiliary variable.

When a study is conducted it is normal for the researchers to pick a sample of controls and approach them for participation. We can refer to these as "first-choice controls" (Law et al. 2002, 2003); subsequent choice controls will be made until the required number of controls is recruited. It has been suggested that you could use participating first-choice controls only. Figure 4.2 shows the results for participation in controls in the UKCCS, fitted by a Lowess smoothed line (Cleveland and Devlin 1988). It is clear that the association between participation and deprivation does not differ by the choice of controls selected. This is intuitively correct, as the control selection is an exchangeable process, where controls selected later in the process possess the same characteristics as those selected earlier.

First-choice controls have been used; for example, Law and colleagues used all first-choice controls without requiring their participation (Law et al. 2003). This is because the exposure measures were derived from postal addresses linked to national census data. These controls should be a representative sample of the target-population; given the initial selection procedures were robust.

4.6.2 Statistical 'Adjustment' for Participation

One approach to dealing with selection bias is to 'adjust' for variables thought to cause, or influence, selection in a statistical model. Some authors have argued that adjusting for selection bias is identical to the process of adjusting for confounding: the variables associated with selection are incorporated into a regression model (e.g. Breslow and Day, 1980).

To investigate this a simulation study was conducted in R (R Development Core Team 2004) to investigate the effect of adjusting for a variable that is related to participation in a case-control study. Target-populations were defined with 10^6 members; all individuals belonging to each population possessed attributes representing A and E. Both variables for each individual were a random draw from a standard normal distribution, with A and E constrained to be correlated ($\rho = -0.8$). For 1,000 of these individuals, selected as cases, O was assigned a value of one which represented the presence of the disease. O was set to zero for the rest of the population; these individuals were eligible to be sampled as controls. The population level relative risk of the exposure (E) for the outcome (O) for each population ranged over a series of plausible risk estimates: between 0.2 and 1.0 for each standard deviation of E.

Two scenarios for the causal relationship between A and O were simulated: (i) The auxiliary variable (A) was independent of the outcome; (ii) The auxiliary variable was causally associated with the outcome. The population level relative risk for O was 1.0 (range 0.96–1.04) and 0.75 (range 0.71–0.78) for each standard deviation of A, for scenarios (i) and (ii) respectively. Three logistic regression models were built to determine the population level relative risks for: E alone; A alone; both E and A.

In both scenarios two control sampling regimes were employed to select 2,000 controls: (a) A case-control study without participation bias – controls randomly sampled from individuals without the disease; (b) A case-control study with participation bias – controls sampled with a probability of selection that was monotonically related to A, the probability being defined as $p = 0.4 - A/10$. All 1,000 cases were selected for all case-control study simulations. The three logistic regression models outlined above were estimated repeatedly for 1,000 independent samples. The median and 95% empirical confidence intervals for each model estimate were obtained, and were plotted against the true, population-level relative risk.

The simulation study showed that, when A was independent of O, the odds ratios obtained by case-control studies employing an unbiased sampling regime estimated the population relative risk with a high degree of accuracy (Fig. 4.3(i) unbiased model E). When A was a true confounder and was adjusted for in the model the unbiased study also recovered the population relative risk consistently across a broad range of risks (Fig. 4.3(ii) unbiased model E + A).

We have already determined that when the auxiliary variable A is not a true confounder, independence between an outcome and exposure may be artefactually produced (Eq. 4.5 and Fig. 4.1e). The case-control study has already conditioned on S rendering any adjustment route, $O \rightarrow S \rightarrow A \rightarrow U \rightarrow E$, blocked. However, when the auxiliary variable is also a true confounder, a route $O \rightarrow A \rightarrow U \rightarrow E$ exists to adjust for selection.

The auxiliary variable was therefore not a confounder in this context (McNamee 2003), and there was no meaningful way to 'adjust' for its complex influence on the outcome. This was supported by the simulation study, which showed that for the scenario, where A was not a true confounder, the biased case-control studies consistently and significantly underestimated the population relative risk (Fig. 4.3(i) biased model E). Furthermore, simulations support

(i) Auxiliary (*A*) not a confounder, but associated with exposure (*E*)

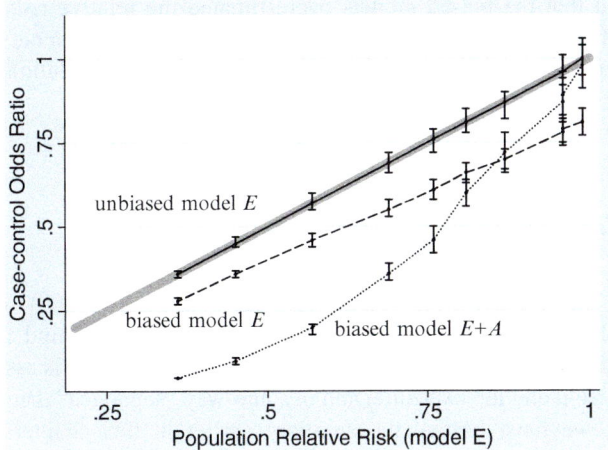

(ii) Auxiliary (*A*) a confounder

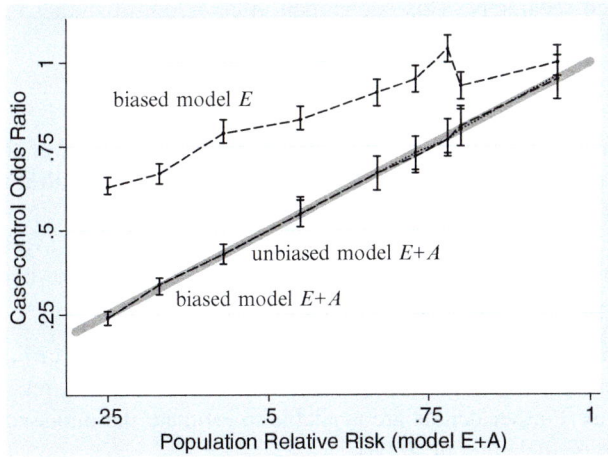

Fig. 4.3 Odds ratios (point) and 95% empirical confidence intervals (*vertical bar*) for biased and unbiased simulated case-control studies (1,000 cases fixed, 2,000 controls, sampled 1,000 times) applied to two populations (10^6 individuals, 1000 cases, sampled once), contrasted to the 'true' population relative risk (*thick solid line*). (**i**) Auxiliary (*A*) not a confounder, but associated with exposure (*E*). (**ii**) Auxiliary (*A*) a confounder

the assertion that attempting to recover the relative risk estimate for the scenario where *A* was not a true confounder, through statistical adjustment for *A*, fails to obtain an odds ratio close to the original relative risk (Fig. 4.3(i) biased model E + A), unless the true relative risk was close to unity. We must, therefore, conclude that we cannot statistically 'adjust' for the auxiliary variable's impact on selection bias.

When A was a true confounder, the conclusion is quite different. The simulation study showed that the biased models overestimated the relative risk (Fig. 4.3(ii) biased model E). In contrast to the first scenario, statistical adjustment by inclusion of A in the model recovered accurately and consistently the population relative risk (Fig. 4.3(ii) biased model E + A).

4.6.3 'Bias Breaking' Model

This model was introduced by Geneletti and colleagues (2009) to provide a statistical solution to selection bias. The basic assumption behind the model is that there is a variable, termed the bias breaking variable, which is associated with both the selection and the exposure, and in some-way "separates" them. This is the variable that we have termed the auxiliary earlier in this chapter. Formalised assumptions are:

(i) The case and control selection procedures are independent processes and can be treated separately. This is common in case-control studies and is a valid assumption as was described earlier.

$$E \perp\!\!\!\perp S | (O, A) \tag{4.6}$$

(ii) This states that, conditional on the outcome within strata of the auxiliary, exposure is independent of selection for the study. This requires the auxiliary to be stratified into categories.
(iii) The bias breaking variable must have additional data available to the researcher, outside of the study, so that a distribution of the bias breaker in relation to the outcome can be obtained.

Where there is no case selection bias, it is possible to use the distribution of A for both cases and controls to estimate the overall distribution of A, regardless of the outcome status. Further details are available to estimate the unbiased estimate of the odds ratio (Geneletti et al. 2009).

4.6.4 Other Statistical Methods

In the survey literature, the issue of differential selection, and the bias that may arise, is known as informative sampling. The issues arising in survey sampling are analogous to the selection of cases and controls in a case-control study.

Informative sampling has a long history in the literature of complex social surveys (see, for example, Rubin 1976). The bias it can cause, if not taken account of, is widely acknowledged (for example, Pfeffermann 1996). One approach to identify this bias is to model the distribution of the sample data as a function of the population distribution and the sampling weights (Pfeffermann and Sverchkov 2003). The density function $f_s(Y_i|x_i)$ of a response variable Y is defined as $f(Y_i|x_i; i \in s)$ where s denotes the sample and $x_i = (x_{1i}, ..., x_{ki})$ represents the values of predictor variables $X_1, ..., X_k$ for observation i. Denoting the population density (before sampling) as $f_u(Y_i|x_i)$ Bayes' theorem yields the result:

$$f_s(Y_i|x_i) = \frac{P(i \in s|Y_i, x_i) f_u(Y_i|x_i)}{P(i \in s|x_i)} \qquad (4.7)$$

Unless $P(i \in s|Y_i, x_i) = P(i \in s|x_i)$ for all possible values of Y the sample and population densities differ and the sampling is said to be informative. In the context of case-control studies $Y = 1$ would correspond to cases and $Y = 0$ to controls. The approaches taken by Pfeffermann and Sverchkov (Pfeffermann 1996; Pfeffermann and Sverchkov 2003) to fit generalised linear models between response Y and predictors $X_1, ..., X_k$ rest on redefining the population density $f_u(.)$ by the sample density $f_s(.)$ assuming known forms for $P(i \in s|Y_i, x_i)$ and $P(i \in s|x_i)$.

These methods are yet to be fully exploited in epidemiological studies though Samuelsen and colleagues discuss the use of stratification and sampling weights in case-cohort studies (Samuelsen et al. 2007). The non-cases are divided into strata according to the values of covariates, and the probability of sampling an individual from each strata is included as an inverse probability weight in the parameter estimation process.

4.7 Conclusions

We have shown how a biased sampling regime within a study may lead to a biased estimate of the relative risk for an exposure. We agree with Hernán and colleagues that authors should be encouraged to approach modelling in a structured way, allowing readers to assess the likelihood of selection biasing the exposure risk estimates, and the potential success of any statistical adjustments (Hernan et al. 2004). Using the case-control sample as the 'oracle' for defining potential causal pathways for variables at the population level, one might erroneously conclude that A is a confounder when it is not. This may be due wholly to the influence of differential participation between cases and controls. The decision to assign an auxiliary variable as a confounder may be complicated by the evidence from the case-control study that suffers from selection bias; an association between A and O may be present. It is worth noting that considering all possible auxiliaries as confounders, when they may not all have a causal relationship with the outcome, seems erroneous even though this practice appears to be commonly employed.

Case-control studies reliant upon individual participation, suffer from selection bias (Law et al. 2002). In the example of Sect. 4.1, a variable identified as causing selection, socioeconomic status, was not a true confounder. As a consequence, it is not possible to recover the population-level relative risks by adjustment within a regression model. Epidemiology may therefore need to revisit the many case-control studies already conducted where the statistical analyses included all perceivable confounders, many of which may have been rather cavalierly labelled as such.

Whilst we are aware that a prospective cohort study may be financially prohibitive, it does provide a solution to this problem. Epidemiology may therefore need to re-evaluate the benefit of many case-controls studies prone to selection bias, against the cost of conducting a large, prospective cohort study.

We believe this example is not an isolated case. Participation rates are dropping globally, ethical constraints are making sample selection increasingly difficult, and methods for selecting individuals use difficult-to-check procedures. It is clear that alternative strategies are required in these situations.

Case-control studies are prone to selection bias induced by differential participation between cases and controls. There are two possible scenarios for the analysis of case-control data where participation bias is anticipated; each has a different outcome:

i. When there is an auxiliary variable that is associated with sampling and it is not a genuine confounder, statistical adjustment will not recover the population-level exposure relative risk.
ii. When the auxiliary variable is a genuine confounder, statistical adjustment will obtain the correctly estimated relative risk for the exposure.

Correctly specifying the causal model is essential to the understanding of how appropriate statistical adjustment may be achieved. DAGs and their development may substantially assist with this task and allow the implementation of novel newly developed methods.

References

Breslow, N. E., & Day, N. E. (1980). Statistical methods in cancer research. Vol 1. The analysis of case-control studies. IARC, Lyon.

Cleveland, W. S., & Devlin, S. J. (1988). Locally weighted regression: An approach to regression analysis by local fitting. *Journal of the American Statistical Association, 83*, 596–610.

Galea, S., & Tracy, M. (2007). Participation rates in epidemiologic studies. *Annals of Epidemiology, 17*(9), 643–653. available from: ISI:000249293100001.

Geneletti, S., Richardson, S., & Best, N. (2009). Adjusting for selection bias in retrospective, case-control studies. *Biostatistics, 10*(1), 17–31. available from: PM:18482997.

Greenland, S., & Brumback, B. (2002). An overview of relations among causal modelling methods. *International Journal of Epidemiology, 31*(5), 1030–1037. available from: PM:12435780.

Greenland, S., Pearl, J., & Robins, J. M. (1999). Causal diagrams for epidemiologic research. *Epidemiology, 10*(1), 37–48. available from: PM:9888278.

Gunby, J. A., Darby, S. C., Miles, J. C. H., Green, B. M. R., & Cox, D. R. (1993). Factors affecting indoor radon concentrations in the United-Kingdom. *Health Physics, 64*(1), 2–12. available from: ISI:A1993KD26400002.

Henderson, M., & Page, L. (2007). Appraising the evidence: What is selection bias? *Evidence-Based Mental Health, 10*(3), 67–68. available from: PM:17652553.

Hernan, M. A., Hernandez-Diaz, S., & Robins, J. M. (2004). A structural approach to selection bias. *Epidemiology, 15*(5), 615–625. available from: PM:15308962.

Law, G. R., Smith, A. G., & Roman, E. (2002). The importance of full participation: Lessons from a national case-control study. *British Journal of Cancer, 86*(3), 350–355. available from: PM:11875698.

Law, G. R., Parslow, R. C., & Roman, E. (2003). Childhood cancer and population mixing. *American Journal of Epidemiology, 158*(4), 328–336. available from: PM:12915498.

McNamee, R. (2003). Confounding and confounders. *Occupational and Environmental Medicine, 60*(3), 227–234. available from: PM:12598677.

Pearl, J. (2000). *Causality: Models, reasoning and inference*. New York: Cambridge University Press.

Pfeffermann, D. (1996). The use of sampling weights for survey data analysis. *Statistical Methods in Medical Research, 5*(3), 239–261. available from: PM:8931195.

Pfeffermann, D., & Sverchkov, M. Y. U. (2003). Fitting generalised linear models under informative sampling. In R. L. Chambers & C. J. Skinner (Eds.), *Analysis of survey data* (pp. 175–195). Chichester: Wiley.

R Development Core Team. (2004). *R: A language and environment for statistical computing*. Vienna: R Foundation for Statistical Computing.

Rubin, D. B. (1976). Inference and missing data. *Biometrika, 63*(3), 581–590. available from: ISI:A1976CP66700021.

Samuelsen, S. O., Anestad, H., & Skrondal, A. (2007). Stratified case-cohort analysis of general cohort sampling designs. *Scandinavian Journal of Statistics, 34*(1), 103–119. available from: ISI:000244852300008.

Schlesselman, J. J. (1982). *Case-control studies: Design, conduct, analysis*. Oxford: Oxford University Press.

Smith, A. G., Fear, N. T., Law, G. R., & Roman, E. (2004). Representativeness of samples from general practice lists in epidemiological studies: Case-control study. *BMJ, 328*(7445), 932. available from: PM:14990513.

The UK Childhood Cancer Study Investigators. (2000). The United Kingdom Childhood Cancer Study: Objectives, materials and methods. UK Childhood Cancer Study Investigators. *British Journal of Cancer, 82*(5), 1073–1102. available from: PM:10737392.

The UK Childhood Cancer Study Investigators. (2002). The United Kingdom Childhood Cancer Study of exposure to domestic sources of ionising radiation: 1: Radon gas. *British Journal of Cancer, 86*(11), 1721–1726. available from: PM:12087456.

Tu, Y.-K., West, R. W., Ellison, G. D. H., & Gilthorpe, M. S. (2004). Why evidence for the fetal origins of adult disease can be statistical artifact: The reversal paradox examined for hypertension. *American Journal of Epidemiology, 161*(1), 27–32.

Chapter 5
Multilevel Modelling

Andrew Blance

5.1 Introduction

Independence (only one observation per individual) amongst the observations is an underlying assumption of single-level analyses (Armitage et al. 2002; Bland 2000). In reality, this assumption is often violated due to clustering of observations. For example, siblings clustered with families or students clustered within classes of a school. Observations which possess such clustering are considered as forming a hierarchical data structure. When a hierarchy is present, a simple (perhaps simplest) solution to the violation of independence is to use the observations within each cluster to produce a single summary or 'global' measure for each top-level (independent) unit and perform subsequent analyses at this level. However, this is not only an inefficient use of the data collected but (more importantly) ignoring the hierarchical structure potentially ignores far more interesting considerations provided by exploring the nature of the hierarchy. In instances such as this, the technique of Multilevel Modelling (MLM) comes into its own, not only dealing with the lack of independence but exploiting it to its advantage.

A discussion detailing the pitfalls of ignoring data hierarchy is outlined. The assumptions and limitations of MLM are outlined and contrasted with those of single-level modelling. An illustration of the effects of clustering introduces variance components. This simplest (null) multilevel model is used to outline the notation used to specify a multilevel model. The initial variance components model is further developed to illustrate random intercepts and (complex) slopes. Markov Chain Monte Carlo (MCMC) methods appropriate for estimating multilevel models are introduced. Model fit diagnostics are considered. Finally, complex (non-strict) hierarchies are outlined. A periodontal example is used throughout the chapter for illustration.

A. Blance (✉)
Division of Biostatistics, Centre for Epidemiology and Biostatistics, Leeds Institute
of Genetics, Health & Therapeutics, University of Leeds, Leeds, UK
e-mail: and.blance@gmail.com

Fig. 5.1 Data hierarchy

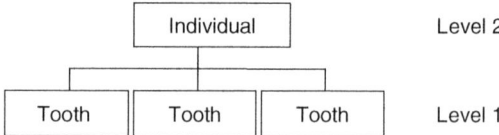

5.1.1 Periodontal Example

As we age, the gum around our teeth recedes resulting in attachment loss. This gives the appearance of longer teeth, hence the saying "long in the tooth". The rate of attachment loss varies from person to person and is influenced by (amongst other things) the standard of oral hygiene. The illustrative example used throughout this chapter consists of observations of (clinical) attachment loss (CAL) measured in millimeters around each tooth, up to 28 teeth per individual (all teeth excluding third molars, i.e. wisdom teeth). The data structure, or hierarchy, can be depicted as in Fig. 5.1.

5.1.2 Independence

Two observations are defined as independent if one is in no way predictable from the other (Armitage et al. 2002; Machin et al. 2007). An alternative way of stating two variables as being independent is to say that the distribution of one is the same for all values of the other. This independence is an *essential* assumption of 'standard' statistical regression methods. Generalised linear models require that outcome observations are independent. Clinical data often violate the assumption that the outcome is independently observed, usually arising from clustering, or nesting of the outcome variable. In the periodontal example, attachment loss measurements for each tooth are clustered/nested within each individual. Knowing the attachment loss of one tooth would tell us something about the attachment losses of the other teeth, owing to the teeth all sharing the same oral environment.

5.1.3 Effect of Ignoring Lack of Independence

In single-level modelling, the standard error (SE) associated with an estimated coefficient is proportional to one over the square root of the number of observations (N): $SE \propto 1/\sqrt{N}$ (Altman 1991). In our periodontal example we have 17,858 observations of attachment loss (potentially 28 teeth per individual and 1,000 individuals). If the 17,858 observations were subject to a single-level analysis the resulting standard errors would be proportional to $(1/\sqrt{17858})$ 1/134. However, if the data were analysed with the number of independent observations correctly taken to be 1,000, the standard errors would be proportional to $(1/\sqrt{1000})$ 1/32. Therefore, ignoring inherent hierarchy in this instance yields standard errors that are an order of magnitude (32/134) smaller than they should be. This also leads to an increase in the potential for Type I errors; incorrectly identifying a covariate as influencing the outcome of interest.

5.1.4 Dealing with Hierarchy

Ignoring the lack of independence, what might be termed the 'Ostrich' approach of burying your head in the sand, is clearly not an acceptable solution. A work-around would be to sample just one lower-level unit per highest level-unit (one attachment loss per individual). Alternatively a subgroup analysis could be performed (e.g. all teeth analysed for each individual separately) yielding as many separate analyses as there are individuals. If and only if the data are balanced (equal numbers of identical teeth per individual), the hierarchy can initially be ignored in estimating coefficients. Correct coefficient standard errors can subsequently be obtained by making the appropriate adjustment to account for the hierarchy. All of these are workarounds to the lack of independence. The statistical analyses are rendered statistically valid. However, they fail to get the most out the data due to a great loss of detailed information. Further, they can lead to more general problems, such as drawing inferences about lower-level units through higher-level analyses, thereby running the risk of committing the ecological fallacy (Bland 2000).

A more optimal solution would be to use statistical methods that yield robust standard errors by dealing with the hierarchy explicitly. These methods can be viewed as belonging to one of two groups: (i) those that treat the hierarchy as a nuisance or, (ii) those which treat the hierarchy as a special feature to be exploited. Examples of the former are Generalised Estimating Equations (Ziegler et al. 1998) and Sandwich Estimates (Qian and Wang 2001; White 1980). An example of the latter is what is now termed multilevel modelling (UK) (Leyland and Goldstein 2001) or hierarchical linear modelling (US) (Raudenbush and Bryk 2002).

5.2 Assumptions and Advantages of MLM

5.2.1 Assumptions Underpinning MLM

MLM requires compliance with the same assumptions of single-level generalised linear modelling (Kirkwood and Sterne 2003; Machin et al. 2007). Namely, a correctly specified link function with appropriate form of explanatory variables in the linear (additive) predictor, appropriately distributed residuals and appropriately structured outcome variance across each covariate. However, providing the non-constant variance structure (*heteroscedasticity*) is modelled explicitly, the 'constant variance' assumption may be relaxed within a multilevel model (Hox 2002).

A multilevel model makes the assumption that cluster units are broadly similar, with differences being attributable to known fixed and random variation. In theory, with sufficient information, all measures of variation can be estimated. In reality there may not be sufficient information collected to determine all fixed and random effects giving rise to variations in the outcome measure. Consequently, inference can only be drawn conditional on the relationship of measured factors associated with the outcome. Explicitly, a fixed effect can only be interpreted whilst 'controlling' for measured confounding factors. The resulting inference of the fixed effects may nevertheless be biased due to unmeasured (and possibly unknown) confounding factors. The same behaviour applies to random effects.

An intuitive way to view a multilevel model is to think of each level as containing a sample of members drawn from a potentially larger population. Since it is necessary for the distributional properties of observations at each level to be estimated, a minimum of 20 top-level units is required. Fewer units at the upper-most level can lead to the distributional properties being poorly estimated, with consequent (negative) implications on the lower-level distributional estimates. The same constraint does not apply to lower levels, since each lower-level unit occurs many times within all higher-level units.

5.2.2 Importance of Centring

MLM is only invariant to linear transformations of the explanatory variables in the absence of random slopes. It is therefore essential that to avoid biased estimates of the random structure of a multilevel model, all covariates that exhibit random variation should be centred about their mean (Hox 2002). Otherwise, covariance estimates are artificially inflated.

5.2.3 Advantages of MLM

Framing random structure firmly within a hierarchical context gives rise to major benefits (Gilthorpe and Cunningham 2000; Quene and van den Bergh 2008). Not least, it provides a naturally intuitive understanding. For example, patients are often the unit of concern, yet observations are frequently made at a lower level. Further, in contrast to techniques that treat clustering as a nuisance to derive robust estimates of the fixed effects, a key feature of MLM is that it provides insights into random effects. The full power of MLM in exploiting random structure will only be realised for research questions posed such that the random effects provide the research answer.

5.3 Constructing Multilevel Models

5.3.1 Variance Components

Partitioning the total variance by its source yields insight as to the relative weights of each source. Consider the 2-level hierarchy of the periodontal example where teeth are clustered within individuals. Figure 5.2 illustrates the variation in attachment loss amongst 140 teeth. The 1,400 observations relate to just 5 individuals as illustrated in Fig. 5.3.

Some of the variation is due to variation *between* individuals and some *within* individuals. Thus the total variance can be partitioned according to that which is attributable to teeth and individual. This is known as variance components and represents the simplest MLM (Snijders and Bosker 1999). The variance components model has no explanatory variables (only the intercept is present) and is often termed the *null model*. Variance components models are mathematically equivalent to 'random effects' ANOVA (Snijders and Bosker 1999). They are useful in establishing the relative proportions of variation across all levels, allowing the variation at each level to be known *a priori* to the introduction of 'explanatory' terms. This in turn allows consideration of the reduction in variation associated with the inclusion of an explanatory term.

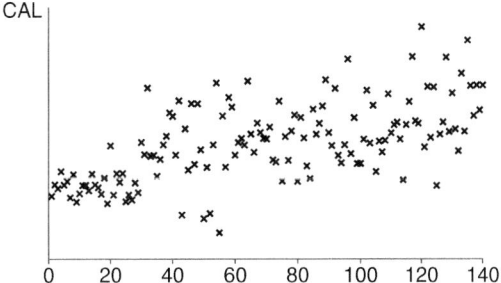

Fig. 5.2 Variation in attachment loss amongst teeth

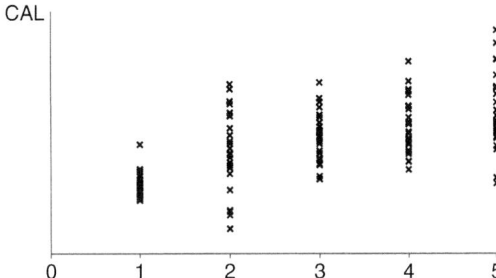

Fig. 5.3 Variation in attachment loss by individuals

Within MLM, the first stage of the analysis is to determine the appropriate multilevel structure. If the variance at a given level does not contribute substantially to the total variance, this level may be obsolete and might therefore be ignored. However, the extent of variation at any specified level may appear insubstantial (or even zero) whilst it remains masked by larger, as yet unmodelled, fixed and random effects. For this reason, it is unwise to discard a particular level simply because its variation is small (or even zero) and not significant, when no other terms have been included in the model. Only where this remains consistently to be true throughout model development would it suggest that the level could be discarded. Thus producing a more parsimonious model, perhaps increasing its interpretability.

5.3.2 MLM Notation

In introducing the theory of MLM, it is useful to outline the notation (algebra) used. Considering a two-level model, the general algebraic formula may be written:

$$y_{ij} = \sum_{m=0}^{N} \beta_{mij} x_{mij} \tag{5.1}$$

where y_{ij} is the outcome measure for the i-th level 1 unit, clustered within the j-th level 2 unit; x_{mij} ($m \geq 1$) is the m-th of N covariates with coefficients β_{mij}; $x_{0ij} = 1$ such that β_{0ij} (the intercept) is the outcome when all explanatory variables are zero.

To aid comprehension of this generic formulation, we start with the simplest of all multilevel models and build the MLM algebra from first principles.

5.3.2.1 Variance Components Notation

A variance components model has only the intercept present. The effect of having no explanatory variables present is that $N = 0$. Thus the variance components model is derived from (5.1) by setting $N = 0$:

$$y_{ij} = \beta_{0ij} = \beta_0 + u_{0j} + e_{0ij}$$

where β_0 is the mean value of the outcome variable y_{ij}, with the total variance partitioned across each level such that: $e_{0ij} \sim N(0, \sigma_{0e}^2)$, the level 1 residuals (e_{0ij}) have zero mean and are normally distributed with variance σ_{0e}^2 across all units; and similarly for $u_{0j} \sim N(0, \sigma_{0u}^2)$ (level 2 residuals), where σ_{0u}^2 is the variance across all units.

5.3.2.2 Periodontal Example

We have two sources of random variation: variation between individuals and variation between teeth (variation within individuals).

$$y_{ij} = \beta_{0ij} = \beta_0 + u_{0j} + e_{0ij}$$

where y_{ij} is the attachment loss (CAL) for the i-th tooth, clustered within the j-th individual; β_0 is the mean value of the attachment loss y_{ij}, with the total variance partitioned across each level such that: $e_{0ij} \sim N(0, \sigma_{0e}^2)$, tooth level residuals (e_{0ij}) have zero mean and are normally distributed with variance σ_{0e}^2 across all units; similarly for $u_{0j} \sim N(0, \sigma_{0u}^2)$ (individual level residuals), where σ_{0u}^2 is the variance across all units. Thus, the total variation is given by $Var(CAL_{ij}) = \sigma_{0u}^2 + \sigma_{0e}^2$.

5.3.3 Random Intercepts Model

A Random Intercept model is a variance components model that includes explanatory covariates (Snijders and Bosker 1999). It is so termed as each level-2 unit (individual) has the same linear relationship between the outcome and explanatory covariate, whilst exhibiting random variation 'around' the collective level-2 mean intercept. Analogous to single-level modelling, covariates are sought for inclusion in the model so as to 'explain' as much variation in the outcome as possible. The effect of each covariate is estimated by a partial regression coefficient. The unexplained variation is important in assessing the adequacy of the model (with larger residual variation reflecting a poorer fit) and the coefficient in assessing the effect of that factor on the outcome. The difference from single-level is that covariates primarily 'operate' at a specific level, with potential for some 'cross-level' interactions, and variation occurs at every level of the hierarchy. The inclusion of a fixed effect may lead to the reduction of variation at more than one level. For example, although smoking status will primarily operate at the subject-level, it may also operate differentially across teeth within the same individual, thereby providing a cross-level interaction between the subject- and the tooth-level.

5.3.3.1 Example of a Random Intercept Model

Consider our periodontal example where we have a 2-level model with only one covariate (age). Consider the relationship between attachment loss (CAL) and age within a longitudinal dataset of clinical measures obtained from repeated full-mouth recordings on a sample of individuals. Suppose we ignore the natural hierarchy and observe a near-linear relationship, as illustrated in Fig. 5.4.

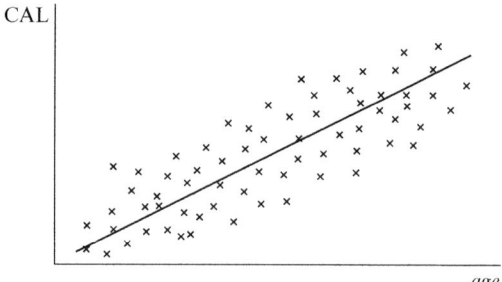

Fig. 5.4 CAL against age; fitted linear relationship obtained from a single-level analysis

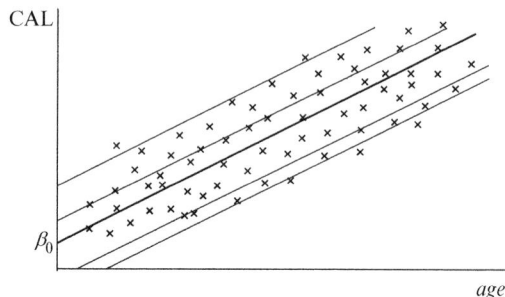

Fig. 5.5 CAL against age; fitted linear relationships obtained from individual single-level regression analysis

Residuals in this single-level illustration are the discrepancies between the observed measures (denoted by each cross) and the predicted measures (denoted by the 'fitted' line) measured along the CAL axis. Clearly, variation in CAL is (partially) 'explained' by age. However, this is not the complete picture; we do not expect all individual' observations to fall on the line, but variation between individuals is masked and merged with variation within individuals, because the data hierarchy has been ignored.

In a multilevel framework, the random variation at level-1 (teeth) is similar to that for the single-level analysis, but there is also additional variation in a 2-level model that allows for level-2 random variation to occur across all level-2 units (individuals), as illustrated in Fig. 5.5. The heavy line represents the estimated average relationship across all subjects with a mean intercept denoted by β_0. In addition, the lighter 'parallel' lines represent the relationship for data belonging to each level-2 unit (individual). The gradient of this relationship (how much CAL changes for one unit change in age) is obtained from the estimated coefficient for the age covariate.

5.3.3.2 Random Intercept Notation

In general, to include covariates that 'operate' at the various levels, such as x_{1j} for the individual-level (i.e. level-2) covariate *age*, and x_{2ij} for the tooth-level covariate *presence/ absence of plaque*, a 2-level random intercept model may be written:

$$y_{ij} = \beta_{0ij} + \beta_1 x_{1j} + \beta_2 x_{2ij} = \left(\beta_0 + \beta_1 x_{1j} + \beta_2 x_{2ij}\right) + \left(e_{0ij} + u_{0j}\right)$$

where the first part ($\beta_0 + \beta_1 x_{1j} + \beta_2 x_{2ij}$) is similar to any single-level model which contains the two covariate effects plus the intercept, whilst the second part ($e_{0ij} + u_{0j}$) is the multilevel random structure for the total variation partitioned across *each* level of the hierarchy. The subscript j is present for the first covariate (x_{1j}) to represent covariate values that vary across individuals (and are constant for all sites within individuals); whereas the subscripts ij are present for the second covariate (x_{2ij}) to represent that these covariate values vary across teeth (within individuals) as well as across individuals (it is not constant for all sites within individuals). The multilevel model thus estimates the parameters of the fixed part of the model ($\beta_0, \beta_1, \beta_2$) alongside the parameters of the random part of the model ($\sigma_{0e}^2, \sigma_{0u}^2$). The random terms ($e_{0ij}, u_{0j}$) are not estimated; only their variances are estimated.

5.3.4 Complex Level-1 Models

Multilevel complex (non-constant) level-1 variation has an analogy in single-level terms, where it is termed heteroscedasticity (Hox 2002). However, within most single-level data structures, non-constant variance is generally deemed a nuisance, requiring a transformation of either the outcome or explanatory variable (or both). Within MLM, non-constant level-1 variance may be modelled explicitly and be of particular interest (Goldstein 2003). This allows MLM to deal with a wider range of complex data structures.

For instance, a natural biological system might yield data that would not be expected to satisfy the constant variance requirement of standard regression, and the only way to address any particular research questions directed at such a system would be to model the full complexity of the variation present. An example might be periodontal measurements, since it has been speculated that CAL suffers both natural biological variations and measurement errors that increase in relation to their 'true' or unobserved value. This may be modelled explicitly within MLM. For instance, if we followed several individuals and plotted their pocket probing depth against age, we might see something that looks like Fig. 5.6.

CAL is bounded below by zero (and above, though this may be less important) and values generally increase with age. Therefore, variability in these outcomes is constrained when they are observed close to zero. Conversely, variation may be greater amongst sites with more disease (when they are measured far from zero). This occurs for multiple teeth within each individual; therefore the non-constant variance observed in Fig. 5.6 occurs for each individual separately.

Complex level-1 variation may occur for three broad reasons. Firstly, constraints within the outcome variable mean that the degree of variation in the outcome changes as a function of a covariate. Secondly, the intrinsic structure of the data due to temporally or spatially distributed outcomes results

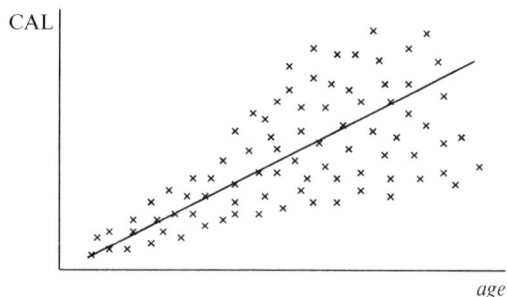

Fig. 5.6 Individual's CAL measurements over several years, with linear fit

in auto-correlation. Thirdly, since regression analyses assume error free covariates, 'spurious' complex level-1 variation may manifest itself as a result of measurement 'error'.

5.3.4.1 Complex Level-1 Notation

If we were to try and model the complex variation in Fig. 5.6, where it is assumed that, for each individual, the within-mouth variation widens with increasing mean CAL (or increasing age), we would express the 2-level model as:

$$CAL_{ij} = \beta_{0ij} + \beta_{1i}age_j = (\beta_0 + \beta_1 age_j) + (e_{0ij} + u_{0j} + e_{1ij}age_j)$$

where the first part $(\beta_0 + \beta_1 age_j)$ is similar to any single-level model that fits the mean covariate relationship, including an intercept term. The second part $(e_{0ij} + u_{0j} + e_{1ij}age_j)$ is the multilevel random structure for the total variation partitioned across each level of the hierarchy, including additional random structure at level-1 that depends upon age. In this instance, age is acting as a proxy/surrogate for mean CAL. The subscript j is present for all references to the covariate *age*, since the covariate value varies across individuals (and is constant for all teeth within individuals). The additional random parameter, e_{1ij}, satisfies the usual assumptions, and represents the level-1 (random) variation which is effectively 'scaled' by the *age* covariate. At level-1, the two random terms (e_{0ij}, e_{1ij}) give rise to two variances and one covariance $(\sigma_{0e}^2, \sigma_{1e}^2, \sigma_{01e})$, where the covariance depicts any underlying relationship (if one exists) between one random term varying 'in tune' with the other.

The multilevel model thus estimates the parameters of the fixed part of the model (β_0, β_1) alongside the parameters of the random part of the model $(\sigma_{0e}^2, \sigma_{1e}^2,$ and σ_{01e} for level-1; σ_{0u}^2 for level-2). The variance 'function' at level-1 now has a complex form: *level-1 variance* $= Var(e_{0ij} + e_{1ij}age_j) = \sigma_{0e}^2 + 2\sigma_{01e}age_j + \sigma_{1e}^2 age_j^2$, since *age* is a fixed covariate. In other words, the level-1 variance structure is a quadratic function of the covariate *age* (Fig. 5.7). Different level-1 variance functions can be obtained by appropriate transformation(s) of the selected covariate(s).

Fig. 5.7 Individual's CAL measurements over several years, with complex level-1 variance

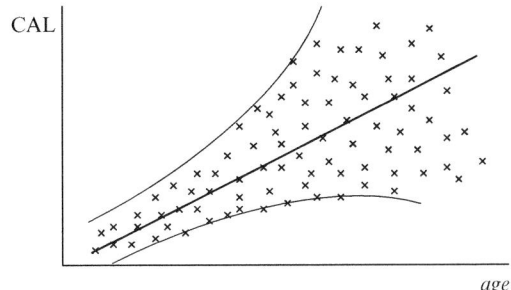

5.3.5 Random Slope Models (or Random Coefficient Models)

A key assumption in single-level regression is that random variation occurs only within the outcome ('around' the intercept) and that fixed variation may be 'explained' by the inclusion of covariates. Within MLM, covariates may also exhibit variation, either random, fixed, or both. Random slopes are where there exists complex (non-constant) random variation at any level above level-1, where covariates exhibit random variation 'around' their (mean) coefficient estimates (Snijders and Bosker 1999).

Complex variation above level 1 can occur as a result of random biological variation or a constraint on the explanatory variables. Random biological variation would arise when not all individuals within a study are alike in their response to various factors, for example due to differences in genetic predisposition or lifestyle. Constraints on explanatory variables again arise due to boundary effects amongst the explanatory variables. However, in this instance it is the influence of the covariate upon the outcome that is attenuated by boundary constraints; the covariate (not the outcome) is bounded (either above or below) and the impact of the covariate on the outcome is less likely to vary near its boundary values.

Perhaps a more intuitive way to understand random slope models is to first consider a 2-level random intercept model with a single covariate describing (initially) the same gradient across all level-2 units (as shown previously in Fig. 5.5). If the gradient varies randomly across (level-2) individuals, the model would become a *random slope* model and there would exist a different linear relationship between the outcome and covariate for each individual, as illustrated in Fig. 5.8, where the heavy line represents the mean slope of all individuals (level-2 units).

However, it is unlikely that the data exhibit a consistent intercept for all individuals. Figure 5.9 indicates the more likely scenario of simultaneous non-zero random slope and non-zero random intercept.

It is worth noting that random covariate effects might occur even when the mean covariate (age) effect is not significant (close to zero), as shown in Fig. 5.10.

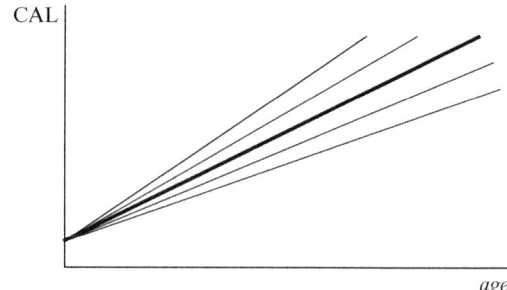

Fig. 5.8 CAL against age; random variation across individuals occurring 'around' the age coefficient mean

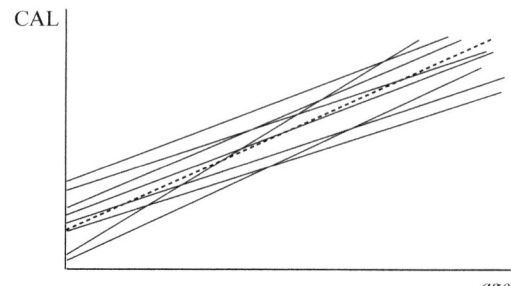

Fig. 5.9 CAL against age; the random slope model may simultaneously exhibit random variation about the intercept

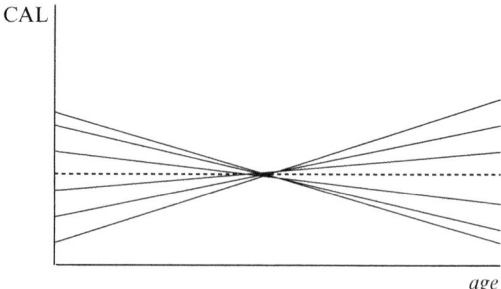

Fig. 5.10 CAL against age; how random covariate effects might occur even when the covariate effect is zero

5.3.5.1 Random Slope Notation

If we were to model the simple random slope model, illustrated in Fig. 5.10, the 2-level model would be:

$$\text{CAL}_{ij} = \beta_{0ij} + \beta_{1j}age_j = \left(\beta_0 + \beta_1 age_j\right) + \left(e_{0ij} + u_{0j} + u_{1j}age_j\right)$$

where the fixed part $(\beta_0 + \beta_1 age_j)$ is akin to any single-level model, and now the random part $(e_{0ij} + u_{0j} + u_{1j}age_j)$ represents the multilevel random structure, with the total variation partitioned across each level of the hierarchy, including additional random structure at level-2 that depends upon *age*. The additional random parameter, u_{1j}, satisfies the usual assumptions (normally distributed with mean zero), but only varies from individual to individual. This term represents level-2 (random) variation, which is effectively 'scaled' by the *age* covariate. At level-2, the two random terms (u_{0j}, u_{1j}) give rise to two variances and one covariance $(\sigma_{0u}^2, \sigma_{1u}^2, \sigma_{01u})$, where the covariance depicts any underlying relationship (if one exists) between one random term changing 'in tune' with the other.

The multilevel model thus estimates the parameters of the fixed part of the model (β_0, β_1) alongside the parameters of the random part of the model $(\sigma_{0e}^2$ for level-1; $\sigma_{0u}^2, \sigma_{1u}^2$, and σ_{01u} for level-2), only now the complex variation occurs at level-2 and not at level-1. The variance 'function' at level-2 again has a complex form: *level-2 variance* $= Var(u_{0j} + u_{1j}age_j) = \sigma_{0u}^2 + 2\sigma_{01u}age_j + \sigma_{1u}^2 age_j^2$, since *age* is not a random variable. Thus, the level-2 variance structure is a quadratic function of the covariate *age*.

Something that is peculiar to multilevel modelling occurs if the covariate, about which we model random slopes, is binary. Consider the covariate *sex* in a similar model to that previously described for *age*: $CAL_{ij} = \beta_{0ij} + \beta_{1j}sex_j = (\beta_0 + \beta_1 sex_j) + (e_{0ij} + u_{0j} + u_{1j}sex_j)$. Then: *level-2 variance* $= \sigma_{0u}^2 + 2\sigma_{01u}sex_j + \sigma_{1u}^2 sex_j^2$, since *sex* is not a random variable. Although the level-2 variance structure appears to be a quadratic function of the covariate *sex*, it is not, since *sex* can only take two values, usually coded 0 and 1, in which case $sex^2 = sex$. Thus: *level-2 variance* $= \sigma_{0u}^2 + (2\sigma_{01u} + \sigma_{1u}^2)sex_j$, and it therefore becomes impossible to determine, simultaneously, the complex variance associated with *sex* (σ_{1u}^2) and the covariance between *sex* and the *intercept* (σ_{01u}). In this situation, we have to constrain one of these two terms to be zero and adopt either $\sigma_{0u}^2 + 2\sigma_{01u}sex_j$ or $\sigma_{0u}^2 + \sigma_{1u}^2 sex_j$ as the variance function at level-2.

Now, the problem is, if we adopt $\sigma_{0u}^2 + 2\sigma_{01u}sex_j$ as the correct expression, we have what appears to be an absurd situation. The model determines a variance for the random intercept and a covariance between the random intercept and random covariate (e.g. *sex*), whilst constraining the variance of the random covariate for *sex* to be zero. However, this parameterisation $(\sigma_{0u}^2 + 2\sigma_{01u}sex_j)$ is correct and the alternative $(\sigma_{0u}^2 + \sigma_{1u}^2 sex_j)$ is only correct in a limited number of circumstances. This is because variance terms can only be positive, whereas the covariance term may be negative also, providing that total variance remains positive. Thus, were *sex* coded such that males were 0 and females were 1, and outcome variation was greater amongst males than females, the expression $\sigma_{0u}^2 + \sigma_{1u}^2 sex_j$ could not capture this situation correctly, since σ_{1u}^2 can only be positive when it would need to be negative. The expression $\sigma_{0u}^2 + 2\sigma_{01u}sex_j$ on the other hand accommodates all situations adequately, since σ_{01u} may be negative.

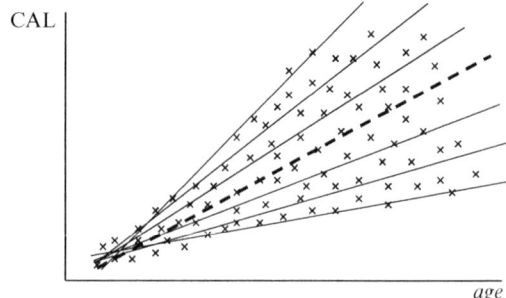

Fig. 5.11 CAL measurements over time; linear fit for each individual, revealing a random slope model

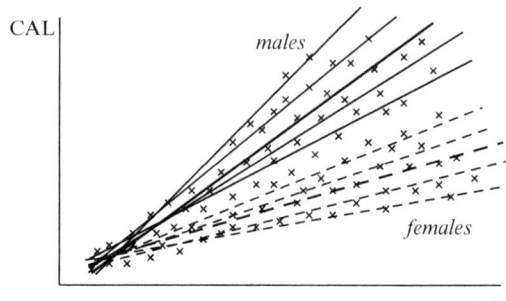

Fig. 5.12 CAL measurements over time; overall linear fit for males (*solid lines*) and females (*dotted lines*) separately, revealing a complex random slope model

5.3.6 Complex Random Slope Models

Complex random slope models are an extension to the random slope model, where the variation in a slope is not entirely random, but may systematically vary as a function of other covariates (Goldstein 2003). For instance, changes in CAL with age may vary randomly across individuals, though this slope may also differ systematically between males and females. Thus, revisiting the relationship presented in Fig. 5.6, if instead of heteroscedasticity (as shown in Fig. 5.7), suppose that within- individual variation in CAL values was constant across all ages for all individuals, but that mean levels of CAL within each individual progressed at different rates. In other words, complex random structure occurs at level-2 and not at level-1 (Fig. 5.11).

Now consider the hypothetical scenario that, on average, males progress faster than females could be visualised by Fig. 5.12.

5.3.6.1 Complex Random Slope Notation

If we were to model the complex random slope model, illustrated in Fig. 5.12, the 2-level model would be:

$$CAL_{ij} = \beta_{0ij} + \beta_{1j}age_j + \beta_2 age_j \times sex_j$$
$$= \left(\beta_0 + \beta_1 age_j + \beta_2 age_j \times sex_j\right) + \left(e_{0ij} + u_{0j} + u_{1j}age_j\right)$$

where the fixed part ($\beta_0 + \beta_1 age_j + \beta_2 age_j \times sex_j$) is akin to a single-level model with an interaction term included ($\beta_2 age_j \times sex_j$), and the random part ($e_{0ij} + u_{0j} + u_{1j} age_j$) is as before, with the total variation partitioned across each level, including additional random structure that depends upon *age*. What is perhaps most striking is how the fixed part includes an interaction term without both covariates present, *sex* is not included as an independent covariate and only within the interaction. This is not so strange within MLM, since there need be no underlying outcome differences by *sex* for there to be any differences in the male and female slopes. Nevertheless, it is likely that a genuine underlying gender difference is frequently observed, hence the more realistic model would be:

$$CAL_{ij} = \beta_{0ij} + \beta_{1j} age_j + \beta_2 age_j \times sex_j + \beta_3 sex_j,$$

where

$$CAL_{ij} = \left(\beta_0 + \beta_1 age_j + \beta_2 age_j \times sex_j + \beta_3 sex_j\right) + \left(e_{0ij} + u_{0j} + u_{1j} age_j\right).$$

The multilevel model estimates the parameters of the fixed part of the model ($\beta_0, \beta_1, \beta_2$, and β_3) along with the parameters of the random part of the model (σ_{0e}^2 for level-1; $\sigma_{0u}^2, \sigma_{1u}^2$, and σ_{01u} for level-2).

Now, it is possible that the degree of random variation is different for males and females, in which case the model could become:

$$CAL_{ij} = \beta_{0ij} + \beta_{1j} age_j \times m_j + \beta_{2j} age_j \times f_j,$$

where

$$CAL_{ij} = \left(\beta_0 + \beta_1 age_j \times m_j + \beta_2 age_j \times f_j\right) \\ + \left(e_{0ij} + u_{0j} + u_{1j} age_j \times m_j + u_{2j} age_j \times f_j\right),$$

such that $m_j = 1$ for males, and zero otherwise; and similarly $f_j = 1$ for females, or zero otherwise. If there were no underlying gender outcome differences being sought, this would be modelled explicitly by constraining the covariate coefficients to be equal ($\beta_1 \equiv \beta_2$). The random parameters, u_{1j} and u_{2j}, depict two random slopes with respect to age, for males and females, respectively. The model estimates the parameters of the fixed part (β_0, β_1, and β_2) along with the parameters of the random part (σ_{0e}^2 for level-1; $\sigma_{0u}^2, \sigma_{1u}^2, \sigma_{2u}^2, \sigma_{01u}, \sigma_{02u}$ and σ_{12u} for level-2), where some covariance terms ($\sigma_{01u}, \sigma_{02u}, \sigma_{12u}$) might be zero or small and not significantly different from zero. In which case, it might be appropriate to constrain these to be zero where model convergence is not readily achieved. Each constraint could be relaxed again in turn if specifically being sought. In any event, the variance structure at level-2 is now very complex. If all variance and covariances are to be estimated, the total level-2 variance structure is: $Var\left(u_{0j} + u_{1j} age_j \times m_j + u_{2j} age_j \times f_j\right)$, which simplifies to (assuming $sex^2 = sex$):

$$level-2\ variance = \sigma_{0u}^2 + 2[\sigma_{01u} + (\sigma_{02u} - \sigma_{01u})sex]age \\ + \left[\sigma_{1u}^2 + \left(\sigma_{2u}^2 - \sigma_{1u}^2\right)sex\right]age^2.$$

5.4 Markov Chain Monte Carlo (MCMC)

Maximum likelihood methods are the usual method employed to obtain estimates of model parameters. The probability of the observed data is written as a function of the unknown parameters (the likelihood function); with the coefficient estimates taking the values of the unknown parameters that maximizes this function. This poses no problems for single-level logistic regression, since the likelihood function can be written explicitly. However, the likelihood function for a multilevel logistic regression cannot be written as an explicit function and thus alternative model fit methods are required. Broadly speaking, there are three strategies for obtaining the estimates sought. Firstly, the likelihood function could be approximated. Maximum Quasi-Likelihood (MQL) and Partial Quasi-Likelihood (PQL) are appropriate examples (Moerbeek et al. 2003). These methods are in general computational amenable but produce (to varying degrees) biased estimates. The second method would be to perform numerical integration. Performing numerical integration over all random parameters can be rather computationally intensive. Finally, a Bayesian approach, for example Markov Chain Monte Carlo (MCMC), could be adopted (Gilks et al. 1996). MCMC is also computationally intensive but will yield unbiased estimates of the random structure.

In addressing the computational demand of MLM, there is always a balance between speed and accuracy that has to be sought. A suggested approach that seems logical is to gain benefit from the increased speed of an approximate maximum likelihood method (for example PQL) during model development. Speed can subsequently be sacrificed for accuracy by using MCMC whenever any doubt arises. In any case, MCMC should at least be used to obtain estimates of a final model.

5.4.1 Overview of MCMC

An initial guess of the model coefficients is made based on a simplified version of the model, usually a standard (biased) multilevel estimation. From this, whilst considering the complex data structure and by adopting the coefficients of all other parameters as correct, the marginal distribution of each coefficient is used to simulate a dataset with properties conforming to the specified model. This yields an updated model estimate for the coefficient being sought, which is then taken as fixed and the same process is applied to the next model coefficient. This is repeated for all model coefficients, in rotation, constantly generating revised estimates.

It has been shown that, providing certain criteria are satisfied, these simulated estimates of model coefficients eventually fit the correct distribution of model coefficients after many repeated simulations. After what is termed a 'burn-in' period, which is where initial (less accurate) simulations are discarded, the MCMC process yields a set of estimates that are useful for making inferences regarding the model. The simulated estimates are representative of a hypothetical population of all possible model estimates, for which the sample data represents only one example. By examining the simulated estimates, it is possible to check if the simulations have converged on the correct values, and that the number of simulations is sufficient to provide meaningful summary information.

The necessary criteria for convergence include 'reasonable' starting values and, in loose terms, a reasonable degree of freedom in how far a new simulation can 'stray' from the previous one. MCMC chains should possess good 'mixing' characteristics; variation around the parameter estimate should be random. That is, no pattern(s) should exist amongst the estimates of a parameter at each iteration of the chain. Good mixing will yield a symmetric (Gaussian) distribution for the kernel density (empirical distribution) of the parameter. For this reason, the MCMC diagnostics should always be considered. Finally, attention should be drawn to the fact that the variance cannot be negative and that the objective of assessment should be in identifying how inherent outcome variability ought to be specified, namely at which level(s) any variance structure exists.

A comprehensive coverage is given by Goldstein (Goldstein 2003), while Browne (Browne 2006; Browne and Draper 2000; 2006) provides in-depth coverage of many aspects of MCMC pertinent to MLM.

5.5 Model Fit Diagnostics

5.5.1 The Fixed Part

The fixed part of the model is checked in the same manner as single-level models. Specifically, the relationship between the outcome and predictor variables should be correctly specified, the residuals should be normally distributed for every value of the predictor variables and the variance of the outcome should be the same at each value of the predictor variables.

5.5.2 The Random Part

Simulated data from the fitted model should 'look' like the observed data. The model is not valid if the simulated data differ (in a non-random way) from the observed data.

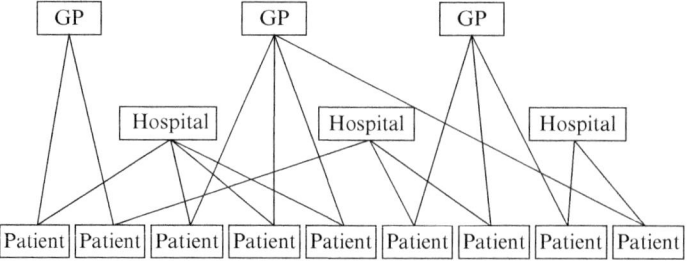

Fig. 5.13 A cross-classified data structure of patients nested within GDPs and nested within hospitals

5.6 Complex Hierarchies

Multilevel methodology can be used for data structures that are not strictly hierarchical, or are not typically thought of as representing a natural hierarchy (Fielding and Goldstein 2006). Examples can be drawn from multivariate data, repeated measures, categorical outcomes, meta-analyses, and cross-classifications. For multivariate data, the lowest level represents the multiple outcomes under consideration. Repeated measures and categorical outcomes work in a similar manner, with occasion/category represented at level 1 for repeated measures and categorical outcomes respectively. Meta-analysis can incorporate covariates (meta-regression) and thus help in addressing the issue of heterogeneity between studies.

An example of a model with no strict hierarchy is General Practitioner (GP) referral for hospital-based treatment. As shown in Fig. 5.13, hospitals are cross-classified with referring GPs. Thus, patients that belong to a particular practice attend different hospitals, and vice versa. This approach can account for differences between hospitals due to organisational procedures, whilst accounting for GP variation in their referral behaviour. Furthermore, the model can incorporate covariates at the patient-level (e.g. age, gender), the hospital-level (e.g. proportion of cases undertaken as day-cases), and the GP-level (e.g. level of qualification, experience).

5.7 Current Areas of Research and Further Reading

The interested reader may wish to consult Hox (2002) or Snijders and Bosker (1999) for fuller coverage. Goldstein (2003) provides readers with useful details of the fit algorithms, while Leyland and Goldstein (2001) provide a text dedicated to MLM in the context of health. An extension of multilevel modelling is to allow the random effects to follow a discrete distribution. This is known as latent class modelling and Chap. 7 in this book provides an introduction to this application. The application of multilevel modelling to longitudinal data can be found in Chap. 12 on latent growth curve modelling and Chap. 13 on growth mixture modelling.

References

Altman, D. G. (1991). *Practical statistics for medical research*. London: Chapman and Hall/CRC.

Armitage, P., Berry, G., & Matthews, J. N. S. (2002). *Statistical methods in medical research* (4th ed.). Malden: Blackwell Science.

Bland, M. (2000). *An introduction to medical statistics* (3rd ed.). Oxford: Oxford University Press.

Browne, W. J. (2006). MCMC algorithms for constrained variance matrices. *Computational Statistics & Data Analysis, 50*(7), 1655–1677.

Browne, W. J., & Draper, D. (2000). Implementation and performance issues in the Bayesian and likelihood fitting of multilevel models. *Computational Statistics, 15*(3), 391–420.

Browne, W. J., & Draper, D. (2006). A comparison of Bayesian and likelihood-based methods for fitting multilevel models. *Bayesian Analysis, 1*(3), 473–513.

Fielding, A., & Goldstein, H. (2006). *Cross-classified and multiple membership structures in multilevel models an introduction and review* (Vol. 791). Nottingham: DfES.

Gilks, W. R., Richardson, S., & Spiegelhalter, D. J. (1996). *Markov chain Monte Carlo in practice*. London: Chapman & Hall.

Gilthorpe, M. S., & Cunningham, S. J. (2000). The application of multilevel, multivariate modelling to orthodontic research data. *Community Dental Health, 17*(4), 236–242.

Goldstein, H. (2003). *Multilevel statistical models* (3rd ed.). London: Arnold.

Hox, J. J. (2002). *Multilevel analysis: Techniques and applications*. Mahwah: Lawrence Erlbaum Associates.

Kirkwood, B. R., & Sterne, J. A. C. (2003). *Essential medical statistics* (2nd ed.). Malden: Blackwell Science.

Leyland, A. H., & Goldstein, H. (2001). *Multilevel modelling of health statistics*. Chichester: Wiley.

Machin, D., Campbell, M. J., & Walters, S. J. (2007). *Medical statistics: A textbook for the health sciences* (4th ed.). Chichester: Wiley.

Moerbeek, M., Van Breukelen, G. J. P., & Berger, M. P. F. (2003). A comparison of estimation methods for multilevel logistic models. *Computational Statistics, 18*(1), 19–37.

Qian, L. F., & Wang, S. J. (2001). Bias-corrected heteroscedasticity robust covariance matrix (sandwich) estimators. *Journal of Statistical Computation and Simulation, 70*(2), 161–174.

Quene, H., & van den Bergh, H. (2008). Examples of mixed-effects modeling with crossed random effects and with binomial data. *Journal of Memory and Language, 59*(4), 413–425.

Raudenbush, S. W., & Bryk, A. S. (2002). *Hierarchical linear models applications and data analysis methods* (2nd ed.). Thousand Oaks: Sage Publications.

Snijders, T. A. B., & Bosker, R. J. (1999). *Multilevel analysis: An introduction to basic and advanced multilevel modeling*. London: Sage.

White, H. (1980). A heteroskedasticity-consistent covariance-matrix estimator and a direct test for heteroskedasticity. *Econometrica, 48*(4), 817–838.

Ziegler, A., Kastner, C., & Blettner, M. (1998). The generalised estimating equations: An annotated bibliography. *Biometrical Journal, 40*(2), 115–139.

Chapter 6
Modelling Data That Exhibit an Excess Number of Zeros: Zero-Inflated Models and Generic Mixture Models

Mark S. Gilthorpe, Morten Frydenberg, Yaping Cheng, and Vibeke Baelum

6.1 Overview

Within biomedical research, count data may appear to possess an 'excess' of zeros relative to standard statistical distributions. There is a plethora of statistical literature addressing how best to model such outcomes. The Zero-inflated Poisson (ZiP) and the zero-inflated binomial (ZiB) are two common modelling strategies proposed. More recently, generic mixture models have also been suggested (Skrondal and Rabe-Hesketh 2004). We discuss these modelling strategies in some depth, introducing the concepts of mixture modelling in simpler terms in this chapter before examining in a wider context in later chapters. Crucial issues surrounding the modelling of counts with an excessive proportion of zeros are addressed, specifically outlining common potential pitfalls, and we provide some helpful tips in model selection and model interpretation.

M.S. Gilthorpe (✉) • Y. Cheng
Division of Biostatistics, Centre for Epidemiology and Biostatistics, Leeds Institute of Genetics, Health & Therapeutics, University of Leeds, Leeds, UK
e-mail: m.s.gilthorpe@leeds.ac.uk

M. Frydenberg
Department of Biostatistics, Faculty of Health Sciences, Institute of Public Health, University of Aarhus, Aarhus, Denmark

V. Baelum
School of Dentistry, Faculty of Health Sciences, University of Aarhus, Aarhus, Denmark

6.2 An Example Taken From Oral Health Research – Dental Caries

In order to examine the ideas we explore in this chapter, we choose for illustration an oral health dataset that is in the public domain and has been analysed extensively already to study different methods for analysing data with excess zeros compared to standard count distributions. The example data are from a prospective study that examined the effect of four interventions to improve the oral health status amongst children. An established indicator of oral health involves counting the number of decayed (d/D), missing (m/M), and filled (f/F) deciduous 'milk teeth' (t) or permanent teeth (T), yielding the measure of *dmft* or *DMFT* (Böhning et al. 1999). The *dmft* count ranges between 0 and 20, whereas the *DMFT* count assumes values between 0 and 32. Amongst relatively healthy individuals, or during the early stages of dentition development, there is potential for an excess number of zero *dmft*/*DMFT* counts.

The example dataset derives from a study conducted in the urban area of Belo Horizonte, Brazil, during the 1990s (Böhning et al. 1999). The effect of four caries prevention methods were examined amongst 797 school children aged 7 years at the start of the study. Data were recorded for the eight deciduous molars; hence the outcome ranges between 0 and 8. The research question was how might different intervention methods prevent caries incidence (new lesions). Interventions were administered in six settings: (1) oral health education; (2) enrichment of the school diet with rice bran; (3) mouthwash with 0.2% sodium fluoride (NaF) solution; (4) oral hygiene; (5) all the interventions combined; and (6) none of the interventions (control). The study was clustered in design, with children nested within schools, which in turn were allocated to one of the intervention groups. The outcome therefore was change in *dmft* count from baseline and was analysed by Böhning et al. (1999) to illustrate that ZiP regression models are useful in evaluating intervention effects on dental caries when data exhibit an excess of zero counts.

The data may be downloaded from the publishers of the original Böhning et al. (1999) article (http://www.blackwellpublishers.co.uk/rss); or from the webpage of the vendor of the software *LatentGOLD4.0*™ (Vermunt and Magidson 2005a) as the data were used as part of a tutorial (http://www.statisticalinnovations.com).

6.3 Zero-Inflated and Generic Mixture Models

A good review of zero-inflated models is given by Ridout et al. (1998), which examines several methods, particularly in relation to the Poisson distribution. The *zero-inflated Poisson* (ZiP) model (Böhning 1998; Lambert 1992; Mullahy 1986) is the most common option, encountered extensively within the biomedical literature. The basic concept behind the ZiP model is that the overall distribution is made up of a mixture of two distributions: one with a central location (mean) of zero and the other with a non-zero central location that is estimated empirically; the proportions of each distribution are determined empirically. In other words, one takes a standard Poisson distribution and combines this with a 'spike' of zeros to make the total overall distribution that consequently possess 'too many' zeros compared to the standard Poisson. The total number of zeros is a combination of those that belong to the 'spike' (otherwise termed the zero 'bin') and those that belong to the Poisson distribution; the proportion of each is estimated as part of the modelling process.

The *zero-inflated binomial* (ZiB) model is another modelling strategy (Hall 2000; Vieira et al. 2000), analogous to the ZiP model, but used in the case of bounded count data (i.e. where the tail of the distribution is no longer infinite but pre-specified). For counts that are bounded above by relatively large numbers, or where the distribution mean is relatively low, there may be little difference between the Poisson and binomial models in their performance in modelling the data, but where the upper bound is smaller (as with the example oral health dataset), or where the distribution mean is half way or farther along the count spectrum, the binomial distribution may provide a more appropriate model. This is because the infinite tail of the Poisson might otherwise provide too many predicted counts beyond the upper bound of the outcomes scale, even though the frequency for each outcome value may be small, and the combined total of all counts exceeding the upper bound might be substantial. In any event, where counts are bounded above and one has doubts about the appropriateness of the Poisson distribution, the binomial distribution may be worth exploring as an alternative. It is important to note, however, that interpretation of binomial model parameters is different to that of Poisson model parameters, as will be discussed in more detail later.

In statistical notation, ZiP/ZiB models are expressed as a mixture of two Poisson/binomial distributions, where one distribution takes the value of zero only and the other may depend upon covariates, yielding the combined response probability (Vermunt and Magidson 2005b):

$$P(y_i|\mathbf{x}_i) = \pi g(y_i; 0) + (1 - \pi) g\left(y_i; f^{-1}[\mathbf{x}'_i \boldsymbol{\beta}]\right)$$

where π is a weight between zero and one; $g(y_i; \mu_i)$ is the Poisson or binomial probability with parameter μ_i; $f[\mu_i]$ is the link function, which takes the form of the natural logarithm for Poisson probability and the *logit* for binomial probability; and $\mathbf{x}'_i \boldsymbol{\beta}$ is the vector of linear predictors (covariates). The standard probability distributions are given by:

$$\text{Poisson: } g(y_i; \mu_i) = \frac{\mu_i^{y_i} \exp(-\mu_i)}{y_i!}$$

$$\text{or binomial: } g(y_i; \mu_i) = \frac{N!}{y_i!(N - y_i)!} \mu_i^{y_i} (1 - \mu_i)^{N - y_i}$$

where y_i is the outcome count, μ_i is the Poisson mean or the binomial distribution parameter, and N is the binomial denominator (the upper bound of the count outcome).

An extension to these models is where one allows for 'over-dispersion', which may occur within a dataset for a number of reasons. The most common cause of over-dispersion is lack of heterogeneity because outcomes are not truly independent. This often occurs due to clustering, i.e. where outcomes are grouped, as frequently occurs in biomedical research. To accommodate this explicitly within the Poisson/binomial distribution, we adapt the distribution parameter to follow another distribution. The over-dispersed Poisson, also known as the *negative binomial*, is derived from the Poisson when its distribution parameter follows a gamma distribution (denoted by Γ) with mean μ_i and variance μ_i^2/v^2:

$$g(y_i; \mu_i) = \frac{\Gamma(y_i + v^2)}{y_i!\,\Gamma(v^2)} \left[\frac{v^2}{v^2 + \mu_i}\right]^{v^2} \left[\frac{\mu_i}{v^2 + \mu_i}\right]^{y_i}.$$

The expected value of y_i is μ_i, and variance is no longer equal to the expected value, but is a factor $1 + \mu_i/v^2$ larger; as $1/v^2 \to 0$, the over-dispersed Poisson distribution reduces to the standard Poisson distribution. Similarly, the over-dispersed binomial, also known as the *beta-binomial*, is derived from the binomial when with its distribution parameter follows the beta distribution (denoted by B) with mean μ_i and variance $\mu_i(1 - \mu_i)/(v^2 + 1)$:

$$g(y_i; \mu_i) = \frac{B(\mu_i v^2 + y_i, (1 - \mu_i)v^2 + (N - y_i))}{B(\mu_i v^2, (1 - \mu_i)v^2)} \frac{N!}{y_i!(N - y_i)!}.$$

The expected value of y_i is $\mu_i N$, and variance is no longer equal to $\mu_i(1 - \mu_i)N$ but is a factor $1 + (N - 1)/(1 + v^2)$ larger; as $1/v^2 \to 0$, the beta-binomial distribution reduces to the standard binomial distribution. For the rest of this chapter, we refer to these extensions to the Poisson/binomial as *over-dispersed* Poisson/binomial.

A further extension to the zero-inflated model is achieved by including covariates in the mixture part of the model, to determine the proportions conditional on these covariates. For the ZiP/ZiB models, this involves replacing the weight π with a function of the covariates:

$$P(y_i|\mathbf{x}_i, \mathbf{z}_i) = \pi\big(h^{-1}[\mathbf{z}'_i \gamma]\big) g(y_i; 0) + \big(1 - \pi\big(h^{-1}[\mathbf{z}'_i \gamma]\big)\big) g\big(y_i; f^{-1}[\mathbf{x}'_i \boldsymbol{\beta}]\big)$$

where $g(y_i; \mu_i)$ and $f[\mu_i]$ are as previously defined, π is now determined by covariates, $h^{-1}[\mathbf{z}'_i \gamma]$ is the inverse of the link function and takes the form of the *logit*, and $\mathbf{z}'_i \gamma$ is a vector of covariates for the class membership model (these covariates need not be identical to those in the distribution part of the model, and caution should be exercised in covariate selection, as will be discussed later). Either the standard or over-dispersed probability distributions apply.

A final extension to the zero-inflated model is where the number of distributions being combined is two or more and no one is constrained to be identically zero (i.e. we no longer have a 'spike' of zeros as one of the distributions being combined). These generic mixture models, also known as *latent class models*, or *discrete latent variable models*, determine a number of *latent classes* or subgroups of the data, the optimum choice of which is made by the researcher, though usually informed by log-likelihood statistics. The model parameters of each latent class, along with their relative contribution to the combined outcome distribution, are determined empirically. The most general probability structure of a mixture model, with class membership informed by covariates, is defined by the function: (Vermunt and Magidson 2005b)

$$d(y_i|\mathbf{x}_i, \mathbf{z}_i) = \sum_{c=1}^{C} P(c|\mathbf{z}_i) d(y_i|c, \mathbf{x}_i)$$

where $d(y_i|\mathbf{x}_i, \mathbf{z}_i)$ is the probability density corresponding to a particular y_i, given a particular set of $\mathbf{x}_i$ covariates that affect the response and given another set of $\mathbf{z}_i$ covariates that affect class membership (again note that the $\mathbf{x}_i$ and $\mathbf{z}_i$ may be the same or different, though the choice of model covariates is not straightforward, as we discuss later); the unobserved variable c intervenes between $\mathbf{z}_i$ and y_i via $P(c|\mathbf{z}_i)$, the probability of belonging to the latent class c given the covariate values; and $d(y_i|c, \mathbf{x}_i)$ is the probability density of y_i given $\mathbf{x}_i$ and c. The class membership model is a multinomial logistic regression model and coefficients are log odds ratios.

Caveat While many generic mixture model options are available, not all are intuitive and interpretable, and in some instances models may not be identifiable. Where a covariate impacts differently within each latent class and where class membership is also predicted by the covariate that operates within each latent class distribution, model interpretation becomes challenging if not impossible, even if the model is identifiable. This is because there is circularity in the conditional interrelationships of covariate parameters in the distribution parts *and* the class membership part of the same model. Where identifiable but not interpretable for purpose of inference, such models may however be used for prediction. As we remain interested in inference, we only consider only two forms of generic mixture model in this chapter where: (i) covariate parameters vary across latent classes that are *not* predicted by the same covariates – which we shall call a *class-dependent* covariate model because the parameter estimates depend upon the class in which they operate; and (ii) covariate parameters are constrained to be equal across classes (the marginal impact of each covariate), whilst class membership *is* predicted by these covariates – which we shall call a *class-independent* covariate model because the distribution parameters operate identically in each latent class whilst these same covariates determine the class structure. The ideal number of latent classes, hence the preferred generic mixture model, is determined by inspection of model-fit criteria. The most commonly adopted model-fit criteria are likelihood-based statistics, which are discussed in the next section.

6.4 Establishing Model-Fit Criteria

The model log-likelihood is a measure of how well the model fits the data. The use of this statistic directly, without any adjustment for parsimony, is not generally favoured as a model-fit criterion alone, since one can nearly always improve upon it (hence improve model fit, ultimately towards the point of a saturated model) by increasing model complexity. One option is to plot changes in the likelihood value against increasing model complexity, e.g. for each increment in the number of latent classes (keeping all other parameter configurations consistent). One then 'eyeballs' the point of complexity at which there is an 'elbow', signifying acceleration in the diminishing return in model improvement for increasing model complexity. This approach is similar to the use of *scree plots* for those familiar with principal component analysis; there is no hard and fast rule employed.

Alternatives strategies to the raw likelihood statistic are penalized versions, such as the Bayesian Information Criterion (BIC) (Vermunt and Magidson 2005b) or Akaike's Information Criterion (AIC) (Vermunt and Magidson 2005b), both of which incorporate a sense of parsimony by accommodating the varying number of model parameters. These statistics effectively provide a trade-off between growing model complexity and how well the model fits the data. There is no consensus, however, on *which* penalized form of the likelihood statistic should be adopted. In general, one should consider a range of likelihood-based statistics for model-fit criteria. In this chapter, we adopt the BIC and AIC, though we also consider model-fit criteria that reflect how well count models perform along the outcome range in terms of predicted counts.

Given the focus of zero-inflated modelling to accommodate an excess numbers of zeros compared to standard distributions, model-fit criteria should perhaps examine how well zero-inflated models do in predicting the total number of zero counts. A transition or contrast from zero to one typically represents the onset of disease in longitudinal data, or elevated disease prevalence in cross-sectional data, which has direct clinical importance. To acknowledge the importance of zero counts, we therefore contrast the number of predicted and observed zeros. However, other count thresholds along the outcome scale may also have clinical importance. For instance, the tail of the distribution (truncated for binomial or infinite for Poisson) typically denotes increasing disease severity. Crossing a 'critical' threshold may represent a cut-off that distinguishes between 'high' and 'low' risk groups (for the purpose of targeted preventions) or in some instances may signify irreversibility or a critical state, such as mortality (e.g. a tooth exfoliates or an individual dies). The entire range of the outcome might have importance for clinical diagnostic or prognostics reasons. Model-fit criteria should therefore seek to capture this.

For an overall assessment of the distribution, we assess the 'root mean squared error' (RMSE) between predicted and observed counts (for the viable range) as a proportion of the number of observations. This is achieved by initially differencing the observed (Obs_i) and predicted ($Pred_i$) counts for the entire scale, squaring these differences and summing, where the 'scale' is either determined by the distribution ($i = 0 \ldots N$, where N is the binomial maximum or an arbitrary observed maximum count for the Poisson, or set by the user, beyond which all predicted Poisson counts are grouped). One then divides by the number of categories set by the choice of scale ($N + 1$), takes the square-root, multiplies by the number of categories ($N + 1$), and divides by the total number of observations, n, to express as a fraction:

$$RMSE = \frac{N+1}{n} \sqrt{\frac{\sum_{i=0}^{N}(Obs_i - Pred_i)^2}{(N+1)}}.$$

Although the RMSE statistic may seem somewhat arbitrary, as indeed it is not directly comparable across different datasets or for different model parameterisations of the same dataset (e.g. Poisson vs. binomial), its construction is such that, in very crude terms, it may be thought of as representing the maximum proportion of 'misallocated' counts. For instance, for an outcome scale of 0–3, if the predicted number of 'zeros' were 3 more than observed, the number of 'ones' 3 less, the number of 'twos' 3 more, and the number of 'threes' 3 less, out of a total of 48 observations, there is crudely speaking 25% misallocated counts (12 misallocated observations out of 48). Calculating RMSE: $3^2 = 9$ occurs four times (36), averaged over four categories (9), square-rooted (3), multiplied by four categories (12), expressed as a fraction of the number of observations (0.25). Were the same predicted counts distributed such that one frequency miscount was 6 over and another 6 under, RMSE: $6^2 = 36$ occurs twice (72), averaged over four categories (18), square-rooted (4.24), multiplied by four categories (16.97), expressed as a fraction of the number of observations (0.35). Thus, where misallocation is evenly distributed, RMSE represents the proportion of misallocated observations; if misallocation is not evenly distributed, RMSE is higher. Hence, the proportion of counts misallocated is no larger than the RMSE. Examples are given for the illustrative dental dataset used later in this chapter.

Caveat Model-fit criteria *per se* do not always provide enough insight as to how well a particular modelling strategy suits the data. This becomes particularly apparent for data exhibiting an excess numbers of zeros compared to standard distributions, as there is the potential for what might be seen as a 'dual' or 'two-stage' process of data generation. In such circumstances, it is feasible that likelihood statistics and predicted counts fail to distinguish between differently parameterised models, as shown for the example dental data in this chapter. Understanding data generation might then usefully inform model choice and hence model interpretation.

6.5 Covariates in the Distribution Part Must Also Be Considered for the Mixture Part

Bias resulting from the omission of an important covariate from the distribution part of a model is well known, but less well known is that bias may also occur when important covariates are omitted from the mixture part. We demonstrate this for ZiP/ZiB models. This may not be immediately obvious, which is perhaps why many researchers have overlooked this problem. However, consider for one moment a hypothetical example of dental data, similar to the Brazilian study, with *dmft* recorded for all deciduous teeth and modelled using a zero-inflated Poisson model with only one covariate (*sex*) and assume this is included only in the distribution part of the model. Accordingly, the proportion of children in the zero-bin must be the same for boys and girls. This is an implicit constraint resulting from not modelling *sex* to predict class membership. The impact on such a model is illustrated by simulation.

We undertook a two-stage simulation process whereby *dmft* data were generated, in the statistical software package *R* (http://www.r-project.org/) using the function *rpois*, to represent 50,000 boys and 50,000 girls: 20% of the boys had a *dmft* count of zero, the remainder taking values from a Poisson distribution with mean 2; and 80% of the girls had a *dmft* of zero, the remainder taking values from a Poisson distribution with mean 1. Data were then modelled using a standard ZiP model (ZiP), i.e. with the covariate *sex* in the Poisson part of the model only. Including *sex* in the ZiP model to predict class membership emulates the two-stage simulation process, so we focus only on how unreliable the standard ZiP model is for this scenario. The log-likelihood, BIC and AIC were obtained by maximising:

$$l(\pi, \mu_F, \mu_M) = \sum_{sex} \sum_{k=0}^{\infty} p_{true}(k, sex) \log(p_{ZiP\_Z}(k, sex; \pi, \mu_F, \mu_M)),$$

where $p_{true}(k, sex)$ is the true probability of observing k for each *sex* based on the true model and $p_{ZiP\_Z}(k, sex; \pi, \mu_F, \mu_M)$ is the same probability under a zero-inflated model with parameters π (proportion in the zero bin), μ_F (mean of the females distribution part), and μ_M (mean of the male distribution part). *LatentGOLD4.0*™ (http://www.statisticalinnovations.com) was used to generate the standard zero-inflated Poisson model and results are presented in Table 6.1.

It is apparent that the standard ZiP model does not perform well for girls. The proportion of children in the zero bin, constrained to be identical for both girls and boys, was estimated to be 22.87%. This was close to the true value of 20% for boys, but was far from the true value of 80% for girls. The distribution mean for girls was also far from true (0.27 opposed to 1.00), though less biased for boys (2.03 opposed to 2.00). The inappropriately specified zero-inflated model yielded considerable deviation from truth in terms of size, shape and central location of the distribution part for girls, yet overall predicted counts were indistinguishable from the simulated data, as seen in Fig. 6.1.

6 Modelling Data That Exhibit an Excess Number of Zeros... 101

Table 6.1 Model fit criteria for the ZiP model undertaken with the simulated data

	Simulated true	ZiP estimated
Log-likelihood	−100,088[a]	−111,700.74
BIC	200,212[a]	223,436.02
AIC	200,184[a]	223,407.48
Zero	0	1,573.74
RMSE	0%	13.7%
Girls		
Proportion in the Zero-bin	80%	22.87%
Distribution mean *dmft* count (95% CI)	1	0.27 (0.26, 0.28)
Boys		
Proportion in the Zero-bin	20%	22.87%
Distribution mean *dmft* count (95% CI)	2	2.03 (1.97, 2.07)

ZiP standard zero-inflated Poisson model with *sex* as a covariate in the non-zero part only (not as a class predictor), *BIC* Bayesian Information Criterion, *AIC* Akaike's Information Criterion, *Zero* the absolute difference between observed and predicted number of zero counts, *RMSE* root mean squared error (see Sect. 3.1) for categories 0–10, *CI* Confidence Interval

[a]True log-likelihood, BIC and AIC are based on the asymptotic likelihood, which was maximised numerically

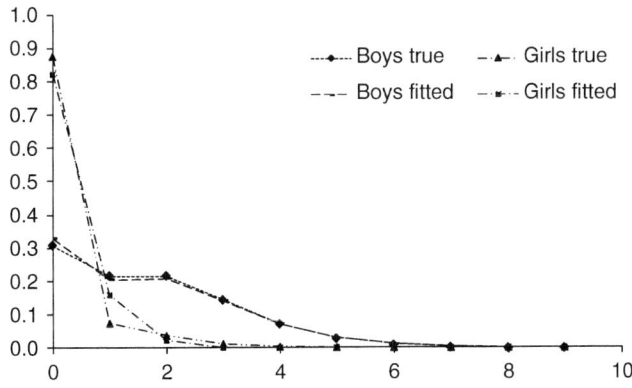

Fig. 6.1 Simulated *dmft* counts for boys and girls: predicted and true distributions for the simulated dataset (including the zero-bin)

Two different model parameterisations (the standard ZiP with *sex* in the distribution part only and the extended ZiP with *sex* in both the distribution and mixture parts) can yield near-identical predicted outcomes, yet each give rise to very different model inferences. If focus was specifically given to the distribution part of the model, the inferred Poisson distribution for girls would look very different to that from the true distribution from which the simulated data were sampled, as illustrated in Fig. 6.2.

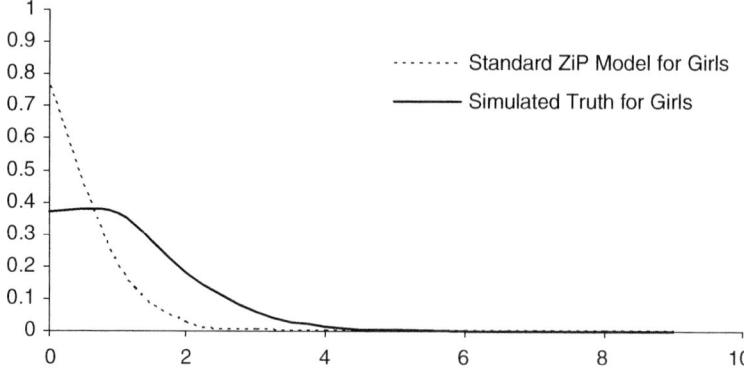

Fig. 6.2 Distributions of the *dmft* counts for girls: the true distribution from which the simulated sample was drawn (*solid line*) and the inferred distribution from the standard Poisson model (both excluding the zero bin)

Despite a deliberately large difference in the simulated number of boys and girls in the zero bin, the standard ZiP model readily accommodated the implied and unnecessary constraint of equal proportions of boys and girls in the zero bin by distorting the distribution part of the model. Were the extended ZiP model evaluated, it would be favoured in this instance due to likelihood-based model fit criteria. However, in many instances researchers do not consider covariates in the mixture part of the model. Many zero-inflated models have been evaluated where covariates are identified as important for the distribution part only, and no consideration is given to these same covariates in the mixture model. The implications of this will vary, but undoubtedly in some instances the most suitable model may have been overlooked, the distribution part may have been biased, and model interpretation may have been misleading. One should thus consider carefully the role of covariates in determining the mixture in zero-inflated models. Considering this problem more generally, if one observes covariate differences in the proportion of total zeros, there may be genuine differences in the mixture proportions. Therefore, exploring bivariate associations between the binary outcome (zero/non-zero) and each covariate could be a good indicator of which covariates ought to be included in the mixture part of the model, at least initially.

Caveat The converse, however, does not necessarily follow, since the absence of any bivariate association between the binary outcome and a covariate does not preclude that covariate from being important to the mixture model. One might err on the side of caution and include all possible covariates in the mixture part, but there is a price to pay in terms of lack of model parsimony, with potentially redundant covariates in the mixture model. The extent by which researchers then seek to trade potential small biases in their models for small improvements in the precision of model estimates is a matter of judgement pertaining to model context and purpose. As a broad guide, one should perhaps discard a covariate from the mixture part of the zero-inflated model only when there are no notable changes to parameter estimates elsewhere in the model.

6.6 Revisiting the Brazilian Caries Dataset

Skrondal and Rabe-Hesketh revisited the Brazilian dataset (modelling follow-up outcomes only), exploring the utility of generic mixture models by relaxing the constraint of there being only two mixtures with one having to be identically zero (Skrondal and Rabe-Hesketh 2004). We re-examine the models by Böhning et al. and by Skrondal and Rabe-Hesketh, for illustrative purposes, and we include a few additional parameterisations of our own.

Issues become apparent that could arise in many similar situations when dealing with data that possess excessive zeros, though it may not always be obvious that there are pitfalls and problems that may lead researchers to settle unwittingly upon the 'wrong' model. Here, we mean 'wrong' in the sense of inappropriate for the context of the data, even though model fit might seem good in terms of both likelihood statistics and predicted outcomes. The unwary might therefore end up with potentially erroneous model interpretations. To understand how this might occur requires a hypothetical consideration of the role of data generation processes and their role in the formulation of modelling strategies. What follows in later sections is therefore not only relevant for dental caries data. In particular, we consider carefully the issue of model selection and interpretation.

Caveat There were a few drawbacks to the original analytical strategy worthy of discussion, to show how study setting and design are as critical as appropriate modelling strategies. Although the allocation of schools was random, there was only one school assigned per intervention arm, which is insufficient to be adequately cluster-randomised. Baseline differences in mean *dmft* across intervention groups may not have been solely due to chance. Without adequate randomisation, causal inferences could not be inferred. Böhning et al. sought to accommodate baseline mean differences in disease levels across schools by including baseline *dmft* as a covariate in their analysis of covariance (ANCOVA) (Böhning et al. 1999). However, this did not overcome the problem. Although ANCOVA accommodates *within-group* heterogeneity in baseline outcomes, a fundamental requirement of ANCOVA is that *between-group* population values must be balanced (usually achieved by randomisation) (Senn 2006). Baseline mean outcome differences amongst groups not attributable to chance could then yield biased results, known as Lord's paradox (Blance et al. 2007; Lord 1967,1969). The original analyses were thus potentially erroneous and the original study findings questionable. Although Skrondal and Rabe-Hesketh modelled the follow-up data from the same study, to illustrate the utility of generic mixture models

(Skrondal and Rabe-Hesketh 2004), baseline group differences would yield problems and the interpretation of model findings remain difficult. It is for this reason that we do not seek to interpret the Brazilian dataset, though we still use the data for methodological illustration.

6.7 Model Selection

Before moving into the realm of model selection and interpretation (in relation to data generation), we first examine some of the more fundamental issues about model generation.

6.7.1 Outcome Distribution

Skrondal and Rabe-Hesketh questioned the use of a Poisson distribution for the Brazilian dataset, since the study counts represented the number of *dmft* ('successes') out of a total of eight deciduous molars ('trials') (Skrondal and Rabe-Hesketh 2004). Model fit then becomes relevant for a finite range of the outcome scale only (counts of 0–8). Using their Generalized Linear Latent and Mixed Models (*GLLAMM*) software, the ZiB model was introduced and compared with the ZiP model. This generally revealed that Poisson models predicted unrealistically long tails and binomial models performed much better. Similarly, our focus will be given to binomial models for the example dataset.

In general, it is important that the familiarity of the Poisson model to most researchers, compared to the binomial model say, does not dictate modelling strategy; especially when it is clear that data are bounded above. One should also consider model interpretation and not be stuck with overly familiar practices. For instance, it seems almost standard practice within the oral health research field to interpret model coefficients in relation to an individual's mean *dmft* (as with a Poisson model), whereas risk ratios for increments along the *dmft* index scale (as with a binomial model) have not gained widespread use. Yet the latter is probably more appealing in terms of what really happens in terms of data generation, since individuals and teeth that are more prone to disease succumb first and the more individuals and teeth that do succumb, the more difficult is it for the remaining individuals and teeth to become unaffected. It is therefore not surprising that binomial outcome models were preferable for the Brazilian dataset, as demonstrated by Skrondal and Rabe-Hesketh (2004), and this may not be just because the data are bounded above.

6.7.2 Over-Dispersion

Within the Brazilian dataset, the *dmft* outcome was derived in a clustered setting of children nested within schools. Since clustering can predispose to outcome over-dispersion (i.e. heavier tails than expected for either the Poisson or the binomial outcome), we explore this explicitly. One could deal with clustering directly within a multilevel model, as described in other chapters, or one could employ a marginal model, such as GEE (Liang and Zeger 1986), but for the purposes of this chapter we maintain focus on the aggregated outcome and accommodate over-dispersion directly. This is because what follows then applies to situations where one typically models aggregated outcomes, as with disease counts within epidemiological studies.

6.8 Hypothetical Data Generation Processes

In order to understand our data better, and to inform modelling strategy, it is important to consider data generation, whether known *a priori* or speculated. Considering caries, for instance, disease onset requires one tooth to become decayed, filled, or extracted for there to be a *dmft* increment from 0 to 1. Thereafter, an increment to this score requires another tooth to suffer a similar fate.

The cariogenic environment of the *individual* (i.e. the level of oral hygiene maintained: the amount and frequency of starch/sugar-rich snacking) does not depend upon whether or not a tooth has already been affected. It might then seem reasonable to assume that underlying latent risks of caries *onset* and *progression* are identical. It is well known, however, that some teeth and some tooth surfaces are more prone to caries development than others (Carlos and Gittelsohn 1965; Leroy et al. 2005; Macek et al. 2003; Parner et al. 2007; Poulsen and Horowitz 1974; Wong et al. 1997). The nature of the cariogenic exposure is also important, since different teeth have different caries risks depending on their morphology and position in the mouth relative to the salivary gland ducts and accessibility for tooth brushing. Moreover, teeth erupt or are shed (exfoliated) at different times, and the 'risk set' thus varies over time, i.e. the period 'at risk' may vary from one tooth to the next. Amongst adults, teeth may also be extracted for reasons that have little to do with caries, thereby initiating the diseased state for reasons unrelated to subsequent caries.

Consequently, distinguishing between disease *onset* and *progression*, one might assume a two-stage process of initial *onset* of disease (i.e. the first occurrence of a caries lesion) followed by subsequent disease *progression* (i.e. new lesions in children with lesions), each with a potentially different underlying risk (Holst 2006). For longitudinal data one might observe differences between the rate of disease *onset* and the rate of disease *progression*; for cross-sectional data one might simply observe an excess in the proportion of zero counts (i.e. the proportion disease-free) compared to standard count distributions. Support for such a dual caries model for longitudinal caries data is found in the now classic water fluoridation studies carried out in Tiel and Culemborg (Groeneveld 1985). These studies show that water fluoridation markedly affects the caries progression rate, whereas the caries incidence is hardly changed. Similarly, as pointed out by Holst, the caries prevalence and extent observed at any given time in a cross-sectional study is a complicated function of two underpinning parameters: the caries incidence and the caries progression rate (Holst 2006). Poulsen et al. compared *Lorenz curves* based on cross-sectional DMFT data for 15-year old Danes in 1980 (97% caries prevalence) and in 1995 (70% caries prevalence) including and respectively excluding the caries-free subjects, and noted that the Lorenz curves differed markedly indicating a skewed distribution of caries risk (Poulsen et al. 2001).

Whether dealing with longitudinal data (*onset* and *progression*) or cross-sectional data (*prevalence* and *extent*), manifest differences in the outcome are potentially consequent on the underlying risk differences in the dual processes of disease initiation and progression. It is therefore important to consider how disease risk varies both *between* and *within* individuals (between teeth/tooth surfaces) and these ideas are illustrated in Fig. 6.3 for hypothetical underlying latent risks of disease over time. Figure 6.3(i) represents the situation where: (A) initially there is no latent risk (e.g. prior to any teeth erupting); (B) individuals experience the risk of disease *onset*, i.e. are on course to yielding a non-zero *dmft* score, though initially will have a zero score; and (C) individuals with disease experience the same underlying latent risk of disease *progression* as for disease *onset*. Since there is a period where some teeth are not at risk of disease, the estimated underlying risk of disease *onset* (the dotted line) appears different to that for the risk of disease *progression*, even though the 'true' underlying latent risks are identical for the 'at risk' period. Figure 6.3(ii) represents the situation where there are three latent sub-types of children, each with varying latent risks of disease *onset* and disease *progression*. For latent class one (LC1), the latent risk of disease *onset* and *progression* are identical. For latent class two (LC2), the underlying risk of disease *onset* is less than that of disease *progression*. The third latent class (LC3) exhibits the opposite in that the underlying risk of disease *onset* is greater than that of subsequent disease *progression*. LC1 and LC2 exhibit near identical underlying latent risks of disease *progression* despite having markedly different underlying risks of disease *onset*. When the period 'not at risk' is included, the estimated underlying latent risks of disease *onset* appear differently from 'true' for LC1 and LC2 and, for this example, the estimated underlying latent risks of disease *onset* and *progression* appear to differ for LC1 and LC2 whilst they seem similar for LC3 – all contrary to 'true'.

Relating these concepts to the types of model we may choose to evaluate the dental caries outcome, i.e. distinguishing between disease *onset* and *progression*, one might assume a two-stage process of initial *onset* of disease (i.e. the first occurrence of a caries lesion) followed by subsequent disease *progression* (i.e. new lesions in children with lesions), each with a potentially different underlying risk. For longitudinal data one might observe differences between the rate

6 Modelling Data That Exhibit an Excess Number of Zeros... 107

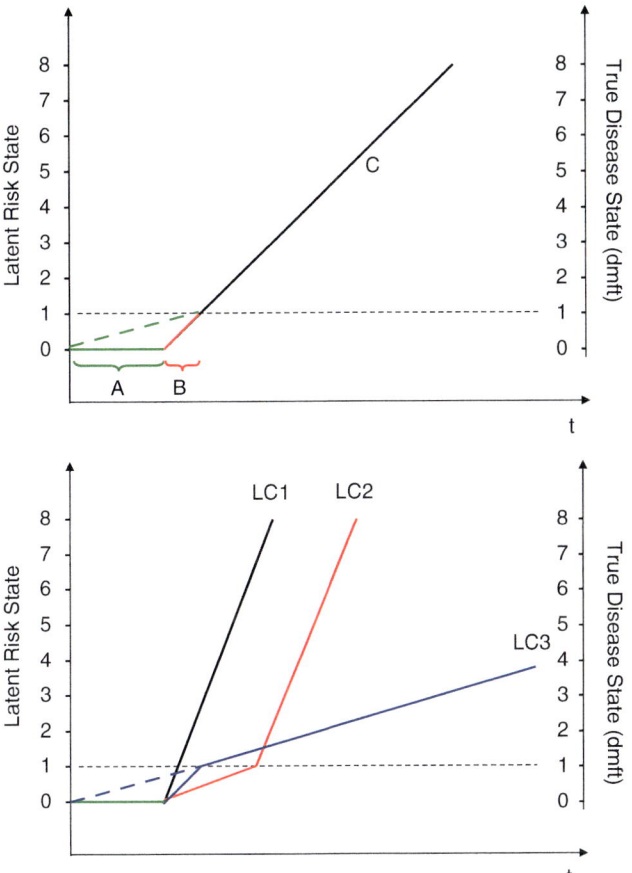

Fig. 6.3 Hypothetical risk models for the *onset* and *progression* of *dmft*. Chart gradients represent the strength of underlying risks for disease *onset* and *progression*; *A* – period with no underlying risk of disease; *B* – period where disease-free individuals are susceptible to disease *onset*; *C* – period where individuals with existing diseases are susceptible to disease *progression*; *LC1* – latent class one: sub-group of individuals with high risk of disease *onset* and *progression*; *LC2* – latent class two: sub-group of individuals with low risk of disease *onset* and high risk of disease *progression*; *LC3* – latent class three: sub-group of individuals with medium risk of disease *onset* and low risk of disease *progression*

of disease *onset* and the rate of disease *progression*; for cross-sectional data one might observe differences between the proportions of observed and expected disease-free (i.e. disease *prevalence*) given the disease *extent* (number of lesions per child) amongst those diseased. Thus, whether dealing with longitudinal data (*onset* and *progression*) or cross-sectional data (*prevalence* and *extent*), manifest differences in the outcome are potentially consequent on the underlying risk differences in the dual processes of disease initiation and development. The ZiP/ZiB models would thus seem most suitable.

Alternatively, if the underlying risks for caries *onset* and *progression* were identical for any one child, but differed across children, generic mixture modelling would seem suitable; this approach encapsulates the concept of 'subtypes' of children. These concepts are not mutually exclusive and where underlying complexity warrants it (i.e. where caries *onset* and *progression* differs both *within* and *between* children), both modelling strategies could be valid simultaneously; it is possible to have generic mixture models with latent classes subdivided into a zero-bin and standard distribution. It is thus valuable to have *a priori* hypotheses of how data may have been generated in terms of underlying differences in caries *onset* and *progression*, in order to select the most appropriate modelling strategy between the zero-inflated and generic mixture models.

6.9 Re-analysing the Brazilian Oral Health Data

We re-examine the dental dataset considering over-dispersion, covariates in the mixture part of zero-inflated models, and generic mixture models with both class dependent and independent covariates. Table 6.2 summarises the observed and predicted counts for all the models considered along with the various model-fit criteria. The best model according to the BIC is the *standard* over-dispersed zero-inflated binomial regression model with covariates in the non-zero part only, i.e. where no covariates predict class membership (oZiB). However, as illustrated by the simulation, this model is problematic. In contrast, according to the AIC, the best two models are the 2-class binomial mixture model with class independent covariates and with class predicted by covariates, and the over-dispersed equivalent (2LCiB_CP and o2LCiB_CP). Considering only zero counts, the best models are the two ZiB models that include covariates as class predictors (ZiB_CP and oZiB_CP). Assessment by the RMSE indicates that the over-dispersed 2-class binomial mixture models with class-*independent* covariates also predicting class membership (o2LCiB_CP) or class-*dependent* covariates not predicting class membership (o2LCdB) are favoured. In general, models with over-dispersion fit better than models without. The favoured zero-inflated model is oZiB_CP and the favoured generic mixture model is o2LCiB_CP, but it is difficult to choose between them using either likelihood statistics or predicted outcomes (Table 6.3).

Due to the study limitations mentioned already, we do not seek to interpret models clinically. Instead we are interested in what factors aid model selection. Predicted probabilities for all 36 types of children (6 interventions × 2 genders × 3 ethnicities) for our two preferred models (oZiB_CP and o2LCiB_CP), have expected counts that are very close ($\rho = 0.98$) and a Bland-Altman plot (Bland and Altman 1999) reveals no systematic bias in their differences, as shown in Fig. 6.4. Choosing between the two models is therefore not assisted by either likelihood statistics or predicted outcomes, so we seek *a priori* knowledge regarding potential data generation processes to inform model selection.

Table 6.2 Binomial regression models: observed and predicted counts of *dmft* along with various model fit criteria assessments

Observed data		Standard regression		Zero-inflated mixture distributions				Generic mixture distributions			
dmft	N	Binomial	oB	ZiB	oZiB	ZiB_CP	oZiB_CP	2LCdB	o2LCdB	2LCiB_CP	o2LCiB_CP
0	231	107.21	217.29	227.88	227.45	230.95	230.45	224.57	227.68	225.17	227.35
1	163	230.82	189.08	120.50	166.17	114.05	156.15	165.74	163.48	173.86	169.70
2	140	233.84	146.75	174.21	149.61	171.77	151.17	132.38	139.25	131.66	137.68
3	116	145.04	104.64	150.21	112.92	152.18	117.24	121.26	117.73	116.01	114.26
4	70	59.90	68.40	84.21	73.50	86.66	76.08	88.71	82.63	84.53	80.15
5	55	16.76	40.22	31.33	40.92	32.44	41.21	45.45	44.12	44.85	43.99
6	22	3.08	20.41	7.53	18.74	7.78	17.95	15.44	17.04	16.57	18.05
7	–	0.34	8.18	1.06	6.42	1.09	5.73	3.15	4.43	3.91	5.07
8	–	0.02	2.02	0.07	1.27	0.07	1.03	0.29	0.64	0.45	0.75
Total	797	797.00	797.00	797.00	797.00	797.00	797.00	797.00	797.00	797.00	797.00
Class size		–	–	23.80%[a]	12.15%[a]	24.74%[a]	15.36%[a]	38.99%[b]	41.59%[b]	47.25%[b]	44.62%[b]
Log-likelihood		−1,546.78	−1,402.61	−1,431.09	−1,398.93	−1,420.33	−1,393.78	−1,389.23	−1,387.60	−1,387.54	−1,386.48
BIC		3,153.68	2,872.03	2,928.99	2,871.36	2,960.92	2,914.49	2,905.39	2,915.49	2,902.01	2,906.57
AIC		3,111.56	2,825.22	2,882.19	2,819.87	2,876.67	2,825.56	2,816.45	2,817.19	2,813.08	2,812.96
RMSE		66.8%	13.8%	27.0%	7.4%	28.4%	8.0%	9.4%	6.9%	9.1%	6.9%
Ranks – BIC, AIC, Zero, RMSE		10:10:10:10	2:6:9:7	8:9:3:8	1:5:5:3	9:8:1:9	6:7:2:4	4:3:8:6	7:4:4:2	3:2:7:5	5:1:6:1

dmft decayed, missing, filled deciduous teeth, *N* frequency, *oB* over-dispersed binomial model, *ZiB* standard zero-inflated binomial model with covariates in the non-zero part only (not predicting class membership), *oZiB* over-dispersed ZiB, *ZiB_CP* zero-inflated binomial model with covariates in the non-zero part and covariates predicting class membership, *oZiB_CP* over-dispersed ZiB_CP, *2LCdB* two-class mixture model with class dependent covariates, *o2LCdB* over-dispersed 2LCdB, *2LCiB_CP* two-class mixture model with class independent covariates and covariates predicting class membership, *o2LCiB_CP* over-dispersed 2LCiB_CP; [a] size of the zero-bin for zero-inflated models, [b] size of the 2nd latent class; *Ranks* rank order of model-fit criterion used to assess different measures of model fit for the Brazilian dental caries follow-up count data; *BIC* Bayesian Information Criterion, *AIC* Akaike's Information Criterion, *Zero* absolute differences between observed and predicted number of zero counts, *RMSE* root mean squared error (see Sect. 6.4)

Table 6.3 Binomial regression models: coefficient estimates (standard errors)

	Standard regression		Mixture distributions				2LCdB		o2LCdB		2LCiB_CP	o2LCiB_CP
	Binomial	oB	ZiB	oZiB	ZiB_CP	oZiB_CP	Class1	Class2	Class1	Class2		
Location 1	−1.00 (0.12)	−1.00 (0.12)	−0.69 (0.11)	−0.83 (0.13)	−0.72 (0.12)	−0.89 (0.26)	−0.47 (0.14)	−2.35 (0.31)	−1.52 (0.29)	−0.44 (0.30)	−0.56 (0.20)	−0.66 (0.24)
Location 2											−2.78 (0.28)	−2.82 (0.31)
Treatment:												
Education	−0.32 (0.13)	−0.27 (0.13)	−0.32 (0.13)	−0.30 (0.13)	−0.34 (0.14)	−0.39 (0.17)	−0.41 (0.15)	−0.21 (0.40)	−0.10 (0.26)	−0.57 (0.27)	−0.55 (0.21)	−0.55 (0.22)
Enrichment	−0.12 (0.13)	−0.12 (0.14)	−0.09 (0.12)	−0.12 (0.14)	−0.08 (0.13)	−0.12 (0.24)	−0.13 (0.14)	−0.27 (0.39)	−0.16 (0.25)	−0.14 (0.19)	−0.11 (0.20)	−0.10 (0.22)
Rinsing	−0.47 (0.14)	−0.50 (0.14)	−0.26 (0.14)	−0.46 (0.16)	−0.19 (0.13)	−0.20 (0.17)	−0.38 (0.15)	−1.50 (0.58)	−0.87 (0.42)	−0.30 (0.18)	−0.20 (0.20)	−0.17 (0.22)
Hygiene	−0.40 (0.15)	−0.43 (0.15)	−0.29 (0.16)	−0.42 (0.16)	−0.26 (0.16)	−0.35 (0.30)	−1.99 (0.24)	2.04 (0.38)	0.83 (0.67)	−2.46 (0.73)	0.43 (0.29)	0.51 (0.32)
All the above	−0.76 (0.15)	−0.77 (0.15)	−0.59 (0.16)	−0.78 (0.16)	−0.46 (0.16)	−0.54 (0.22)	−2.64 (0.34)	1.58 (0.34)	−1.12 (0.35)	−0.62 (0.21)	−0.44 (0.24)	−0.46 (0.24)
Sex:												
Male	0.17 (0.08)	0.17 (0.09)	0.13 (0.08)	0.17 (0.09)	0.11 (0.09)	0.17 (0.14)	0.24 (0.10)	0.07 (0.17)	0.06 (0.18)	0.27 (0.12)	0.19 (0.12)	0.20 (0.13)
Ethnicity:												
White	0.13 (0.09)	0.12 (0.09)	0.11 (0.09)	0.12 (0.10)	0.12 (0.09)	0.17 (0.25)	0.14 (0.10)	0.15 (0.19)	0.02 (0.19)	0.25 (0.12)	0.25 (0.14)	0.28 (0.14)
Black	−0.18 (0.14)	−0.19 (0.14)	−0.14 (0.15)	−0.21 (0.14)	−0.08 (0.15)	−0.03 (0.26)	−0.12 (0.18)	−0.07 (0.37)	−0.31 (0.25)	0.07 (0.31)	0.19 (0.24)	0.22 (0.23)
Model parameters:												
Od		0.17 (0.02)		0.12 (0.02)		0.10 (0.03)			0.12 (0.03)	0.00 (0.04)		0.02 (0.02)

oB over-dispersed binomial model, *ZiB* standard zero-inflated binomial model with covariates in the non-zero part only, *oZiB* zero-inflated binomial model with covariates in the non-zero part *and* covariates predicting class membership, *oZiB_CP* over-dispersed ZiB_CP, *ZiB_CP* two-class mixture model with class dependent covariates, *o2LCdB* over-dispersed 2LCdB, *2LCiB_CP* two-class mixture model with class independent covariates *and* covariates predicting class membership, *o2LCiB_CP* over-dispersed 2LCiB_CP, *Treatment* reference group is 'no treatment', *Sex* reference group is 'female', *Ethnicity* reference group is 'dark skinned', *Od* over-dispersion parameter ($1/\nu^2$, see Sect. 6.3). The shaded models are the two preferred models – one a zero-inflated model, the other a generic mixture model

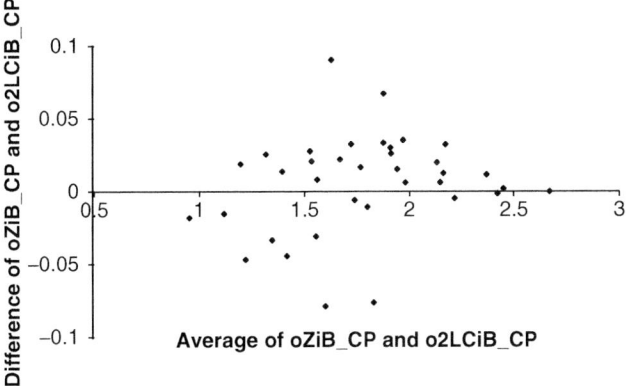

Fig. 6.4 Bland-Altman plot of contrast between two over-dispersed Binomial models (oZiB_CP and o2LCiB_CP)

The Brazilian dataset is too small and insufficiently robust to provide evidence to support or rebut the hypothesised two-stage data generation process. Nevertheless, findings from such a relatively simple evaluation might inform a modelling strategy and steer a preference between zero-inflated or generic mixture models, particularly where model-fit criteria and predicted outcomes make no such distinction. Regarding the dental caries data, if we assume that disease follows a two-stage process it would be more suitable to adopt a zero-inflated model; if we had evidence that caries *onset* and *progression* have similar underlying risks within individuals and differences occur only between individuals, then generic mixture models would be more suitable. Despite the lack of evidence either way from the Brazilian dataset, given extensive *a priori* clinical knowledge of caries *onset* and *progression* that supports a dual process, we opt for the zero-inflated model (oZiB_CP) as our preferred model.

6.10 Summary

Böhning et al. rightly argued that one needs to consider the problem of excess zeros in dental data and they advocated the use of the zero-inflated Poisson model for the Brazilian oral health dataset. However, the Poisson distribution is not always ideal for bounded data. Within the Brazilian dataset, counts represented the number of successes (*dmft*) out of a finite number of trials (eight deciduous molars) and consequently the binomial distribution was more suitable. Where data are also inherently clustered, over-dispersion needs to be modelled explicitly and adopting data-specific model-fit criteria may be useful in evaluating the performance of models with respect to predicted outcomes where there is clinical importance for certain thresholds. The estimated proportion of zeros is an obvious marker of model performance when evaluating data with excessive zeros compared to standard count distributions. We also propose the use of a root mean squared error (RMSE) between observed and predicted counts for the entire viable outcome range. However, data-specific model-fit criteria do not generally agree with the likelihood-based criteria, endorsing the cautious use of log-likelihood statistics in isolation.

For cross-sectional analyses of a randomised study, one anticipates that membership of the zero bin is balanced across all treatment groups at baseline (due to randomisation), but there is no reason for other covariates to have balanced zero counts. In non-randomised studies, inadequately randomised studies, or within longitudinal studies where the analyses are of follow-up data, the assumption of balanced zeros across intervention groups is no longer viable. For zero-inflated models, it is thus necessary to consider covariates in the mixture model, especially if identified as necessary in the distribution part.

As different model parameterisations can yield near-identical predicted outcomes and model fit statistics, whilst yielding potentially diverse model inferences, it becomes necessary to consider data generation to inform model selection and model interpretation. This could be particularly valuable where different covariates affect *onset* and *progression* differently. In epidemiology, for instance, it is proposed that childhood cancers are triggered by infection and that the infectious agents are transmitted via population mixing (Kinlen et al. 1990). A small community may be free from an infectious assault (a period of 'not at risk'), but once circumstances change due to factors associated with population mixing, the community may become exposed to the infectious agents (start of exposure) and the rate of spread of infection then depends upon other factors associated with population mixing. The underlying risk of cancer is affected by exposure to infectious agents and factors specific to the infected individuals. Different factors are associated with population mixing and would potentially have a different impact upon the *onset* and *progression* of rates of cancer in each community. Where the number of cancers across several small areas within a region is modelled assuming a zero-inflated Poisson distribution, different population mixing measures could be evaluated. A measure that captures elevated risk to a community of exposure to incoming infectious agents should be associated with elevated rates of communities belonging to the distribution part of the zero-inflated model. Similarly, a measure that captures elevated risk to a community of infectious agents spreading within communities should be associated with elevated rates of communities having higher prevalence rates of cancers (conditional on the community belonging to the distribution part). It may thus be possibly to evaluate more carefully the infectious agent hypothesis using zero-inflated models and evaluating measures of population mixing in terms of where their impact lies in the model parameterisation of a zero-inflated model.

Introducing the flexibility of generic mixture models might at first seem to evade the problem of needing to explore covariates for the mixture part of the model, since the implicit constraint on zero counts imposed by zero-inflated models with no covariates in the mixture part is circumnavigated (unless one latent class is determined empirically to have a central location of zero). However, the problem is shifted from an issue surrounding a single threshold (zero/one) to the entire outcome range, and one might reasonably ask if generic mixture models should not also have class prediction by all available covariates. We might be satisfied in some instances that class predictors are appropriate, though not essential, providing the model is identifiable and interpretable. The problem of deciding between zero-inflated or generic mixture model (especially when there are no discernable model differences in terms of likelihood statistics and predicted outcomes) is then best guided by *a priori* hypotheses on data generation. If one believes in a two-stage data generation process, the zero-inflated model is firmly favoured. Where the outcome is *change* in disease status, interpretation is attributable to differences in the underlying risks of *onset* and *progression*. For cross-sectional data, consistency with this notion is sought via inspection of *prevalence* and *extent* of disease. Whilst caution must be exercised, since such interpretations are only 'consistent with' and 'supportive of' hypothesised historical data generation processes, modelling strategies and model selection may nevertheless be enhanced by *a priori* hypotheses surrounding data generation; possibly more than by model-fit criteria *per se*.

6.11 Conclusions

When dealing with biomedical count data that exhibit an excess of zeros, model selection is not straightforward. It is crucial to consider appropriate outcome distributions and explore context-specific model-fit criteria. For zero-inflated models, one should consider covariates in the mixture model if identified as necessary in the distribution part. Difficulties in distinguishing between models based solely on likelihood statistics and predicted counts need to be informed by *a priori* hypotheses of data generation. Zero-inflated models reflect whether or not there are or have been risk differences in the *onset* and *progression* of disease, whereas generic mixture models identify sub-types of individuals; both model strategies can be employed simultaneously. Model selection is not about model fit *per se*, but also about interpretation and robustness in the model truly reflecting the context in which the data were generated.

6.12 Further Reading

A couple of textbook chapters of interest regarding caries incidence include: "*The epidemiology of dental caries*" by Burt BA, Baelum V, Fejerskov O. Pp. 123–145; and "*The role of dentistry in controlling caries and periodontitis globally*" by Baelum V, van Palenstein Helderman W, Hugoson A, Yee R, Fejerskov O. Pp. 575–605; in: Fejerskov O, Kidd E eds *Dental caries. The disease and its clinical management* Blackwell Munksgaard, 2008. There are a plethora of other biomedical examples where data exhibit an excess of zeros compared to standard count distributions, especially within the epidemiology of rare diseases, which often involves spatial modelling with the incidence of disease per small geographical area of interest and many small areas yielding zero counts. For books dedicated to this there is Andrew Lawson's handbook of spatial analyses: "*Statistical Methods in Spatial Epidemiology*" Lawson, AB; Wiley, 2006. For spatial modelling in general: "*Zero-inflated models with application to spatial count data*" by Agarwal DK, Gelfand AE, Citron-Pousty S; Springer Netherlands, 2004; and "*The SAGE Handbook of Spatial Analysis*" by Fotheringham AS, Rogerson PA eds; Sage, 2009.

References

Blance, A., Tu, Y. K., Baelum, V., & Gilthorpe, M. S. (2007). Statistical issues on the analysis of change in follow-up studies in dental research. *Community Dentistry and Oral Epidemiology, 35*(6), 412–420. available from: PM:18039282.

Bland, J. M., & Altman, D. G. (1999). Measuring agreement in method comparison studies. *Statistical Methods in Medical Research, 8*(2), 135–160. available from: PM:10501650.

Böhning, D. (1998). Zero-inflated Poisson models and C.A.MAN: A tutorial collection of evidence. *Biometrical Journal, 40*(7), 833–843.

Böhning, D., Dietz, E., & Schlattmann, P. (1999). The zero-inflated Poisson model and the decayed, missing and filled teeth index in dental epidemiology. *Journal of the Royal Statistical Society, Series A, 162*, 195–209.

Carlos, J. P., & Gittelsohn, A. M. (1965). Longitudinal studies of the natural history of caries. II. A life-table study of caries incidence in the permanent teeth. *Archives of Oral Biology, 10*(5), 739–751. available from: PM:5226906.

Groeneveld, A. (1985). Longitudinal study of prevalence of enamel lesions in a fluoridated and non-fluoridated area. *Community Dentistry and Oral Epidemiology, 13*(3), 159–163. available from: PM:3860338.

Hall, D. B. (2000). Zero-inflated Poisson and binomial regression with random effects: A case study. *Biometrics, 56*(4), 1030–1039. available from: http://www.blackwell-synergy.com/loi/biom.

Holst, D. (2006). The relationship between prevalence and incidence of dental caries. Some observational consequences. *Community Dental Health, 23*(4), 203–208. available from: PM:17194066.

Kinlen, L. J., Clarke, K., & Hudson, C. (1990). Evidence from population mixing in British New Towns 1946–85 of an infective basis for childhood leukaemia. *Lancet, 336*(8715), 577–582. available from: PM:1975376.

Lambert, D. (1992). Zero-inflated Poisson regression, with an application to defects in manufacturing. *Technometrics, 34*(1), 1–14. available from: ISI:A1992GZ77700001.

Leroy, R., Bogaerts, K., Lesaffre, E., & Declerck, D. (2005). Multivariate survival analysis for the identification of factors associated with cavity formation in permanent first molars. *European Journal of Oral Sciences, 113*(2), 145–152. available from: PM:15819821.

Liang, K. Y., & Zeger, S. L. (1986). Longitudinal data analysis using generalized linear models. *Biometrika, 73*, 13–22.

Lord, F. M. (1967). A paradox in the interpretation of group comparisons. *Psychological Bulletin, 68*, 304–305.

Lord, F. M. (1969). Statistical adjustments when comparing preexisting groups. *Psychological Bulletin, 72*, 337–338.

Macek, M. D., Beltran-Aguilar, E. D., Lockwood, S. A., & Malvitz, D. M. (2003). Updated comparison of the caries susceptibility of various morphological types of permanent teeth. *Journal of Public Health Dentistry, 63*(3), 174–182. available from: PM:12962471.

Mullahy, J. (1986). Specification and testing of some modified count data models. *Journal of Econometrics, 33*(3), 341–365. available from: ISI:A1986F205600002.

Parner, E. T., Heidmann, J. M., Vaeth, M., & Poulsen, S. (2007). Surface-specific caries incidence in permanent molars in Danish children. *European Journal of Oral Sciences, 115*(6), 491–496. available from: PM:18028058.

Poulsen, S., & Horowitz, H. S. (1974). An evaluation of a hierarchical method of describing the pattern of dental caries attack. *Community Dentistry and Oral Epidemiology, 2*(1), 7–11. available from: PM:4153274.

Poulsen, S., Heidmann, J., & Vaeth, M. (2001). Lorenz curves and their use in describing the distribution of 'the total burden' of dental caries in a population. *Community Dental Health, 18* (2), 68–71. available from: PM:11461061.

Ridout, M., Demétrio, C. G. B., & Hinde, J. (1998) Models for count data with many zeros. *Proceedings article for an International Biometric Conference* (pp. 179–192). Cape Town. http://www.kent.ac.uk/IMS/personal/msr/webfiles/zip/ibc_fin.pdf.

Senn, S. (2006). Change from baseline and analysis of covariance revisited. *Statistics in Medicine, 25*(24), 4334–4344. available from: PM:16921578.

Skrondal, A., & Rabe-Hesketh, S. (2004). *Generalized latent variable modeling: Multilevel, longitudinal and structural equation models.* London: Chapman & Hall.

Vermunt, J. K., & Magidson, J. (2005a). *Latent GOLD 4.0 User's Guide.* Belmont Massachusetts: Statistical Innovations Inc.

Vermunt, J. K., & Magidson, J. (2005b). *Technical guide for Latent GOLD 4.0: Basic and advanced.* Belmont Massachusetts: Statistical Innovations Inc. http://www.statisticalinnovations.com/products/LGtechnical.pdf.

Vieira, A. M. C., Hinde, J. P., & Demetrio, C. G. B. (2000). Zero-inflated proportion data models applied to a biological control assay. *Journal of Applied Statistics, 27*(3), 373–389. available from: ISI:000086354400009.

Wong, M. C., Schwarz, E., & Lo, E. C. (1997). Patterns of dental caries severity in Chinese kindergarten children. *Community Dentistry and Oral Epidemiology, 25*(5), 343–347. available from: PM:9355769.

Chapter 7
Multilevel Latent Class Modelling

Wendy Harrison, Robert M. West, Amy Downing, and Mark S. Gilthorpe

7.1 Overview

Multilevel latent class models can reveal new insights into clustered data. For instance, within observational studies, latent class analysis of multilevel data allows groups or clusters of patients to be identified (e.g. according to casemix or different pathways through the healthcare system) and allows sub-groups of organisations to be derived (e.g. according to the treatments available, quality of care, or differences in patient outcomes). It is also feasible to generate organisation-level latent classes with similar patient casemix and differences between these casemix-adjusted latent classes can then be evaluated, whereby factors that differ across the organisational classes are then tested for their association with differences in clinical outcomes. This allows areas of healthcare provision to be targeted for intervention and evaluation to improve patient care. The same methods can be adopted in a cluster-randomised setting, where the multilevel latent class methodology improves on the cluster-randomisation, generating organisational classes that are balanced in terms of patient casemix – a form of pseudo-randomisation of observational data.

W. Harrison • R.M. West • M.S. Gilthorpe (✉)
Division of Biostatistics, Centre for Epidemiology and Biostatistics, Leeds Institute of Genetics, Health & Therapeutics, University of Leeds, Leeds, UK
e-mail: m.s.gilthorpe@leeds.ac.uk

A. Downing
Cancer Epidemiology Group, Centre for Epidemiology and Biostatistics,
University of Leeds, Leeds, UK

7.2 An Epidemiological Study of Colorectal Cancer Mortality

To illustrate the methodology, we consider a practical example based on routinely collected data for patients registered with colorectal cancer. Many factors may influence survival from colorectal cancer, including place of diagnosis and treatment centre (hospital within Trust), stage at diagnosis, and risk factors such as age at diagnosis, sex, and socioeconomic background (SEB); the latter reflects how patients vary in terms of exposure to diet and smoking (Davy 2007; Duncan et al. 1999; James et al. 1997; Macdonald et al. 2007), or healthcare seeking behaviours that lead to varying stages of disease progression at diagnosis (Adams et al. 2004; Ionescu et al. 1998). Patients are nested within hospitals and therefore Trusts. Within our example, we seek to identify different sub-types of both patients and Trusts. We model simultaneously how patients might vary and how Trusts differ in performance, to seek out which factors might be associated with patient survival.

7.2.1 The Linked Dataset

Patients with colorectal cancer (ICD-10 (World Health Organisation 2005) codes C18, C19 and C20) diagnosed between 1998 and 2004 and resident in the Northern and Yorkshire regions were identified from the Northern and Yorkshire Cancer Registry and Information Service (NYCRIS) database. Patient age, sex, tumour stage at diagnosis (using the Dukes classification (Dukes 1949)), diagnostic centre (Trust), and whether or not the patient received treatment were extracted. Socioeconomic background (SEB) was defined at the 2001 enumeration district level of residence (super output area) using the Townsend Index (Townsend et al. 1988) and matched to patients using their postcode of residence.

We adopted the outcome of mortality (alive/dead) at 3 years after diagnosis, as this was considered to be clinically meaningful and facilitated ready comparison with other studies. Whilst interest lies in investigating potential treatment centre characteristics associated with colorectal cancer survival, this can be complex to assess, as patients may be treated at different Trusts throughout their care. In our data, 90% were treated initially within the same Trust as they were diagnosed, though only 75% remained within this Trust throughout. We nevertheless choose to analyse by Trust of diagnosis in order to include all patients, whether treated or not, and maintain a reasonable proportion of patients whose treatment was initially received within the same Trust as they were diagnosed. As 78 patients had diagnostic centres found to be external to Trusts within the Northern and Yorkshire region, these were excluded, yielding 24,455 patients available for analysis.

7.3 Research Question, Aims and Objectives

We seek to answer two distinct research questions with the example dataset:

i. *"What is the relation between 3-year mortality and socioeconomic background (SEB) of patients and what factors affect this relationship?"*

This research question is an example within epidemiology of seeking to determine the impact of an exposure or risk factor (SEB in this instance) on an outcome (3-year survival) where it is impossible to conduct a randomised controlled trial. When seeking to determine the outcome–exposure relationship, adjustment for potentially confounding factors is crucial. Achieving this is not always straightforward, as we will discuss.

ii. *"How does Trust performance vary after accommodating patient (casemix) differences?"*

This research question seeks to assess variation in Trust performance (in terms of mean 3-year survival rates) over and above differences anticipated due to patient casemix. Some Trusts may perform better or worse than others in terms of their median survival rates due to their patient casemix (which likely varies geographically), or due to underlying differences in the effectiveness of Trust function and healthcare delivery, or both. It is important to identify good and poor performing Trusts in order to identify good clinical practice.

Before addressing each research question, we discuss the scope of potential models available within a multilevel latent-class framework, because each research question requires a slightly different multilevel latent class model to deliver the appropriate analytical strategy.

7.4 The General Concept of Multilevel Latent-Class Models

The concept of latent classes was introduced in Chap. 6. Within a multilevel dataset it is possible to have a latent-class structure at *each* level of the data hierarchy. Considering latent classes at more than one level permits several complex model configurations, each relating to different assumptions, with slightly different interpretations, not all of which have analogues to continuous latent-variable models or standard multilevel models. As mentioned in Chap. 6, some parameterisations may not be identifiable, and some identifiable models may not be interpretable. These issues only become more complex in a multilevel setting.

7.4.1 Building a Multilevel Latent Class Model

To extend our thinking slowly, we may begin by considering multilevel latent-class structures as if built one level at a time. For instance, with the two-level colorectal cancer dataset (patients nested within Trusts), we may consider initially that patients belong to different latent classes (i.e. sub-groups of individuals that are homogeneous *within* groups, though heterogeneous *between* groups in their 3-year mortality). Conditional on belonging to a given patient-level class, the Trusts in which they are treated may then be grouped according to *similarities* or *differences* in terms of patient outcomes.

If grouped according to *similarities*, a Trust class might contain Trusts that have roughly the same mean levels of 3-year survival, whilst the proportion of patients within each patient-level class might differ. Trust classes are then homogeneous with respect to patient outcomes, whilst heterogeneous in terms of patient-class profiles. This modelling strategy is appropriate for research question (i).

If grouped according to outcome *differences*, Trust classes might contain Trusts that have the same proportions of patients within each patient class, where patient classes differ in terms of mean 3-year survival. Trust-level classes are then homogeneous with respect to patient-class profiles (i.e. casemix), whilst heterogeneous in terms of patient outcomes (survival). This modelling strategy is appropriate for research question (ii).

In practice, within the estimation process, there is no sense of ordering in terms of at which level the latent classes are formed ahead of other levels, because this happens simultaneously, i.e. patient-level classes are determined *simultaneously* with Trust-level classes. Models are an optimum solution for all classes, at all levels, conditional on covariates considered in the model; estimation procedures seek to maximise the likelihood function in a single process.

The simplest scenario is where the continuous latent variable at the upper level is replaced by a categorical latent variable. The usual constraint of normally distributed upper-level residuals is then no longer applicable. Within a standard multilevel model of the colorectal cancer data, the mean outcome for each Trust (the proportion of patients who survive 3 years) is assumed to be normally distributed and the model estimates an overall Trust mean 3-year survival fraction and its variance. If a categorical latent variable were adopted instead, Trust classes are determined such that each Trust is assigned to a class according to probabilities that sum to one over all Trust classes. The model estimates the mean 3-year survival for each Trust class and also the size of each Trust class (i.e. summation of individual Trust probabilities for each Trust class); and no assumptions are made regarding the distribution of Trust class means or Trust class sizes.

7.4.2 Model Covariates – Standard Regression Covariates and Class Predictors

As was seen in Chap. 6, covariates can be entered into a latent-class model in the usual way, as within a standard regression model, i.e. as 'predictors' of the outcome variation. The same covariates may also enter the model as 'predictors' of the latent-class structure. In either scenario, causality should not be inferred. The term 'predictor' is unfortunate in that it may mislead users to infer causality when it only implies an association between outcome variation and the covariate in question. With this in mind, the nomenclature favoured here is that covariates in the regression part of model (referred to as the distribution part of the model in Chap. 6) are referred to as 'covariates', whilst the covariates (same or different) in the class membership part of the model (distinguishing between a zero bin and the distribution in Chap. 6) will be referred to as 'class predictors', though causality must not be inferred.

Chapter 6 also indicated that there may be circumstances in which it is preferable or even necessary to include covariates in both the fixed part of the model and as class predictors. As with multilevel modelling, covariates may operate at any level. Similarly for multilevel latent-class models, covariates may predict class membership at any level. For the two-level colorectal cancer dataset, we can simultaneously predict patient- and Trust-class membership, though certain covariates will operate at the patient-level (e.g. age, sex, socioeconomic background) whilst other covariates will operate at the Trust-level (e.g. Trust size, number of specialists). Patient-level covariates can seek to predict either patient- or Trust-class membership, though for our illustration we allow patient covariates to predict patient-class membership only. Similarly, Trust-level covariates can predict class membership at both levels, though for our illustration we do not consider any Trust-level covariates.

In addition, covariates can be included as inactive within the model. These covariates are not used to predict class membership, though once the patient- and Trust-classes have been identified their distribution across these classes is observed and interpreted. For example, it may be of interest to determine the proportion of patients treated within each patient class. In our illustration, we include treatment, position of the tumour, and type of tumour (determined using the ICD-10 code) as inactive covariates.

7.4.3 Class Dependent/Independent Intercepts

When adopting a multilevel latent class structure, the central location of each class is estimated for all levels of the hierarchy simultaneously, i.e. each latent class at any level has its own intercept or mean probability. This is very broadly analogous to random intercepts within a continuous latent variable multilevel model. Discrete latent variable intercepts at a lower level, however, may be either *class dependent* or *class independent* in relation to class structures at higher levels. Consider, for instance, the two-level colorectal cancer dataset, where patients are nested within Trusts. With say M_P classes at the patient level ($M_P \geq 2$), and M_T classes at the Trust level ($M_T \geq 2$), M_P intercepts may exhibit relative differences that are either identical or different within each Trust class. Where they are identical, patient-class intercepts differ by the same degree, irrespective of which Trust class their treatment centre is assigned to:

patient-class intercepts are thus Trust class *independent*. Where patient classes vary across Trust classes, they are Trust class *dependent*. Model interpretation differs between these two latent-class multilevel models and the choice of model is driven by context.

Let us consider the context of the illustrative dataset. Individuals tend to vary in many ways, such as in their willingness to seek medical advice if feeling ill, or in their diet, or their levels of daily exercise. It is therefore likely that some patients are more homogenous in their experience of disease and other characteristics, some of which may be related either to their risk of developing disease or to their bodies' ability to cope with illness once disease has developed. Similarly, some Trusts are more likely to share common practices and procedures, offering standard treatment pathways for patients of a particular kind, whereas others may differ slightly due to local factors, such as size and the numbers of medical specialists (consider for instance differences between teaching hospitals, city general hospitals, and 'cottage' hospitals). The Trust-class *independent* configuration enables identical contrasts to be made amongst patient classes within Trust classes, in a relative sense, i.e. the patient classes with 'best' and 'worst' mortality differ in relative terms identically for each Trust class. If the Trust class *dependent* configuration were adopted, contrasts in survival amongst patient classes in one Trust class could, relatively speaking, mean different things according to which Trust class were considered. In both instances, Trust classes may differ in their overall 3-year mortality. For illustration and ease of interpretation within the colorectal cancer dataset, we adopt the class *independent* configuration for model intercepts – this is not essential, though helpful in this context. In other circumstances (especially for different datasets) the class *dependent* configuration might be more appropriate.

7.4.4 Class Dependent/Independent Covariate Effects

Similar to the concept surrounding random intercepts, random covariate effects may be modelled as Trust class *dependent* or *independent*. Within standard multilevel models, covariate effects are usually referred to as *fixed effects* and we adopt this nomenclature here. Consider the two-level colorectal cancer dataset with C_F subject-level covariates in the fixed part of the model (e.g. age, sex, socioeconomic background). In standard multilevel models, the C_F covariates could have estimated regression coefficients that remain fixed for all Trusts (hence the term *fixed effects*). Alternatively, an extension would be that these covariates could randomly vary across Trusts, thereby yielding *random effects*, sometimes referred to as *random slopes*.

In a multilevel latent class model, if there are M_T Trust classes, we might constrain each subject-level covariate to have identical estimated parameter values for each of the M_T Trust classes (Trust class *independent*), or we may wish to relax this constraint and explore any number of these covariate parameters (e.g. C_R)

to have different estimated values for each Trust class (i.e. to be Trust class *dependent*). This latter option is akin to random slopes in the standard multilevel model, but where the *random effects* (represented by a continuous latent variable) are effectively categorised and multiple *fixed effects* parameter values are estimated for each Trust latent class.

Not all covariate fixed effects would necessarily be modelled this way, and so the number of patient-level covariates that are Trust class *dependent* could be fewer than the total number of patient-level covariates, i.e. $C_R \leq C_F$, yielding $C_R \times M_T$ parameters to be estimated. This can nevertheless be much less parsimonious than the standard multilevel model, since the latter has only one continuous latent variable variance to be estimated per covariate random slope, opposed to multiple fixed effects parameter values for each Trust class. This is why it is necessary to consider carefully the pros and cons of class *dependent* vs. *independent* covariate effects. Furthermore, interpretation again differs between these two types of multi-level latent-class models and choice is driven by context.

Considering the context of the colorectal cancer dataset, we initially adopt the class *dependent* configuration to allow for *random effects*, though for parsimony we switch to class *independent* covariate effects if there is little evidence that a covariate parameter value varies substantially across classes. A combination of configurations is possible and may be more parsimonious. For instance, one covariate might have two distinct parameter values across six latent classes, such that parameter estimates are constrained to take one value for three classes and another value for the other three classes. Although technically possible, a complex *a priori* grasp of how the data are generated should prevail to warrant such complex model structures.

7.4.5 Class Dependent/Independent Class Sizes

Class size may also be class *dependent* or *independent*. Consider again the 2-level colorectal cancer dataset with M_P patient-level and M_T Trust-level latent classes. There are $M_P \times M_T$ latent classes and each may have a different proportion of the total number of patients (Trust class *dependent*). Some patient classes may possess no patients at all because the number of patient classes per Trust class is fixed in the model parameterisation, yet in practice some Trust classes might favour fewer patient classes, so some are 'empty'. Alternatively, it is possible to constrain class sizes such that the proportion of each patient class remains the same for each Trust class (Trust class *independent*). The total number of patients per Trust class can still vary. Model interpretation differs according to which strategy is adopted, which is again driven by context.

Considering the colorectal cancer dataset, model strategy (i) requires that patient class sizes are Trust class *dependent*, to reflect that each Trust class may be made up of differing proportions of patient classes. Model strategy (ii) requires patient classes to be Trust class *independent*, to reflect that each Trust class is required to have exactly the same profile of patient classes (and hence patient casemix characteristics).

7.4.6 Latent-Class Misclassification Error

Patients are assigned probabilistically to classes, i.e. they have a probability of belonging to each patient class (which sums to one, as each patient must be fully assigned to all patient classes) and they also have a probability of belonging to each Trust class (which also sums to one). Depending upon whether class dependent or independent, patient-class probabilities may either be constrained to be the same for each Trust class or they may vary across Trust classes. With modal assignment, each patient is entirely placed into a patient class and Trust class according to the highest membership probability at each level. The proportion of patients deemed to be 'misclassified' is the discrepancy between the number of patients assigned modally and the number assigned probabilistically (the latter need not be an integer, as it is a sum of probabilities between zero and one). This discrepancy, termed *classification error* (CE), is usually expressed as a percentage. We observe a CE value at both the patient and Trust levels. One purpose of including class membership covariates might be to reduce CE.

A low CE indicates that latent classes are more 'real', in that they correspond to groups where individuals or Trusts are almost entirely assigned to a single class. A lower CE may be favoured because it results in greater interpretability of the latent classes when considering individuals or Trusts, i.e. the latent subgroups comprise complete patients and entire Trusts. In contrast, a large CE indicates that latent classes are more 'virtual', i.e. a construct of probabilistic assignment only, as they differ substantially from model assignment. In this case, the latent classes may be regarded as purer, more 'distilled' classifications than are observed for individual patients or Trusts. The latent classes thus describe well-differentiated 'traits' or 'characteristics', and whilst all patients and Trusts possess one or more of these traits and characteristics, for a large CE, rarely will any one class correspond to a distinct subgroup of patients or Trusts.

It therefore depends upon the context and purpose of the model as to whether or not one worries about CE values, low or high. It is perhaps important to be mindful of the magnitude of classification errors in order that in some instances one might prefer models where classification errors are not too large, or not too close to zero, depending upon whether one is more interested in obtaining distinct subgroups or merely a well-differentiated characterisation of traits. Being able to interpret meaningfully the latent-class structure is crucial, and as indicated in Chap. 6, latent class model selection should not be determined solely by likelihood statistics.

7.4.7 Model Construction

The statistical software *LatentGold* (Vermunt and Magidson 2005a) was used for all latent variable models. The number of latent classes at the patient and Trust levels is sequentially increased from one to identify the optimum model according to a number of model-fit criteria, including the Bayesian Information Criterion (BIC) (Schwarz 1978), the Akaike Information Criterion (AIC) (Akaike 1974) and change in log-likelihood (LL). Both the BIC and AIC incorporate a sense of model parsimony by accommodating the varying number of model parameters (Vermunt and Magidson 2005b) while the LL does not. Use of the BIC implies that the true model is among those compared, although this may not be the case as modelling inherently simplifies the data; whereas use of the AIC may suggest a more complex model than necessary, as it may over-fit the data. Although the LL improves with an increasing number of classes at both levels, improvements grow more slowly to reveal a diminishing return for increased model complexity.

We evaluate a standard multilevel model (continuous upper-level latent variable) as well as the latent-class multilevel model to contrast the standard approach with the latent-class approach. We select models that minimise all three criteria, while providing a useful model and informative results.

7.5 Modelling Outcome-Exposure Relationships with Observational Data

To address research question (i), we take stock of the generic problems in analysing outcome-exposure relationships with observational data. Whilst discussed in terms of our illustrative dataset, issues raised here affect all epidemiological datasets.

7.5.1 Statistical Adjustment for 'Confounders' on the Causal Path

Previous studies investigating the association between cancer mortality and known potential risk factors, e.g. age, sex and socioeconomic background (SEB), have typically considered stage of disease (where available) as a potential confounder. When assessing the impact of a single risk factor, appropriate statistical adjustment is commonly sought for *all* known potential confounders, if recorded. If the primary risk factor under investigation causally precedes an alleged confounder, statistical adjustment may be inappropriate, as discussed in Chap. 4 and illustrated using directed acyclic graphs (DAGs) (Pearl 2000). Problems arise because statistical adjustment for an alleged confounder on the causal path from exposure to outcome can suffer bias (Kirkwood and Sterne 2003) known as the reversal paradox (Stigler 1999). This has been shown to be a potentially serious problem in epidemiology (Hernandez-Diaz et al. 2006; Tu et al. 2005).

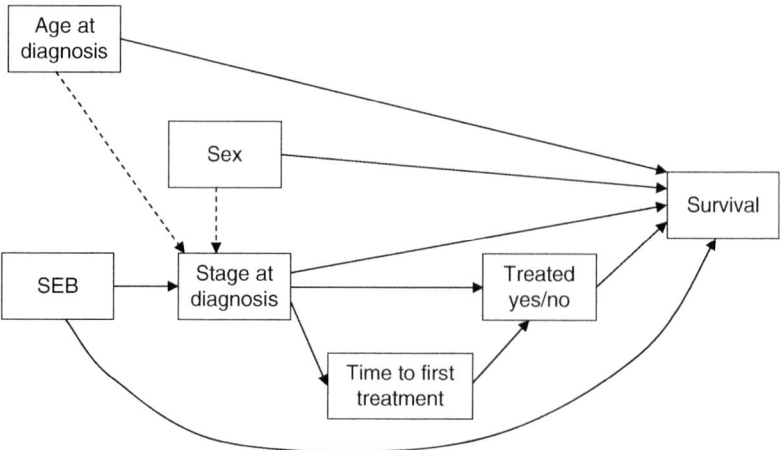

Fig. 7.1 Directed acyclic graph showing the relationship amongst all available variables at the population level

When considering SEB as the main exposure variable, it has been suggested that SEB may influence late presentation (Ionescu et al. 1998; Kogevinas et al. 1991), which may then influence stage at diagnosis. Therefore, SEB causally precedes stage at diagnosis. Figure 7.1 shows the proposed relationships amongst all available variables at the population level by use of a DAG. If stage is adjusted for by inclusion in a regression model examining the relationship between SEB and mortality, this may introduce bias and lead to inappropriate model interpretation. This may explain why findings into the impact of SEB on cancer mortality vary, with some studies finding a significant relationship between worsening SEB and increased cancer mortality (Coleman et al. 1999; Pollock and Vickers 1997; Schrijvers et al. 1995), whilst others have found no such association (Lyratzopoulos et al. 2004; Wrigley et al. 2003). It depends upon whether or not any statistical adjustment for alleged confounding has indeed removed the impact of genuine confounding (for which the alleged confounding is merely a proxy), introduced bias due to the reversal paradox, or an unknown combination of both.

7.5.2 Measurement Error and Incomplete Data

Standard regression analyses may give rise to biased results when model covariates (such as stage at diagnosis) are measured with error, or have missing values (Carroll et al. 2006; Fuller 1987), and this bias is exacerbated within product interaction terms (Greenwood et al. 2006), e.g. when investigating the role of SEB across different levels of stage at diagnosis. Stage, widely used as a potential confounder, often suffers from a large proportion of incomplete data (24% missing in NYCRIS in 2008) (UKACR Quality and Performance Indicators 2008: Final 2008). The Dukes classification of colorectal cancer identifies four distinct grades of tumour ranging from stage A to D. Tumours are graded according to pathology, and variability in the quality of pathology can lead to patients being classified incorrectly (Quirke and Morris 2006); classification is thus prone to error. There is also potential bias in the grading of stage as the quality of pathology can sometimes lead to patients being 'under-staged' (Morris et al. 2007a). For example, for the tumour to be classified at stage C, lymph nodes must be involved. The number of lymph nodes retrieved, however, is highly variable and if few nodes are available this limits the likelihood of identifying node involvement, so the tumour may instead be classified at stage B. This has an impact on the treatment received, as patients diagnosed with a stage B tumour may not receive beneficial chemotherapy (Morris et al. 2007b). Additionally, the recording of stage has changed somewhat over time. If a tumour is initially graded at stage C, but clinical evidence of metastatic disease is then found, the current policy in the NYCRIS region is to 'up-stage' the tumour to stage D. This may not have occurred in previous years, leading to additional potential bias in longitudinal data.

Including stage as a covariate and exploring its statistical interactions with any risk factor therefore has the potential to introduce large bias, even where the reversal paradox does not occur. Where stage lies on the causal path between exposure and outcome, as it appears to between SEB and survival, the additional uncertainty of bias from inappropriate statistical adjustment also needs to be considered.

7.5.3 *Indices of Socioeconomic Background (SEB)*

When investigating the relationship between patients' socioeconomic circumstances and cancer mortality, individual measures of deprivation are rarely available, especially when using routine data. Indices of socioeconomic background (SEB), such as the Townsend Index (Townsend et al. 1988) and the Index of Multiple Deprivation (Noble et al. 2004), are all that is usually routinely available. These indices are measured at the small-area level, such as electoral ward or super-output area. This can lead to the ecological fallacy (Robinson 1950) if area-based findings are extrapolated to individuals living in each area. For this reason, another level should ideally be introduced – the small-area level – and this would be cross-classified with Trusts, i.e. patients from one small area might attend different treatment centres and similarly patients from one Trust may be drawn from different small areas of residence.

Theoretically, it is possible to conduct a cross-classified multilevel latent-class model (where small areas may also be grouped into latent classes). Our primary interest, however, is illustration of the multilevel latent class methodology, and our primary research question also pertains to the population or sub-populations (i.e. latent classes), not individuals. We therefore adopt the simplified approach of attributing small-area scores of SEB to individual patients and adopt a strict two-level hierarchy only, omitting the cross-classified small-area level completely. Similar analyses have recently been undertaken to investigate the association between SEB and mortality from breast cancer, while including area of residence at the upper level (Downing et al. 2010).

7.5.4 Model Construction for Research Question (i)

Deriving multiple patient latent classes divides patients into sub-groups such that the relationship between survival and SEB might vary within each latent class. The latent classes then correspond to specific patient features that can be labelled post-hoc according to outcome (e.g. 'good' or 'poor' survivors) or covariates (e.g. 'early-' or 'late-' stage disease at diagnosis). Adopting multiple latent classes for the Trusts effectively groups diagnostic or treatment centres, though the relationship between mortality and SEB varies only across patient classes, not Trust classes.

The continuous measures of patient age at diagnosis and Townsend score (SEB) exhibited non-linear relationships with 3-year survival. Generalised additive models (GAMs; discussed in more detail in Chap. 15), identified the higher order terms required for each; the statistical software used was *R 2.9.0* (Venables and Smith 1990). For both terms, the non-linearity was explored and threshold values identified, to simplify the number of higher order terms required. Patient age at diagnosis was centred on the study mean of 71.5 years and Townsend score was centred on the population mean of zero (the study mean was -0.040). Models were also adjusted for sex.

Stage was included as a class predictor rather than as a fixed-effect covariate, meaning the resultant patient classes had a graduated mortality risk analogous to that observed for different stages of disease. This allowed the relationship between mortality and various risk factors to be explored across patient classes, introducing an implicit 'interaction' with stage at diagnosis, without the risk of exacerbated bias due to measurement error. Additional variables were included as inactive covariates, which allowed them to be interpreted within the classes but did not allow them to predict class membership.

7.5.5 Results

Table 7.1 shows the results of the standard multilevel-regression analysis. The reference group in these study data comprised males of mean age (71.5 years) with stage A at diagnosis and a Townsend score of zero. In the study population, 12,856 patients (52.2%) died within 2 years. There was a substantial association between being female and decreased odds of death, and between increasing deprivation or increasing age and increasing odds of death.

Table 7.1 Multilevel regression results from standard analysis: odds of death within 3 years with stage included as a class predictor

Model statistics	Prevalence
Overall	52%
Reference group	49%
Model covariates	OR (95% CI)
Female	0.86 (0.81–0.91)
Townsend (per SD more)	1.18 (1.16–1.21)
Age (per 5 years older)	1.33 (1.30–1.35)
Age squared (per 5 years older)	1.01 (1.01–1.01)

CI Confidence Interval; there were 12,856 (52%) deaths within 3 years in the entire study population; the reference group comprised males, aged 71.5 years classified as Stage I at diagnosis, and attributed a Townsend score of zero

All multilevel latent class models revealed an improved fit compared with standard multilevel regression analysis according to all model-fit criteria considered. Although the model-fit criteria identified different optimum models (the LL and BIC identified the model with three patient classes and one Trust class while the AIC identified the model with four patient classes and three Trust classes) the preferred model was that with three patient classes and two Trust classes, because this sufficiently differentiated patient characteristics, while four patient classes and either extra or fewer Trust classes added little insight to patient and hospital variation. For the final model, patient CE was 22% and Trust CE was 8%.

Table 7.2 summarises the preferred multilevel latent class model, with patients apportioned into either a large good-prognosis group, a small reasonable-prognosis group, or an even smaller poor-prognosis group. Patient class 1 contained 42% of cases of which 10% died within 3 years, compared with patient class 2 with 31% of cases of which 69% died within 3 years, and patient class 3 with 27% of cases of which 99% died within 3 years.

The impact of deprivation differed insubstantially across the patient classes. In classes 1 and 2 (good and reasonable prognosis), living in a more deprived area was clearly associated with increased odds of death. In class 3 (poor prognosis), the association was less clear, with the odds ratio indicating only slightly decreased odds of death and with a wide confidence interval. This indicates that the role of SEB in 3-year colorectal mortality operates somewhat differently for differently staged individuals, with SEB having less impact for those with late-stage disease. The mean Townsend scores also differed across the classes, indicating that individuals in class 2 (reasonable prognosis) generally lived in more deprived areas than individuals in either of the other two classes.

The impact of sex differs substantially across the classes. In class 3 (poor prognosis), females had an increased risk of death compared to males, whereas in class 1 (good prognosis), females had a decreased risk of death and in class 2 (reasonable prognosis), females also had a decreased risk of death. This difference

Table 7.2 Results for the subject classes in the 3-patient-, 2-Trust-class multilevel regression model: odds ratio of death within 3 years

Model covariates	OR (95% CI)			Wald test (p-value)
	Class 1	Class 2	Class 3	
Female	0.60 (0.46–0.77)	0.84 (0.61–1.15)	1.75 (0.48–6.30)	0.022
Townsend (per SD)	1.21 (1.07–1.37)	1.59 (1.31–1.92)	0.99 (0.55–1.77)	0.048
Age (per 5 years)	2.18 (0.83–5.75)	2.53 (2.00–3.21)	0.58 (0.22–1.53)	0.011
Age squared (per 5 years)	1.00 (0.96–1.03)	1.01 (1.00–1.02)	1.06 (0.96–1.16)	0.340
Model summary statistics				
Class size	42%	31%	27%	
Overall prevalence	10%	69%	99%	
Reference group prevalence	6%	69%	97%	
Model class profiles				
Stage A	23%	6%	0.5%	
Stage B	47%	19%	8%	
Stage C	27%	30%	16%	
Stage D	0.5%	12%	69%	
Missing	3%	32%	7%	
Patients treated	98%	76%	69%	
ICD-10 C18 (colon)	58%	57%	62%	
ICD-10 C19 (rectosigmoid jct.)	11%	10%	11%	
ICD-10 C20 (rectum)	31%	34%	27%	
Tumour on left side	69%	67%	61%	
Tumour on right side	28%	25%	29%	
Tumour across both sides	3%	8%	11%	

OR Odds Ratio, *CI* Confidence Interval; there were 12,856 (52%) deaths in the entire study population; the reference group comprised males, aged 71.5 years classified as Stage I at diagnosis, and attributed a Townsend score of zero

in risk profile by sex across classes indicates that the role of sex in 3-year colorectal mortality operates differently for differently staged individuals, with women faring better than men with early-staged disease, and the reverse with late-stage disease. The proportions of females differed across the classes (class 1: 42%; class 2: 33%; class 3: 25%), indicating that the majority of females had a decreased risk of death compared with males.

The impact of age in the model differed substantially across classes. In class 2 (reasonable prognosis), older age was clearly associated with increased odds of death, as too in class 1 (good prognosis), though the association was reduced. In contrast, in class 3 (poor prognosis), the odds ratio indicates a decreased odds of death for older age. The mean age also differed across the classes (class 1: 71.6 years, SD 8.6 years; class 2: 76.6 years, SD 8.4 years; class 3: 71.5 years, SD 8.8 years), indicating that individuals in class 2 (reasonable prognosis) were, on average, older than the individuals in either of the other two classes.

The stage profile differed across the patient classes. Class 1 (good prognosis) corresponded to early stage diagnosis with 69% of the stage A/B patients versus 28%

of the stage C/D patients. Class 2 (reasonable prognosis) corresponded to more evenly balanced staging at diagnosis with 25% of the stage A/B patients and 43% of the stage C/D patients. This class also contained 32% of patients with missing stage. Class 3 (poor prognosis) corresponded to late stage diagnosis with only 8% of the stage A/B patients versus 85% of the stage C/D patients. Of particular note is the proportion of stage D patients in each class, with a negligible proportion (0.5%) in class 1 (good prognosis), class 2 (reasonable prognosis) containing 12%, and class 3 (poor prognosis) containing 69%. A higher proportion of patients was treated in class 1 (98%) compared to either class 2 (76%) or class 3 (69%), which may be due to their stage at diagnosis. Treatment relates to curative treatment only, and early-stage patients are more likely to receive curative, rather than palliative treatment (National Institute of Clinical Excellence 2004). The proportions of patients diagnosed with each type of tumour, based on the ICD-10 codes, was similar across the patient classes. The proportions of patients diagnosed with tumours in any of the defined positions of the body were also similar across the patient classes. There is no indication from these data that either the type or position of the tumour is associated with survival.

We do not investigate the Trust classes here, as patient class differentiation was our primary focus. In this model, no adjustment has been made for patient casemix so we cannot make any inference at this stage as to the performance of the hospitals within each Trust class.

7.5.6 Discussion

The multilevel latent class regression model substantially improved fit for the illustrative dataset compared to the standard multilevel model. As both patients and Trusts were categorised into latent classes, this led to an improved interpretation of the data. We are therefore able to investigate how risk factors associate with mortality within sub-groups, rather than only for all patients or Trusts, as in the standard multilevel model. New insights were available that were not previously apparent using the standard multilevel model. For instance, although the standard analysis found age, sex and SEB differences in survival, multilevel LCA showed that within latent classes, age and sex differences varied according to patient class and SEB varied according to patient sub-type; Trusts, whilst heterogeneous, did not have a huge impact on the association between patient factors and 3-year mortality.

By not modelling stage as a covariate, we have attempted to avoid the reversal paradox and minimise bias due to measurement error and incomplete data. As the patient classes correspond to stage at diagnosis, we have been able to determine how the covariates associate with mortality within different stage groupings, without using product interaction terms. Categorising missing values in stage allows the modelling to take account of incomplete data and assign patients to the most suitable patient class according to how their outcome corresponds to other patients. There are some limitations:

First, with stage included as a class predictor, bias is minimised, though it will not be completely eradicated. Patient classes may, however, be derived without stage as a class predictor and the same differentiation across patient classes may then be observed. For patients presenting with early- or mid-stage disease, their characteristics may help determine their chances of dying from colorectal cancer, whilst for patients presenting with late-stage disease, their characteristics are less likely to be associated with mortality. Second, it would be more sophisticated to explore survival as a continuous measure, e.g. using Cox's proportional hazards regression. This was not undertaken as this would have introduced even further complexity. Third, as already suggested, SEB is really measured at the area-level and so should be considered as a separate level, effectively cross-classified with the Trust level. This too could be accommodated, but to achieve these more complex models – cross-classified Cox proportional hazards regression – one needs more powerful software, e.g. WinBUGS (Lunn et al. 2000) or eventually MPlus (Muthén and Muthén 2007), once developed for cross-classified modelling.

We have considered a number of model-fit criteria when assessing our 'best-fit' model and we have chosen the model that minimises these criteria while providing a useful and informative summary of the data. Alternative models could, however, have been selected. Our chosen model has a low classification error at the Trust level (8%), meaning that the classes are more 'real' and we can differentiate between the Trusts, categorising them into good or poor performance groups. At the patient level, the classification error was higher (22%), meaning that these classes are more 'virtual'. Some patients will fall into one class entirely, whilst others may 'belong' substantially to more than one patient class.

7.5.7 A Multilevel Latent-Class Model Approach to Casemix Adjustment

To address research question (ii), we wish to 'adjust' for patient casemix in order to assess the relative (ranked) performance of Trusts. We contrast this approach to that of adopting Trust standardised mortality ratios (SMRs).

7.5.8 Model Construction for Research Question (ii)

For research question (ii), there is no concern surrounding the role of confounding, hence we are not seeking confounder adjustment, since we do not seek to inference the role of any exposure(s); rather, we seek to optimise outcome prediction by modelling patient characteristics in order to accommodate casemix differences. Consequently, all available covariates for which there is complete data (age, sex, and SEB) are considered. In addition, stage at diagnosis (coded A to D for increasing severity and missing coded X) is also considered, despite its extent of missing data (13.1%), because stage plays a crucial role in affecting survival outcomes and it is easy to code the missing data as a separate category. Although additional patient variables are available, these all have substantial incomplete data that would bring into question their utility were a missing category introduced, and these additional patient variables were therefore not used as outcome predictors. If it were deemed necessary to include these other variables, imputation techniques might be adopted, though that distracts from the salient issue here of illustrating the multilevel latent class methodology.

The modelling strategy adopted was thus to determine patient-level latent classes having first included patient-level covariates, with Trust-level variation accommodated via a continuous latent variable; the optimum number of patient classes was determined by considering model parsimony, though more patient classes might be preferred to discriminate amongst patient subtypes. With patient-level subtype structure ascertained, Trust classes were sought where the continuous latent variable was replaced by a categorical latent variable. The optimum number of Trust classes was again determined considering parsimony, though also with a mind on utility; a minimum of two Trust classes is necessary to exhibit discretised Trust-class differences in patient outcomes, though in some instances more classes might be necessary to differentiate amongst certain Trusts, as discussed later. Having incorporated available patient-level covariates, and having modelled patient class uncertainty associated with unavailable patient-level covariates, the resulting Trust class differences in patient outcomes were thus adjusted for patient casemix. Trust classes then exhibited a graduated patient outcome (3-year survival), which was used to generate ranks of Trust performance: Trusts were ordered based on their probability weights of belonging to the better survival Trust class.

For the comparison of methods, SMRs for each Trust were derived and a scaled difference from 'SMR = 1' determined for each Trust by dividing by the square root of the Trust size. For both the SMRs and the multilevel latent class models, 200 bootstrapped datasets were generated from the original dataset and each analysed individually in the same manner to generate 95% confidence intervals (CIs) from sample percentiles. Trusts were ranked in order of 'best' to 'worst' survival determined by the multilevel latent class model and contrasted to ranks generated from the Trust SMRs.

7.5.9 Results

Table 7.3 summarises the 'ideal' MLLC model determined by the procedures described. Patients were assigned to two latent classes of similar size, one with

Table 7.3 Results for the subject classes in the 2-patient-, 2-Trust-class multilevel latent class regression model: odds ratio of death within 3 years

Model summary statistics	Class 1	Class 2
Class size	54.3%	45.7%
Overall prevalence	63.0%	39.3%
Reference group prevalence	23.2%	7.0%
Model covariates	OR (95% CI)	
Stage = B	2.40 (1.63–3.54)	0.55 (0.21–1.43)
Stage = C	7.72 (4.61–12.94)	1.74 (0.75–4.06)
Stage = D	20.19 (8.88–45.89)	Infinite[a]
Stage = X	6.30 (1.89–20.97)	33.41 (7.93–140.68)
Female	0.94 (0.78–1.14)	0.58 (0.38–0.88)
Townsend (per SD)	1.32 (1.21–1.43)	1.03 (0.81–1.31)
Age (per 5 years)	1.51 (1.42–1.60)	2.53 (1.31–4.90)
Age squared (per 5 years)	1.005 (0.997–1.012)	0.984 (0.960–1.008)

OR Odds Ratio, *CI* Confidence Interval. There were 12,856 (52.2%) deaths in the study population. The reference group comprised males, aged 71.5 years, classified as Stage A at diagnosis, and attributed a Townsend score of zero

[a]The odds ratio could not be estimated as there were zero patients who survived 3 years in this subcategory

reasonable prognosis (PC1: 54.3% of cases, of which 63.0% died within 3 years), and one with better prognosis (PC2: 45.7% of cases, of which 39.3% died within 3 years). Trusts were similarly assigned to two latent classes. The largest Trust class, with 53.1% of patients, had better prognosis (TC1: 51.3% of patients died within 3 years; TC2: 53.2% of patients died within 3 years).

Table 7.4 summarises the number of deaths within each patient class by stage. Allocating patients to classes according to their largest class probability (modal assignment), all patients in PC1 diagnosed either at stage B or C died within 3 years; in PC2, all patients diagnosed at stage A, B or C survived. This difference is anticipated, as stage at diagnosis is an important predictor of survival. Most of the early- or mid-stage patients died within 3 years in PC1 compared to PC2, and there was a clear graduation in survival with increasing stage at diagnosis from early- to late-stage within both classes.

Trust ranks and their bootstrapped 95% CIs, according to both methods considered, are summarised in Table 7.5; a low ranking value indicates a better survival rate than expected. Differences in the median rank of Trust performance between the MLLC model approach and the Trust SMRs are well within their estimated 95% CIs. Figure 7.2 provides a graphical representation of these results, in order of increasing median probability of belonging to the best survival Trust class for the MLLC methodology.

For the final model, patient CE was 35% and Trust CE was 17%. The large patient-level CE indicates that patient classes are more a 'distilled' classification of patient traits than well-defined subgroups or subtypes of individuals. The Trust-level CE indicates that Trusts also comprise shared traits, though it is feasible that some Trust classes comprise more a distinct subgroup of Trusts.

7 Multilevel Latent Class Modelling

Table 7.4 Deaths within 3 years, by stage, in each of the 2-patient classes for the 2-patient, 2-Trust multilevel latent class regression model

Stage at diagnosis	Modal class 1, died within 3 yrs		Modal class 2, dies within 3 yrs	
	No	Yes	No	Yes
A	1,099	550	1,210	0
B	0	1,955	4,829	0
C	0	2,736	3,437	0
D	437	3,202	0	1,962
X	413	2,360	359	91
TOTAL	1,949	10,803	9,835	2,053

Table 7.5 Trust ranks from the multilevel latent class model and the calculation of Trust SMRs

Trust	Median probability of belonging to best survival Trust class	Median rank (95% CI)	
		ML LC	SMR
1	1.000	1 (1–9.5)	6 (2–11)
2	0.999	3 (1–11)	4 (1–10.5)
3	0.997	4 (1–11)	3 (1–10.5)
4	0.996	4 (1–15)	8 (3–14.5)
5	0.993	5 (1–12.5)	5 (1–13)
6	0.956	8 (2–16)	9 (2–17)
7	0.912	9 (3–17)	5 (1–17)
8	0.908	9 (2–17)	6 (1–18)
9	0.897	9 (3–18)	5 (1–18)
10	0.816	10 (3–17)	8 (1–18)
11	0.575	11 (3.5–18)	11 (3–17)
12	0.476	13 (5.5–18)	12.5 (3–18)
13	0.372	12 (4–18.5)	11.5 (5.5–17)
14	0.359	12 (3–19)	12 (7–17)
15	0.152	14 (5.5–19)	15 (4.5–18)
16	0.070	14 (4–19)	13 (7–18)
17	0.070	15 (7.5–19)	16 (7.5–18)
18	0.003	18 (7–19)	15 (10–18)
19	0.002	18 (13.5–19)	19 (18–19)

7.5.10 Discussion

The simplest multilevel latent class model, where the continuous latent variable at the upper level is replaced by a categorical latent variable, estimates the mean outcome for each Trust class and the size of each Trust class (summation of Trust probabilities for each Trust class) with no assumptions made regarding the distribution of means or class sizes. The upper-level discrete latent variable allows for individual Trusts to be assigned probabilistically to the discrete latent trust classes,

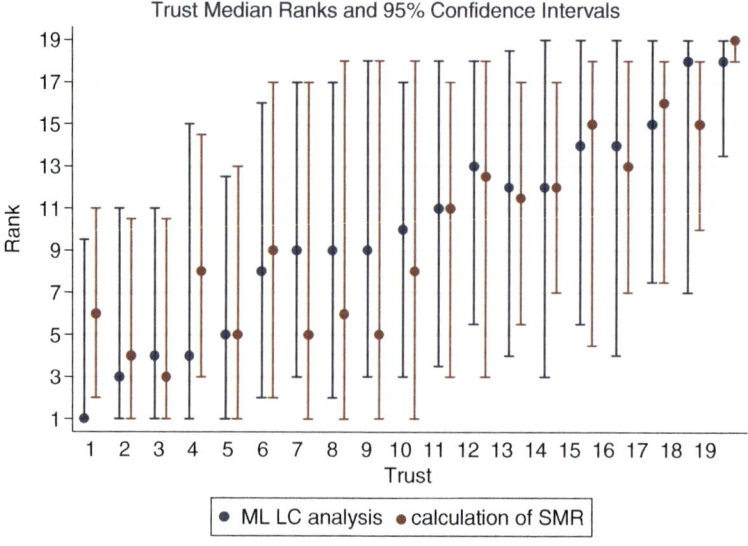

Fig. 7.2 Trust Median Ranks and 95% Confidence Intervals, ordered by the multilevel latent class (ML LC) analysis

providing less restricted weighting of Trust relative performance than the standard normal assumption. This likely improves the accuracy of estimated patient differences across Trust classes, which in turn improves the estimated patient casemix adjustment for individual Trusts. The multilevel latent-class model is also more likely to capture contextual effects due to inherent data hierarchy than by merely estimating Trust ranks according to their SMRs.

Continuous and discrete latent variables, if combined, may prove more parsimonious, with variation within each Trust class captured by the continuous latent variable, potentially leading to fewer Trust classes to describe efficiently the overall Trust-level variation. If determination of Trust ranks is important, however, the estimation of Trust outcomes is more straightforward if the categorical latent variable only is used at the Trust level, as this avoids having to derive the normally distributed random effects within each Trust class. Improvements in patient casemix modelling might be feasible were more patient variables considered, but this could incorporate incomplete data, which can cause bias. Within a latent-class framework the uncertainty surrounding unrecorded or unused patient characteristics is modelled explicitly – with 'fuzzy' matching.

In fixing patient-level latent-class composition and modelling patient casemix differences, the residual Trust-class differences in outcome reflect variations in Trust performance. This paves the way for the analysis of treatment centre characteristics (in addition to patient casemix characteristics), whereby differences in the patient pathway of care are modelled explicitly to evaluate organisational features in relation to patient outcomes (survival or which treatments are received). Such strategies permit hypothesis generation around which healthcare delivery and organisational features might warrant intervention to bring about improvements in patient care. Preliminary investigation of observational data using these methods could inform prospective cluster-randomised trials targeted at changing service organisation and healthcare delivery.

The probabilities of Trust class membership in Table 7.5 are marked, with most Trusts belonging entirely or predominantly to one Trust class, with only a few Trusts exhibiting a mixed assignment to both Trust classes. This is unsurprising, as there is only a modest difference between the two classes in median survival, and probabilistic assignment differentiates between the two by providing a class weighted combined survival rate. It is not feasible, however, for a Trust to be assigned a class weighted survival rate below that of the poorer survival class, or above that of the better survival class. This is an implicit constraint on the estimated weighted survival for Trusts allocated entirely to one of the two classes (e.g. Trust 1). To alleviate this, one could incorporate a continuous Trust-level latent variable alongside the discrete Trust-level latent variable, though the estimation of Trust survival rates then becomes more complex. Alternatively, more Trust-level classes could be sought, increasing the number until no Trust had a probabilistic assignment of exactly one to classes at the extremities of the range of Trust outcome means.

The main advantage of the multilevel latent class approach is that it introduces the concept of mixtures at the upper levels, leading to improved accuracy of the estimated outcome differences across Trust classes, hence improved 'casemix adjustment' for individual Trusts. Trust level covariates may then be included, capturing additional casemix complexity. This simplified illustration demonstrates a principle that could readily extend to a number of more sophisticated model scenarios (e.g. time-to-event analysis, multiple treatment centres, cross-classified structures).

7.6 Concluding Remarks

Multilevel latent class analysis has considerable utility. It improves upon standard multilevel models by yielding better fit and providing enhanced insight. The introduction of latent classes allows for investigation into how the risk factors considered are associated with survival within patient classes and within Trust classes, rather than for all patients and across all Trusts.

7.7 Further Reading

The book *Multilevel Modelling of Health Statistics* (Leyland AH, Goldstein H. Wiley Series in Probability and Statistics) gives a valuable introduction to techniques used in the analysis of hierarchical data, including those for modelling repeated measurements. Binomial regression and Poisson regression are discussed, together with multivariate multilevel models and multinomial regression, before ending with a chapter on software. The book *Multilevel Analysis Techniques and Applications* (Hox J. Lawrence Erlbaum Associates, Mahwah NJ. 2002) builds from a basic two-level regression model. It contains a thorough discussion of estimation methods and model comparison and includes more advanced methods such as bootstrapping estimates and Bayesian estimation methods. The analysis of longitudinal data is also included, as are logistic regression modelling and cross-classified multilevel models. Sample size and power analysis is considered and the book ends with a move towards latent curve modelling. The book *Generalized Latent Variable Modeling: Multilevel, Longitudinal, and Structural Equation Models* (Skrondal A, Rabe-Hesketh S) focuses on latent variable modelling and includes multilevel regression, factor models, structural equation models and longitudinal models. A general model framework is introduced and estimation methods are examined in detail. A very useful aspect of this book is the applications section where real research is introduced and analysed. Multiple outcome measures are considered here: dichotomous, ordinal, counts, durations and survival, comparative and mixed responses.

References

Adams, J., White, M., & Forman, D. (2004). Are there socioeconomic gradients in stage and grade of breast cancer at diagnosis? Cross sectional analysis of UK cancer registry data. *BMJ, 329* (7458), 142.
Akaike, H. (1974). A new look at the statistical identification model. *IEEE Trans Auto Control, 19*, 716–723.
Carroll, R. J., Ruppert, D., Stefanski, L. A., & Crainiceanu, C. M. (2006). *Measurement error in nonlinear models* (2nd ed.). London: Chapman & Hall.
Coleman, M., Babb, P., Damiecki, P., et al. (1999). *Cancer survival trends in England and Wales, deprivation and NHS region* (SMPS, Vol. 61, pp. 119–212). London: The Stationery Office.
Davy, M. (2007). Socio-economic inequalities in smoking: An examination of generational trends in Great Britain. *Health Statistics Quarterly, 34*, 26–34.
Downing, A., Harrison, W. J., West, R. M., Forman, D., & Gilthorpe, M. S. (2010). Latent class modelling of the association between socioeconomic background and breast cancer survival status at 5 years whilst incorporating stage of disease. *Journal of the Epidemiology and Community Health, 64*(9), 772–776. Published Online First: 19 August 2009.
Dukes, C. E. (1949). The surgical pathology of rectal cancer. *Journal of Clinical Pathology, 2*, 95–98.
Duncan, C., Jones, K., & Moon, G. (1999). Smoking and deprivation: Are there neighbourhood effects? *Social Science & Medicine, 48*(4), 497–505.
Fuller, W. A. (1987). *Measurement error models*. New York: Wiley.
Greenwood, D. C., Gilthorpe, M. S., & Cade, J. E. (2006). The impact of imprecisely measured covariates on estimating gene-environment interactions. *BMC Medical Research Methodology, 6*, 21.
Hernandez-Diaz, S., Schisterman, E. F., & Hernan, M. A. (2006). The birth weight "paradox" uncovered? *American Journal of Epidemiology, 164*(11), 1115–1120.

Ionescu, M. V., Carey, F., Tait, I. S., & Steele, R. J. (1998). Socioeconomic status and stage at presentation of colorectal cancer. *Lancet, 352*(9138), 1439.

James, W. P., Nelson, M., Ralph, A., & Leather, S. (1997). Socioeconomic determinants of health. The contribution of nutrition to inequalities in health. *BMJ, 314*(7093), 1545–1549.

Kirkwood, B., & Sterne, J. (2003). *Medical statistics* (2nd ed.). Oxford: Blackwell.

Kogevinas, M., Marmot, M. G., Fox, A. J., & Goldblatt, P. O. (1991). Socioeconomic differences in cancer survival. *Journal of Epidemiology and Community Health, 45*, 216–219.

Lunn, D. J., Thomas, A., Best, N., & Spiegelhalter, D. (2000). WinBUGS – A Bayesian modelling framework: Concepts, structure and extensibility. *Statistics and Computing, 10*, 325–337.

Lyratzopoulos, G., Sheridan, G. F., Michie, H. R., McElduff, P., & Hobbiss, J. H. (2004). Absence of socioeconomic variation in survival from colorectal cancer in patients receiving surgical treatment in one health district: Cohort study. *Colorectal Disease, 6*(6), 512–517.

Macdonald, L., Cummins, S., & Macintyre, S. (2007). Neighbourhood fast food environment and area deprivation-substitution or concentration? *Appetite, 49*(1), 251–254.

Morris, E. J. A., Maughan, N. J., Forman, D., & Quirke, P. (2007a). Identifying stage III colorectal cancer patients: The influence of the patient, surgeon and pathologist. *Journal of Clinical Oncology, 25*(18), 2573–2579.

Morris, E. J. A., Maughan, N. J., Forman, D., & Quirke, P. (2007b). Who to treat with adjuvant therapy in Dukes B/Stage II colorectal cancer? The need for high quality pathology. *Gut, 56*, 1419–1425.

Muthén, L. K., & Muthén, B. O. (2007). *Mplus user's guide* (5th ed.). Los Angeles: Muthén & Muthén.

National Institute of Clinical Excellence. (2004). *Guidance on cancer services: Improving outcomes in colorectal cancers – Manual update*. London: National Institute of Clinical Excellence.

Noble, M., Wright, G., Dibben, C., et al. (2004). *The English indices of deprivation 2004 (revised)* (p. 2004). Yorkshire: Office of the Deputy Prime Minister.

Pearl, J. (2000). *Causality: Models, reasoning and inference*. Cambridge: University Press.

Pollock, A. M., & Vickers, N. (1997). Breast, lung and colorectal cancer incidence and survival in South Thames Region, 1987–92: The effect of social deprivation. *Journal of Public Health Medicine, 19*, 288–294.

Quirke, P., & Morris, E. (2006). Reporting colorectal cancer. *Histopathology, 50*, 103–112.

Robinson, W. S. (1950). Ecological correlations and the behaviour of individuals. *American Sociological Review, 15*, 351–357.

Schrijvers, C. T. M., Mackenbach, J. P., Lutz, J.-M., Wuinn, M. J., & Coleman, M. P. (1995). Deprivation, stage at diagnosis and cancer survival. *International Journal of Cancer, 63*, 324–329.

Schwarz, G. (1978). Estimating the dimension of a model. *The Annals of Statistics, 6*(2), 461–464.

Stigler, S. M. (1999). *Statistics on the table*. Cambridge: Harvard University Press.

Townsend, P., Phillimore, P., & Beattie, A. (1988). *Health and deprivation: Inequality and the North*. London: Croom Helm.

Tu, Y. K., West, R., Ellison, G. T., & Gilthorpe, M. S. (2005). Why evidence for the fetal origins of adult disease might be a statistical artifact: The "reversal paradox" for the relation between birth weight and blood pressure in later life. *American Journal of Epidemiology, 161*(1), 27–32.

UKACR Quality and Performance Indicators 2008: Final [online]. (2008). [cited 2-2-2009] [last updated 2008]. Available from http://82.110.76.19/quality/UKACR%20report2008_final.pdf.

Venables, W. N., & Smith, D. M. An introduction to R [online]. Austria: The R Foundation, 1990. Available from http://www.r-project.org/.

Vermunt, J. K., & Magidson, J. (2005a). *Latent GOLD 4.0 User's Guide*. Belmont, Massachusetts: Statistical Innovations Inc.

Vermunt, J. K., & Magidson, J. (2005b). *Technical guide for Latent GOLD 4.0: Basic and advanced*. Belmont, Massachusetts: Statistical Innovations Inc.

World Health Organisation. (2005). *The International Statistical Classification of Diseases and Health Related Problems ICD-10: Tenth Revision* (2nd ed.). Geneva: World Health Organisation.

Wrigley, H., Roderick, P., George, S., Smith, J., Mullee, M., & Goddard, J. (2003). Inequalities in survival from colorectal cancer: A comparison of the impact of deprivation, treatment, and host factors on observed and cause specific survival. *Journal of Epidemiology and Community Health, 57*(4), 301–309.

Chapter 8
Bayesian Bivariate Disease Mapping

Richard G. Feltbower and Samuel O.M. Manda

8.1 Introduction

The geographical distribution of disease is an important aspect of epidemiological research, providing a useful indication of the heterogeneity of disease incidence as a way of developing and testing aetiological hypotheses. However, incidence of rare diseases aggregated over small geographical areas provide problems for presentation and modelling. For example, deriving or mapping relative risks (RR) for areas with very small populations is likely to produce artificially inflated estimates. Similarly, plotting estimated significance values, which is not something one would generally recommend, associated with disease risk will tend to accentuate those areas which are more densely populated compared to more rural areas. Bayesian methods have therefore been proposed (Besag et al. 1991) to deal with sparse data arising, for example, through small incidence or mortality rates within the context of an ecological analysis; this approach improves the precision and stability of risk estimates. These methods also provide a framework to model simultaneously the spatial and non-spatial (or heterogeneity) effects on disease risk.

By way of introducing these concepts, it is worth reminding ourselves how in the classical 'frequentist' model risk estimates are generally derived when undertaking an ecological analysis investigating geographical disease epidemiology. A Poisson regression model is fitted to the observed numbers of disease cases in each area. The expected number of cases in each area is parameterised as the product of the expected cases and the underlying risk. A log-linear model is then based on the

---

R.G. Feltbower (✉)
Division of Epidemiology, Centre for Epidemiology and Biostatistics, Leeds Institute of Genetics, Health & Therapeutics, University of Leeds, Leeds, UK
e-mail: r.g.feltbower@leeds.ac.uk

S.O.M. Manda
Biostatistics Unit, South Africa Medical Research Council, Pretoria, South Africa

mean of the Poisson distribution, specified by the sum of two parts: the logarithm of the expected cases, which is just an offset term, and the logarithm of the underlying risk (McCullagh and Nelder 1989). The expected number of cases is typically obtained from the age-gender specific incidence rates for the entire region under study. However, when considering how risk estimates differ across areas, especially if the disease of interest is rare (such as the case with childhood cancer or diabetes where incidence rates are of the order 3–20 per 100,000 person years) then it is not uncommon to observe areas which exhibit zero counts. Similarly, if the population of a rural area is extremely sparse with an associated expected disease count of just greater than zero, we may actually observe at least one case. In these scenarios, our estimate of disease risk – the standardised incidence (or mortality) ratio SIR (or SMR) – for certain areas will be zero or artificially inflated, thus our inferences concerning epidemiology will be seriously flawed.

The rest of the chapter will cover an introduction to Bayesian smoothing approaches, where we will consider multivariate spatial models when we wish to model more than one disease simultaneously. An example investigating the epidemiological similarities and correlation between childhood leukaemia and Type 1 diabetes (T1D) over small areas will be used to illustrate these techniques, where we compare classical and Bayesian approaches to spatial disease modelling.

8.2 Bayesian Smoothing

The rationale behind using Bayesian techniques to underpin disease mapping is that for any given area i say, all neighbouring areas j are likely to share similar environmental exposures and therefore one would expect disease rates and RR estimates for area i to resemble those of all adjacent areas. The Bayesian approach uses this principle to borrow strength or information from neighbouring areas to provide more robust risk estimates for each area within the study region of interest. This also overcomes the problem of relying on the unlikely assumption that disease risks are independent across geographical areas, a concept which is difficult to justify when there may be significant evidence of clustering or extra-Poisson variation.

Bayesian 'spatial' smoothing is traditionally used to refer to RR estimates which have been derived according to the local distribution of RR in areas which are close or adjacent to one another. This is in contrast to 'non-spatial' smoothing which uses the global distribution of RR for all areas within the study region (Clayton and Kaldor 1987). A further advantage of spatial smoothing techniques is the ability to remove or reduce the effect of arbitrary geographical boundaries, since geo-political areas are unlikely to be related to the disease of interest. Thus, any artefactual variation exhibited in the data by methods of data aggregation is reduced.

8.2.1 The Besag Model

A conventional way of applying spatial modelling was set out by Besag et al. (1991) within the context of image analysis. The principles which underpin Besag's statistical model allow us to differentiate between the relative contribution of the spatial and non-spatial effects on disease risk. The non-spatial or heterogeneity random effects appear in the model as extra-Poisson variation and arise through the variation among the underlying populations at risk due to omitted covariates. The spatial random effects control for unmeasured spatial covariates. That are similar across close or adjacent geographical areas.

The model is defined such that the observed disease counts O_i in each area i, with associated expected counts E_i, are assumed to take a Poisson distribution, i.e. $O_i \sim Poisson(E_i RR_i)$ for $i = 1, \cdots, N$ areas, where RR_i is the relative risk of disease in area i. The maximum likelihood estimate of the relative risk of disease in area i equals O_i/E_i, which is the SIR_i.

We might wish to extend this model by including area-level covariates such as socio-economic status, whilst accounting for both the spatially structured and unstructured (heterogeneity) random effects for the relative risks across areas. Referring to the model of Besag et al. (1991), the logarithm of the RR for each area i is modelled so that:

$$\log(RR_i) = \alpha_0 + \beta^T x_i + u_i + v_i \quad (8.1)$$

where α_0 represents the intercept of the log relative risk; x_i represents the covariate for each area with associated parameter β; u_i represent the independent heterogeneity effects between areas (Clayton and Kaldor 1987) and are synonymous with extra-Poisson variation; v_i represent the spatially dependent random effects which are defined by a range of different structures describing adjacency or closeness in space. This class of models is referred to as convolution models and generally we may define a normal prior distribution (Besag et al. 1991) for the non-spatial heterogeneity effects such that $u_i \sim Normal(0, \sigma_u^2)$.

We may assume that the spatially correlated random effects v_i arise through a combination of independent random effects errors e_i that are normally distributed i.e. $e_i \sim Normal(0, \sigma_{e_i}^2)$ as set out by Langford et al. (1999) and Leyland et al. (2000). Here we assume that the components v_i may be written as

$$v_i = \frac{\sum_{j \in \Theta_i} e_j}{n_i} \quad (8.2)$$

where Θ_i represents the set of areas sharing a common boundary with area i, with n_i denoting the number of neighbours for area i. Thus, through the averaging of the independent random effects, e_j defines the effect of area j on the disease risk in area i. In this context Eq. 8.1 effectively then becomes a multilevel model, with each area i

occurring at the second level and it's neighbours in Θ_i being at the third level where the first level is the observed disease incidence. Multilevel modelling concepts are covered in more detail in chapters 5 and 7. Alternatively, instead of an adjacency model defined in the above example, the distance between the centroids of two areas could be taken as the combined effect of the neighbouring areas.

In the preceding construction, the total variation in disease risk (8.1) for each area i is the sum of variance of the heterogeneity and spatial effects and is dependent on the number of neighbours n_i i.e.

$$Var(logRR_i) = \sigma_u^2 + \frac{\sigma_e^2}{n_i} \qquad (8.3)$$

The proportion of variation attributable to the heterogeneity (non-spatial) and spatial random effects can therefore be easily calculated, the latter being scaled by an appropriate summary of the count of the number of neighbours for any area; for example, the modal number of neighbouring areas (Feltbower et al. 2005).

8.2.2 Bayesian Multivariate Spatial Models

Further benefits of using Bayesian techniques can be gained by jointly modelling more than one disease outcome, for example through an improvement in the precision and efficiency of parameter estimates for the other disease (Leyland et al. 2000). By considering the simple extension of modelling two disease counts jointly, we can define a Bayesian bivariate spatial model which allows us to test common epidemiological or aetiological features among different conditions, and also calculate the degree of correlation within small areas. In addition, this approach enables us to describe the association of both diseases with covariates of interest.

Langford et al. (1999) and Leyland et al. (2000) describe how the multivariate (bivariate) spatial model is defined within a multilevel context. These models also provide a framework to identify diseases which may share common risk factors, or indeed differences in risk between diseases and disease-specific risk factors (Knorr-Held and Best 2001; Dabney and Wakefield 2005). Alternative multivariate spatial models involve modelling common and specific latent factors within 'shared component' models (Knorr-Held and Best 2001; Held et al. 2006), although the application of these are not covered in this chapter.

8.2.3 Markov Chain Monte Carlo (MCMC) Simulation Methods

Empirical Bayes methods for disease mapping were originally developed and described more than 20 years ago by Clayton and Kaldor (1987). Empirical Bayes methods rely on the conditional distributions given the overall observed data and hyperparameters that are estimated marginally from the data using maximum likelihood (ML) or iterative generalised least squares (IGLS) methods. Thus, these hyperparameters are simply entered into the estimation of the random effect means. Compared to a fully hierarchical Bayesian approach using MCMC based methods, such as Gibbs sampling (Smith 1993), maximum-likelihood (ML) based estimation methods have the advantage of being fast to compute and easier to identify convergence of the final estimates. However, since ML methods do not account for the uncertainty in the hyperparameters, the variability in the random effects is underestimated, which might lead to erroneous inferences.

Modern computing power however has now largely meant that MCMC techniques have superseded the empirical Bayes approach when describing and modelling disease rates across geographical areas. The two main advantages of the fully Bayesian approach are that prior information can be incorporated into the modelling process and the full posterior distribution can be derived. Further details of MCMC techniques can be found in Gilks et al. (1996) and are also covered in chapter 9.

8.3 Methods for Illustrative Example

We illustrate the methods outlined in this chapter using an example taken from a paper describing the epidemiological similarities and spatial correlation between acute lymphoblastic leukaemia (ALL) and T1D (Feltbower et al. 2005).

8.3.1 Incidence Data

We extracted data on children aged under 15 and diagnosed with ALL and Type 1 diabetes (T1D) between 1986 and 1998 from two population-based disease registers covering the former Yorkshire Regional Health Authority in the north of the United Kingdom (UK) (Feltbower et al. 2003; McKinney et al. 1998). The registers cover a geographical area of 12,000 km^2 and a childhood population of 700,000. We limited the case series to a period centred at the time of the 1991 national UK census to ensure the inclusion of relevant socio-demographic denominator data. ALL and T1D were chosen as there is growing epidemiological evidence suggesting that both diseases may be linked to infectious exposure (Greaves 1997; Parslow et al. 2001; Feltbower et al. 2004).

Patients' addresses and postcodes (equivalent to zip codes) at the time of diagnosis were validated and linked to one of 532 Electoral Wards in existence in Yorkshire, UK, at the time of the 1991 UK Census. These small geographical areas have a median childhood population count of 750 (interquartile range 400–2,030).

8.3.2 Population Data

Population estimates from the 1991 UK Census were used to calculate age-sex standardised incidence rates.

8.3.3 Covariates

We compared separately the risk for both diseases from three socio-demographic factors previously linked to disease onset, measured at Ward level. These included: (i) population mixing, measured using the Shannon index (Stiller and Boyle 1996; Parslow et al. 2001), describing the diversity of origins of incomers into each Ward for the childhood population (ages 0–14); (ii) person-based childhood population density (Parslow et al. 2001), which is a population weighted average of population density (persons per hectare), and more appropriate for investigating infectious aetiology as it reflects the population density at which a typical person lives; and (iii) deprivation, measured using the Townsend Score (Townsend et al. 1988) which was derived from the following census variables: unemployment, household overcrowding, car ownership and housing tenure.

Incidence rate ratios (IRR) and 95% confidence (credible) intervals are presented according to categories used in previous epidemiological publications for comparative purposes (Parslow et al. 2001; Stiller and Boyle 1996) and are based on the rankings of the values across all Wards for each covariate. They were defined as follows:

- Population mixing: <10th percentile, 10th–90th percentiles (reference group) and >90th percentile. This grouping enables effects to be detected at the extremes of the range, as there is little variation in the value of the Shannon Index for the majority of Wards.
- Population density: three equal groups in size of Wards (lowest density taken as the reference group).
- Deprivation: five equal groups in size of Wards (least deprived taken as the reference group).

8.3.4 Classical (Frequentist) Poisson Regression Approach

For each disease, a Poisson regression model was fitted to the observed numbers of cases in each Ward using the log of the number of expected cases as the offset derived from age-sex specific incidence rates for Yorkshire between 1986 and 1998. This was implemented within a classical framework. All three socio-demographic variables (population density, mixing and deprivation) were included separately in the Poisson model, whilst no other confounding factors were added to this initial model. The effect on SIRs of including all three covariates was then assessed.

Evidence of any extra-Poisson variation, or overdispersion, was undertaken using negative binomial regression. All frequentist statistical analyses were performed using Stata version 8.

8.3.5 Bivariate Spatial Model

We modelled the two disease counts jointly, examining the effects from each covariate using Bayesian spatial and non-spatial smoothing. By extending Eq. 8.1 for the case of two diseases, we can denote the disease-specific RR as:

$$\begin{aligned} \log(R_{i1}) &= \alpha_{01} + \beta'_1 x_i + u_{i1} + v_{i1} \\ \log(R_{i2}) &= \alpha_{02} + \beta'_2 x_i + u_{i2} + v_{i2} \end{aligned} \quad (8.4)$$

Where α_{0h} is an intercept of the log relative risk for disease h ($h = 1,2$) in ward i; x_i is a covariate vector with the corresponding parameter β_h;
u_{i1} and u_{i2} are the independent unstructured random effects (representing global smoothing);
v_{i1} and v_{i2} are the spatially structured random effects (representing local smoothing).

8.3.6 Model Estimation and Sensitivity Analysis

We assume the four random effect terms u_{i1}, u_{i2}, e_{i1}, and e_{i2} arise from a multivariate normal distribution with zero mean vector and covariance matrix X (Langford et al. 1999; Leyland et al. 2000), though we chose to adopt a hierarchical Bayesian approach (Congdon 2003) rather than use IGLS estimation. All fixed effect parameters were given vague but proper Normal (0, 1,000) prior distributions.

However, for the covariance matrix D describing the four random effects, a sensitivity analysis was performed consisting of both informative and vague specifications for the scale matrix in the parameterization of the Wishart distribution for the precision matrix D^{-1}.

Posterior estimation of all the model parameters was carried out using the Gibbs sampling algorithm implemented in the software package WinBUGS (Lunn et al. 2000). The variance and covariance between the spatial effects v_{i1} and v_{i2} and the total risk variation ($u_{i1} + v_{i1}$) and ($u_{i2} + v_{i2}$) were computed empirically at each iteration of the Gibbs sampler.

For each model considered, three parallel Gibbs sampler chains from independent starting positions were run for 50,000 updates. All fixed effects and covariance parameters were monitored for convergence to stationary distributions. Trace plots of sample values of each of these parameters showed that they were converging to the same distributions. A burn-in period of 15,000 updates was used as convergence of the three chains was shown to have been reached after this period had elapsed, since Gelman-Rubin reduction factors (Gelman and Rubin 1992) were all estimated near 1.0. For posterior inference, we used a combined sample of the remaining 35,000 iterations. Finally, the effect on the degree of spatial correlation between both diseases was examined with and without adjustment for each sociodemographic factor previously linked to the spatial distribution of disease incidence.

Numerous diagnostic tests have been developed such as the Deviance Information Criterion (DIC), which is a natural extension of the Akaike Information Criterion (AIC) derived from the chains produced by the MCMC run. The DIC is a composite assessment combining both overall model fit with complexity and penalises additional parameters to encourage parsimony.

8.4 Results of the Illustrative Example

299 children with ALL and 1,551 with T1D were included in the dataset. Figures 8.1 and 8.2 showing the spatially smoothed SIR illustrate the variation in disease rates across wards, especially in the South-Eastern part of the region below the Humber estuary. Lower rates of ALL and T1D were seen in the more urban county of West Yorkshire, whereas higher disease rates were observed in the more rural county of North Yorkshire. The median (and interquartile range) for the number of cases distributed across all 532 Wards was 0 (0–1) and 2 (1–4) for ALL and T1D respectively.

8.4.1 Classical (Frequentist) Approach

Table 8.1 shows the unadjusted and adjusted IRRs for each covariate, for ALL and T1D separately. Generally, we infer higher rates of ALL and T1D in areas of low population mixing; however, in areas with high mixing, significantly lower rates of ALL were observed, although no similar association in incidence was seen for diabetes.

An inverse association was present for population density for each condition with lower rates associated with higher levels of population density. However, this association disappeared for T1D and was reversed for ALL once the effects from population mixing and deprivation were taken into consideration. There was some evidence of a negative association between deprivation and diabetes, although no clear relationship was evident between deprivation and ALL.

Although all three variables included in the model were positively correlated, we saw no evidence of multi-collinearity. Variance inflation factors were all less than 2.5. Population mixing exhibited the least degree of correlation of any of the

8 Bayesian Bivariate Disease Mapping

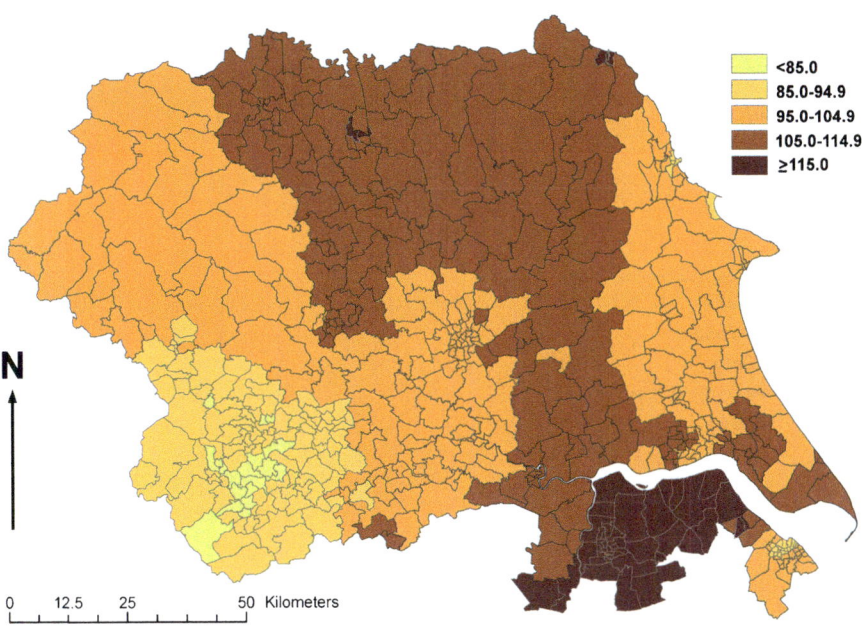

Fig. 8.1 Spatially smoothed standardised incidence ratios for childhood type 1 diabetes diagnosed between 1986 and 1998 across electoral wards in Yorkshire, UK

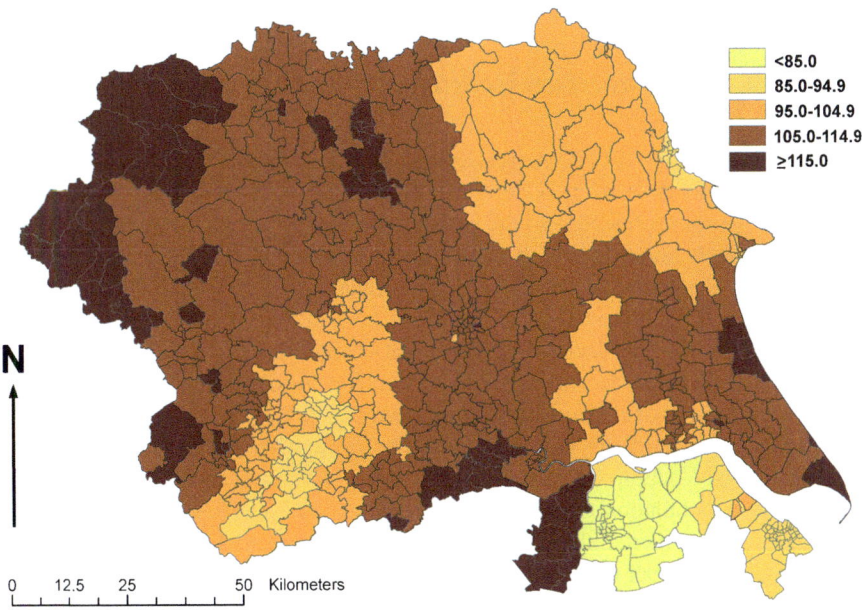

Fig. 8.2 Spatially smoothed standardised incidence ratios for childhood acute lymphoblastic leukemia diagnosed between 1986 and 1998 across electoral wards in Yorkshire, UK

Table 8.1 Incidence rate ratios (IRR) and 95% Confidence Intervals (CI) derived using the classical (frequentist) approach for Type 1 diabetes

Covariate	Unadjusted estimates		Adjusted[a] estimates	
	IRR	95% CI	IRR	95% CI
Population density				
Low	1.00		1.00	
Medium	0.92	0.77–1.09	1.01	0.83–1.23
High	0.75	0.63–0.88	0.95	0.76–1.19
Population mixing (Shannon Index)				
<10th percentile	1.50	1.11–2.02	1.29	0.94–1.78
10th–90th percentile	1.00		1.00	
>90th percentile	1.01	0.88–1.16	0.94	0.82–1.08
Townsend deprivation score				
1 Least deprived	1.00		1.00	
2	1.05	0.86–1.29	1.07	0.87–1.32
3	1.03	0.84–1.26	1.06	0.87–1.30
4	0.86	0.71–1.04	0.90	0.73–1.12
5 Most deprived	0.76	0.63–0.91	0.81	0.65–1.02

[a]Each covariate is adjusted for each of the other two covariates

covariates; for example, areas with high levels of mixing had an equal number of areas in the medium and highest population density categories. A graphical comparison between the observed counts and predicted counts from a simulated model showed good symmetry for each disease.

8.4.2 Bayesian Bivariate Modelling Approach

By modelling the effects of both disease counts together as a bivariate outcome, and assuming dependent random effects between diseases with no adjustment for covariates, we found that 50% of the variation occurred through the spatial component for diabetes and ALL, with the remainder occurring through heterogeneity effects. A modest degree of positive spatial correlation was found between diseases of 0.33 (95% CI −0.20 to 0.74).

Compared to the classical univariate model (Tables 8.1 and 8.2), the parameter estimates largely remained the same after allowing for dependent random effects and the contribution of each covariate on its own (Table 8.3). The spatial correlation between diseases fell from 0.33 to 0.18 (95% CI −0.62 to 0.82), 0.14 (−0.50 to 0.78) and 0.06 (−0.59 to 0.69), respectively, after separately accounting for population mixing, population density, and deprivation. Adding the spatial component of variation into a model already containing the heterogeneity component significantly improved model fit using the DIC.

After adjusting for all three covariates simultaneously (Table 8.4), the spatial correlation fell to 0.12 (−0.63 to 0.73), whilst the parameter estimates were similar to the adjusted IRRs presented in Tables 8.1 and 8.2 from the classical approach.

Table 8.2 Incidence rate ratios (IRR) and 95% CI derived using the classical (frequentist) approach for acute lymphoblastic leukaemia

Covariate	Unadjusted estimates		Adjusted[a] estimates	
	IRR	95% CI	IRR	95% CI
Population density				
Low	1.00		1.00	
Medium	0.92	0.62–1.38	1.14	0.72–1.79
High	0.83	0.56–1.23	1.21	0.73–2.03
Population mixing (Shannon Index)				
<10th percentile	1.36	0.67–2.74	1.27	0.59–2.75
10th–90th percentile	1.00		1.00	
>90th percentile	0.74	0.54–0.99	0.64	0.47–0.89
Townsend deprivation score				
1 Least deprived	1.00		1.00	
2	1.28	0.78–2.11	1.47	0.89–2.43
3	1.24	0.77–2.00	1.38	0.85–2.24
4	1.11	0.70–1.77	1.10	0.67–1.81
5 Most deprived	0.92	0.59–1.44	0.88	0.52–1.47

[a]Each covariate is adjusted for each of the other two covariates

Furthermore, there was little change in the proportion of variation attributable to spatial and non-spatial effects between the unadjusted and adjusted models in Tables 8.3 and 8.4. Performing a sensitivity analysis based on different prior specifications of the scale matrix showed that the fixed effect estimates and random effect variances remained largely the same, although the unadjusted spatial correlation fell to around 0.10.

A small positive spatial correlation of 0.10 (−0.55 to 0.78) and 0.13 (−0.32 to 0.55) was observed between the unstructured random effects (u_{i1} and u_{i2}) and the overall residuals ($u_{i1} + v_{i1}$ and $u_{i2} + v_{i2}$), indicating the presence of a modest correlation between the 'net' risks of each disease which was not explained by the three covariates in the model.

8.5 Discussion

In this chapter, we have shown that mapping the spatial distribution of diseases using Bayesian smoothing techniques can help to both visualise and assess the level of spatial and non-spatial variation across geographical areas. For instance, in our example with ALL and diabetes in Yorkshire, UK, we observed lower rates of disease in the more populated county of West Yorkshire and elevated rates in the less populated county of North Yorkshire.

We were also able to test for evidence of a common environmental aetiology between ALL and T1D by considering a bivariate outcome within a hierarchical framework. The similarity in risk between diseases could be quantified across small

Table 8.3 Fixed and random effects estimates (median and 95% credible intervals) from a Bayesian bivariate model with dependent errors

	[a]Population density		[a]Population mixing		[a]Deprivation	
	Diabetes	Leukemia	Diabetes	Leukemia	Diabetes	Leukemia
Random effects						
Heterogeneity	0.02 (0.00–0.04)	0.04 (0.01–0.11)	0.02 (0.00–0.04)	0.04 (0.01–0.12)	0.01 (0.00–0.04)	0.04 (0.01–0.08)
Spatial	0.01 (0.00–0.02)	0.06 (0.02–0.17)	0.02 (0.01–0.04)	0.06 (0.01–0.15)	0.01 (0.00–0.04)	0.05 (0.01–0.12)
Proportion of total variation	45% (13–79%)	59% (20–86%)	57% (18–85%)	57% (16–84%)	52% (15–87%)	56% (25–83%)
Spatial correlation	0.14 (−0.50–0.78)		0.18 (−0.62–0.82)		0.06 (−0.59–0.69)	
Fixed effects						
Population density						
Low	1.00	1.00				
Medium	0.93 (0.77–1.09)	0.99 (0.63–1.44)				
High	0.76 (0.64–0.90)	0.88 (0.59–1.28)				
Population mixing						
<10th			1.47 (1.05–1.94)	1.34 (0.60–2.48)		
10th–90th			1.00	1.00		
>90th			1.03 (0.90–1.20)	0.74 (0.53–0.99)		
Deprivation						
1 (lowest)					1.00	1.00
2					1.06 (0.85–1.32)	1.37 (0.79–2.19)
3					1.04 (0.85–1.26)	1.30 (0.73–2.07)
4					0.86 (0.71–1.04)	1.17 (0.70–1.84)
5 (highest)					0.76 (0.64–0.91)	0.98 (0.59–1.57)

[a]Models defined by the inclusion of each covariate separately without adjustment for any other fixed effects

Table 8.4 Fixed and random effects estimates (median and 95% credible intervals) from a Bayesian bivariate model with dependent errors and all three covariates considered simultaneously

	All covariates entered into the model as fixed effects	
	Diabetes	Leukemia
Random effects		
Heterogeneity	0.02 (0.00–0.06)	0.04 (0.01–0.10)
Spatial	0.01 (0.06–0.24)	0.05 (0.01–0.11)
Proportion of total variation	48% (9–85%)	52% (20–85%)
Spatial correlation	95% CI = (−0.63–0.73)	
Fixed effects		
Population density		
Low	1.00	1.00
Medium	1.02 (0.83–1.25)	1.18 (0.71–1.90)
High	0.97 (0.75–1.22)	1.29 (0.74–2.40)
Population mixing		
<10th	1.30 (0.94–1.72)	1.32 (0.58–2.49)
10th–90th	1.00	1.00
>90th	0.95 (0.81–1.08)	0.65 (0.46–0.87)
Deprivation		
1 (lowest)	1.00	1.00
2	1.08 (0.87–1.32)	1.53 (0.93–2.45)
3	1.06 (0.87–1.31)	1.43 (0.87–2.15)
4	0.91 (0.73–1.15)	1.17 (0.73–1.90)
5 (highest)	0.82 (0.65–1.01)	0.92 (0.55–1.48)

geographical areas, such that we observed a positive and statistically non-significant joint spatial correlation of 0.33 (95% CI −0.20 to 0.74). We found that the spatial correlation was attenuated once we allowed for the effects of deprivation, in contrast to less attenuation after adjusting for either population mixing or population density.

Our Bayesian smoothing approach also revealed substantial heterogeneity in incidence across Wards, accounting for half of the observed variation for each condition. The parameter estimates for all three fixed effects using a classical (frequentist) approach were almost identical to the Bayesian results, and the ability to specify prior knowledge made no difference to the results.

As with all ecological analyses, inferences derived from the results should be made with some degree of caution because estimated fixed effects at the community level may not directly resemble those at the individual level. More importantly, in modelling disease outcomes for rare conditions, such as childhood cancer and childhood diabetes, Poisson regression is prone to overdispersion where the sample variance is higher than the mean. This can often occur when counts of disease cluster within certain geographical areas, and may be difficult to ignore if we are interested in a common aetiological factor, although this extra-Poisson variation can be easily incorporated in both a Bayesian and frequentist modelling framework. Furthermore, the small disease counts across wards was difficult to overcome and we could not have determined the spatial correlation between diseases in a classical manner without smoothing incidence rates across wards using Bayesian methods.

8.6 Conclusions

A Bayesian smoothing approach in modelling the spatial correlation between diseases therefore brings a number of advantages and is particularly appropriate for these types of data. Equally, the methodology can be easily applied to other studies investigating the co-occurrence of disease incidence or mortality. Spatio-temporal modelling techniques are now emerging which allow for changing rates of disease over time, enabling much more extensive datasets spanning large time periods to be analysed. They can also be used to investigate similarities and differences in risk profiles between diseases using a shared-component model.

8.7 Further Reading

A number of books have appeared in recent times that are devoted to the field of spatial epidemiology. In particular, Lawson et al. (2003) and Lawson (2008) cover basic disease mapping and a review of multivariate disease mapping. Recently, flexible multivariate models such as Generalised Hierarchical Multivariate Conditional Autoregressive (GMCAR) and Order-free Coregionalized Lattice Models are emerging and they offer a unified approach (Jin et al. 2005). They are based on theoretical work on multivariate Gaussian Markov random fields (Mardia 1988). In addition, generalized spatial structural equation models, which handle the case of multivariate latent spatial factors, are being developed. The new class of models are versatile and practical and can account for associations between different diseases within areal units as well as the spatial association between areal units.

Acknowledgement We are grateful to Oxford University Press for permission to reproduce tables which originally appeared in the following article: American Journal of Epidemiology, Vol 161, Issue 11 , pp 1168–1180, 2005, "Detecting small-area similarities in the epidemiology of childhood acute lymphoblastic leukemia and diabetes mellitus, Type 1: a Bayesian approach."

References

Besag, J., York, J., & Mollie, A. (1991). Bayesian image restoration, with two applications in spatial statistics (with discussion). *Annals of the Institute of Statistical Mathematics, 43*, 1–75.

Clayton, D., & Kaldor, J. (1987). Empirical Bayes estimates of age-standardized relative risks for use in disease mapping. *Biometrics, 43*, 671–681.

Congdon, P. (2003). *Applied Bayesian models.* Chichester: Wiley.

Dabney, A. R., & Wakefield, J. C. (2005). Issues in the mapping of two diseases. *Statistical Methods in Medical Research, 14*, 83–112.

Feltbower, R. G., McKinney, P. A., Parslow, R. C., Stephenson, C. R., & Bodansky, H. J. (2003). Type 1 diabetes in Yorkshire, UK: Time trends in 0–14 and 15–29 year olds, age at onset and age-period-cohort modelling. *Diabetic Medicine, 20*, 437–441.

Feltbower, R. G., McKinney, P. A., Greaves, M. F., Parslow, R. C., & Bodansky, H. J. (2004). International parallels in leukemia and diabetes epidemiology. *Archives of Disease in Childhood, 89*, 54–56.

Feltbower, R. G., Manda, S. O. M., Gilthorpe, M. S., Greaves, M. F., Parslow, R. C., Kinsey, S. E., Bodansky, H. J., & McKinney, P. A. (2005). Detecting small-area similarities in the epidemiology of childhood acute lymphoblastic leukemia and diabetes mellitus, type 1: A Bayesian approach. *American Journal of Epidemiology, 161*, 1168–1180.

Gelman, A., & Rubin, D. B. (1992). Inference from iterative simulations using multiple sequences. *Statistical Science, 7*, 457–472.

Gilks, W. R., Richardson, S., & Spiegelhalter, D. J. (1996). *Markov Chain Monte Carlo in practice*. London: Chapman and Hall.

Greaves, M. (1997). Etiology of acute leukemia. *The Lancet, 349*, 344–349.

Held, L., Natario, I., Fenton, S. E., Rue, H., & Becker, N. (2006). Towards joint disease mapping. *Statistical Methods in Medical Research, 14*, 61–82.

Jin, X., Carlin, B. P., & Banerjee, S. (2005). Generalised hierarchical multivariate CAR models for areal data. *Biometrics, 6*, 539–557.

Knorr-Held, L., & Best, N. G. (2001). A shared component model for detecting joint and selective clustering of two diseases. *Journal of the Royal Statistical Society A, 164*, 73–85.

Langford, I. H., Leyland, A. H., Rasbash, J., & Goldstein, H. (1999). Multilevel modelling of the geographical distributions of diseases. *Journal of the Royal Statistical Society C, 48*, 253–268.

Lawson, A. B. (2008). *Bayesian disease mapping: Hierarchical modeling in spatial epidemiology*. Boca Raton: CRC Press.

Lawson, A. B., Browne, W. J., & Vidal Rodeiro, C. L. (2003). *Disease mapping with WinBUGS and MLwiN*. London: Wiley.

Leyland, A. H., Langford, I. H., Rabash, J., & Goldstein, H. (2000). Multivariate spatial models for event data. *Statistics in Medicine, 19*, 2469–2478.

Lunn, D. J., Thomas, A., Best, N., & Spiegelhalter, D. (2000). WinBUGS – A Bayesian modelling framework: Concepts, structure, and extensibility. *Statistics and Computing, 10*, 325–337.

Mardia, K. V. (1988). Multi-dimensional multivariate Gaussian Markov random fields with application to image processing. *Journal of Multivariate Analysis, 24*, 265–284.

McCullagh, P., & Nelder, J. A. (1989). *Generalized linear models* (2nd ed.). London: Chapman and Hall.

McKinney, P. A., Parslow, R. C., Lane, S. A., Lewis, I. J., Picton, S., Kinsey, S. E., & Bailey, C. C. (1998). Epidemiology of childhood brain tumors in Yorkshire, UK 1974–1995: Changing patterns of occurrence. *British Journal of Cancer, 78*, 974–979.

Parslow, R. C., McKinney, P. A., Law, G. R., & Bodansky, H. J. (2001). Population mixing and childhood diabetes. *International Journal of Epidemiology, 30*, 533–538.

Smith, A. F. M. (1993). Bayesian computations via the Gibbs sampler and related Markov Chain Monte Carlo methods. *Journal of the Royal Statistical Society B, 55*, 3–23.

Stiller, C. A., & Boyle, P. J. (1996). Effect of population mixing and socioeconomic status in England and Wales, 1979–85, on lymphoblastic leukemia in children. *BMJ, 313*, 1297–1300.

Townsend, P., Phillimore, P., & Beattie, A. (1988). *Health and deprivation: Inequality and the North*. London: Croom Helm.

Chapter 9
A Multivariate Random Frailty Effects Model for Multiple Spatially Dependent Survival Data

Samuel O.M. Manda, Richard G. Feltbower, and Mark S. Gilthorpe

9.1 Introduction

In the analyses of clustered failure-time data, independent and identically distributed random effects (*frailties*) are used to account for possible correlation structures between observations in the same cluster (Clayton 1991; Sastry 1997; Abrahantes et al. 2007). These developments arose from a seminal article by Vaupel et al. (1979), who introduced the notion of unobserved heterogeneity or *frailty* for univariate survival data amongst subjects. A standard model assumes a univariate random effect, which is a constant term common to the individuals in a cluster; thus these models are sometimes referred to as *shared frailty* models. Hougaard (2000) discusses a number of the specifications and the resulting inferences for shared frailty models.

The univariate random frailty models have a number of undesirable properties including the limitation that correlations amongst the observations in a cluster are positive. Additionally, all observations in a cluster are constrained to have the same frailty effect value, which might be unrealistic when there are different types of failure-time events in a cluster (Abrahantes et al. 2007). However, a greater limitation of the univariate random frailty model with independent and identically distributed random frailties is that, although they may partially account for unmeasured and unobserved covariates, they do not explicitly allow

---

S.O.M. Manda (✉)
Biostatistics Unit, South Africa Medical Research Council, Pretoria, South Africa
e-mail: samuel.manda@mrc.ac.ta

R.G. Feltbower
Division of Epidemiology, Centre for Epidemiology and Biostatistics, Leeds Institute
of Genetics, Health & Therapeutics, University of Leeds, Leeds, UK

M.S. Gilthorpe
Division of Biostatistics, Centre for Epidemiology and Biostatistics, Leeds Institute
of Genetics, Health & Therapeutics, University of Leeds, Leeds, UK

for possible spatial dependence in hazard rates among clusters that are spatially arranged (Banerjee et al. 2003). The latter may arise, for instance, through lesser variation in hazard rates in neighbouring densely urban populated areas, as opposed to sparsely populated rural areas, or through similarities in the underlying cultural and traditional beliefs affecting timing of events.

Thus, it becomes necessary to include both the effect of area under investigation and the effect of surrounding areas in modelling spatially observed time-to-event data. In this chapter, we focus on the ideas developed in Banerjee et al. (2003) by using spatially correlated survival models for failure-time data which are *spatially* arranged. However, rather than model the spatial dependence using a conventional conditional autoregressive (CAR) normal model (Besag et al. 1991), we instead use a multiple membership multiple classification (MMMC) model (Browne et al. 2001) to capture both the unstructured heterogeneity *and* spatially structured random effects. Further, we consider an extension of the univariate spatially correlated survival model (the 2-way spatial frailty effect model) to include multiple frailty effects of order $2 \times K$, where K is the number of possible failure type events that can happen to a subject. The resulting $2 \times K$ spatial random effects are modeled using a $2K$-multivariate normal model (Leyland et al. 2000). By incorporating information from all types of failure events, the resulting fixed and random parameter estimates have improved efficiency. Furthermore, similarities and differences can be made on the effect of risk factors (Manda et al. 2009), in addition to identifying event-specific risk factors, which otherwise would have been masked by well known common factors (Manda and Leyland 2007). The methods presented in this chapter are therefore somewhat similar to those in Chap. 8, where we modelled joint aggregated count data.

The proposed multivariate frailty model for correlated survival data is illustrated with an analysis of timing of first childbirth and timing of first marriage amongst women aged between 15 and 49 years across health districts in South Africa. We investigate differential patterns of early childbearing and marriage rates using key covariates – age of woman, education, type of residence and race – while accounting for possible variation in the hazard rates due to the effects of unobserved and unmeasured covariates, which may induce spatial dependence in hazard rates among women in the same health district. The excess fitted hazard risks are mapped in order to highlight parts of the country with persistent excess hazard risks for early child bearing and marriage, thereby generating in-depth epidemiological investigations on what could be causing the interjectory between the districts.

9.2 Basic Survival Model with Random Frailty Effects

We adopt a counting process construction for modelling survival data (Andersen and Gill 1982). In the set-up considered here, it is supposed there are I clusters and that the ith cluster has n_i subjects; each subject could experience any number of the K possible failure events. For event of type $k(k = 1, \ldots, K)$, subject $ij(i = 1, \ldots, I;$ $j = 1, \ldots, n_i)$ has an observed process $N_{ijk}(t)$, which counts the number of such events that have occurred to the subject by time t. In addition, a process $Y_{ijk}(t)$, which indicates whether or not the subject was at risk for the event of type k at time t, is also observed. The intensity process $\lambda_{ijk}(t)$ of event of type k for subject ij is a product of the risk indicator and the event hazard function $h_{ijk}(t)$; i.e. $\lambda_{ijk}(t) = Y_{ijk}(t)h_{ijk}(t)$. We also measure a (possibly time-varying) p-dimensional vector of risk factors $x_{ij}(t)$, where p is the number of risk factors being investigated. Thus, for subject ij, the observed data are $D = \{N_{ijk}(t), Y_{ijk}(t), x_{ij}(t); t \geq 0; k = 1, \ldots, K\}$ and are assumed independent. Furthermore, suppose $dN_{ijk}(t)$ is the increment of $N_{ijk}(t)$ in the infinitesimal interval $[t, t+dt)$ and F_{t-} are the available data just before time t, such that the increment $dN_{ijk}(t)$ is constrained to take only values 0 and 1. This constraint implies that the mean increase of $N_{ijk}(t)$ during the infinitesimal interval $[t, t+dt)$ is given by $\lambda_{ijk}(t)dt = \Pr(dN_{ijk}(t) = 1|F_{t-})$.

The effect of the risk factors on the baseline intensity function of type k for subject ij at time t is given by the Cox proportional hazards model:

$$\lambda_{ijk}\left(t|\lambda_{0k}(t), \beta_k, x_{ij}(t), w_{ik}\right) = Y_{ijk}(t)\lambda_{0k}(t)\exp(\beta_k^T x_{ij}(t) + w_{ik}) \quad (9.1)$$

where β_k is the failure-specific p-dimensional parameter vector of regression coefficients; w_{ik} is the failure-specific random effect that captures the risk of the unobserved or unmeasured risk variables; and λ_{0k} is the baseline intensity of type k event. Under non-informative censoring, the likelihood of the observed data D over all the subjects and event types is proportional to:

$$\prod_{i=1}^{I}\prod_{j=1}^{n_i}\prod_{k=1}^{K}\prod_{t\geq 0}^{T} \lambda_{ijk}(t|\lambda_{0k}(t), \beta_k, x_{ij}(t), w_{ik})^{dN_{ijk}(t)} \exp(-(\lambda_{ijk}\left(t|\lambda_{0k}(t), \beta_k, x_{ij}(t), w_{ik}\right)dt) \quad (9.2)$$

which, by taking increments $dN_{ijk}(t)$ as independent random variables, is a Poisson likelihood, where the means of the derived Poisson variables are given by $\lambda_{ijk}\left(t|\lambda_{0k}(t), \beta_k, x_{ij}(t), w_{ik}\right)dt = Y_{ijk}(t)\exp(\beta_k x_{ij}(t) + w_{ik})d\Lambda_{0k}(t)$. The function $d\Lambda_{0k}(t)$ is the increment in the integrated baseline hazard function of type k event in interval $[t, t+dt)$. The baseline hazard function is modeled as piecewise constant, where in each interval the increment $d\Lambda_{0k}(t) = dt\lambda_{0k} = dt \exp(\theta_{0k}(t))$, where $\theta_{0k}(t)$ is the piecewise log baseline hazard function.

The model described in Eq. 9.1 is the univariate shared frailty model for clustered survival data. A common approach is to model the cluster-specific event-specific random effects w_{ik} with independent and identically distributed normal and log-gamma random variables (Hougaard 2000). This specification has been based on computational easiness; however, nonparametric frailty effects are possible (Manda 2011). The univariate model in (9.1) has been extended to include both random intercepts (frailties) and random covariate effects (random coefficients) (Sargent 1998), and a number of estimation methods for such models are given in Abrahantes et al. (2007). However, these extensions are still using independent and identically distributed random variables, which now are multivariate in nature. The focus here is on models that account for possible spatial correlation in hazard among clusters that are spatially arranged. In particular, we extend the spatial survival models as described in Banerjee et al. (2003) to situations where individuals in a cluster can experience multiple failure-time events of different types. The models considered here could be termed *multivariate spatially correlated survival* models.

9.3 Multivariate Model for Correlated Cluster Frailty Eefects

As discussed in Sect. 9.1, in many epidemiological contexts it is very unlikely that health outcome risks are independent across geographical areas. For any given area *i* say, all the neighbouring areas are likely to share similar environment exposures and therefore one would expect hazards rate estimates for the area *i* to resemble those of all the adjacent areas.

In order to incorporate explicitly the spatial dependency in the data, the event-specific spatial random effect w_{ik} is split into two components – u_{ik} and v_{ik} – representing the unstructured and spatially structured random effects, respectively, in area *i*. Banerjee et al. (2003) considered the spatially structured random effect using the conditional autoregressive (CAR) normal model. Here, we adopt a multiple memberships multiple classifications (MMMC) model (Browne et al. 2001), where we use two classifications: an *area* classification, which captures non-spatial variation (classification level 2); and *neighbour* classification (classification level 3), which captures effects due to neighbouring areas.

For our application, suppose that m_i is the number of neighbours of district *i*. Within the framework of MMMC spatial modelling, the hazard risks for the timing of childbearing and the timing of marriage among women in South Africa were modelled as log-hazards:

$$\log \lambda_{ij1}(t) = \log(Y_{ij1}) + \log d\Lambda_{01}(t) + \beta_1^T x_{ij}(t) + u_{1\,district(i)}^{(2)}$$
$$+ \sum_{l \in Neighbours(i)} w_{l1} u_{l1}^{(3)} \qquad (9.3a)$$

$$\log \lambda_{ij2}(t) = \log(Y_{ij2}) + \log d\Lambda_{02}(t) + \beta_2^T x_{ij}(t) + u_{2\,district(i)}^{(2)}$$
$$+ \sum_{l \in Neighbours(i)} w_{l2} u_{l2}^{(3)} \qquad (9.3b)$$

where now $u_{ik} = u_{k\,district(i)}^{(2)} (district(i) \in (1, 2, \ldots, I))$ are the disease-specific unstructured random effects and $v_{ik} = \sum_{l \in Neighbours(i)} w_{lk} u_{lk}^{(3)}$ (Neighbour $\in (1, 2, \ldots, m_i)$) are the spatially structured random effects. The error $u_{lk}^{(3)}$ represents the effect of the lth district on other districts' hazard rates of type *k* event. The effect is captured by the weight w_{lk} indicating the relevance of the lth district to the ith district (Leyland et al. 2000). The weight could be a scaled representations of distance between two districts. The simplest model has weight given as $w_{lk}^{(3)} = 1/m_i$

if district i and j are neighbours and 0 otherwise. Thus, all districts that border a particular district are part of neighbour classification for that district. The direct district effects $u_{k_{district(i)}}^{(2)}$ are modeled as $u_k^{(2)} \sim Normal(0, \sigma_{uk(2)}^2)$ and the neighbouring district effects $u_{lk}^{(3)}$ by $u_{lk}^{(3)} \sim Normal(0, \sigma_{uk(3)}^2)$. Thus the spatial structured effect v_{ik} is normally distributed with mean 0 and variance $\sigma_{uk(3)}^2/m_i$. Thus, the between district spatial dispersion is inversely proportional to the number of neighbours a district has. We model the event-specific time-intercepts θ_{0tk} with a random walk prior $\theta_{0tk} \sim Normal(0, \sigma_0^2)$; $\theta_{0tk} \sim Normal(\alpha_{0(t-1)k}, \sigma_0^2)$ for time t ($t \geq 2$).

In order to model possible dependence in the two types of failure events, the four random effects are modelled using a multivariate normal prior distribution (Leyland et al. 2000; Manda and Leyland 2007). For simplicity, suppose ϕ_i is the overall district-level spatial vector with elements $\phi_i = (u_1^{(2)}, u_2^{(2)}, u_1^{(3)}, u_2^{(3)})$, a vector of unstructured direct district effects and neighbouring district effects for the timing of first childbirth and marriage, respectively. The random effects vector ϕ_i will usually have mean vector $\theta_\phi = (0,0,0,0)$ and covariance matrix Σ_ϕ, having diagonal elements $(\sigma_{u1(2)}^2, \sigma_{u2(2)}^2, \sigma_{u1(3)}^2, \sigma_{u2(3)}^2)$ and (upper) off-diagonal elements $(\sigma_{u1(2)u2(2)}, \sigma_{u1(2)u1(3)}, \sigma_{u1(2)u2(3)}, \sigma_{u2(2)u1(3)}, \sigma_{u2(2)u2(3)}, \sigma_{u1(3)u2(3)})$. This specification provides interpretation for variances and covariances between disease risk profiles within and between districts. For instance, the overall disease-specific district variance is given by $\sigma_{uj(2)}^2 + \sigma_{uj(3)}^2/m_i$ and the covariance between the two disease-specific direct-unstructured effects within a district is $\sigma_{u1u2(22)}$ and between the two disease-specific neighbour effects within a district is given by $\sigma_{u1u2(33)}/m_i$ from which the respective correlation coefficients are: $\sigma_{u1(2)u2(2)}/\sqrt{\sigma_{u1(2)}^2 \sigma_{u2(2)}^2}$ and $\sigma_{u1(3)u2(3)}/\sqrt{\sigma_{u1(3)}^2 \sigma_{u2(3)}^2}$ the later being a conditional correlation ince the number of neighbouring district has been omitted.

Our modelling approach also allows the computation of relative contributions of spatial and unstructured heterogeneity to the total variation of the random effects. As the unstructured and structured variances are marginal and condition, for ease of comparison, the relative contributions are obtained empirically using the sample values of the unstructured and spatial random effects (Feltbower et al. 2005).

9.4 Maternal Health in South Africa

Improvement in maternal health is one of the goals of the Millennium Development declaration (Human Sciences Research Council (HSRC) 2009). Under this goal, governments were asked to make concentrated efforts at reducing maternal mortality ratios and at increasing universal access to reproductive health services, both of which are affected by early childbearing and marriage. Early childbearing, especially among teenage mothers, exposes the mother and child to higher risk of adverse health (Sharma et al. 2003; Gupta and Mahy 2003; Magadi 2004).

On the other hand, early marriage, in the absence of using contraceptives, increases the risk of early childbearing. Thus, rising ages at first childbirth and at first marriage are important domains of public health policy-making, as they both play roles in fertility levels, maternal and child health, and women's status in a society (Kalule-Sabiti et al. 2007; Palamuleni 2011).

Improvements in social and economic conditions among the women in South Africa, and in many parts of the world, have attributed to reduction in rates of teenage childbearing and marriage (Department of Health 2002; Kalule-Sabiti et al. 2007). However, both rates have been shown to vary according to women's educational level, employment status, ethnicity, and period of birth (Kalule-Sabiti et al. 2007). There is evidence of differences in the rates by provinces, with the most economically advanced provinces (Gauteng and Western Cape) having the lowest rates of childbearing; and the predominately rural and underdeveloped provinces such as Limpopo, Eastern Cape and Mpumalanga have the highest childbearing rates (Statistics South Africa 2010). On the other hand, the more economically advanced provinces have higher rates of early marriage than provinces that are less economically advanced (Palamuleni et al. 2007).

Thus, an understanding of the factors, whether individual or ecological, affecting the risks of early childbearing and marriage among women, especially in the sub-Saharan Africa, could contribute to reductions in the maternal mortality ratios and to increases in universal access to reproductive health services. A study carried out in some sub-Saharan African countries showed that risk factors for first childbirth and first marriage are similar (Lloyd and Mensch 2006), but they used separate univariate proportional hazards models. Presently, there is a scarcity of research studies in South Africa and the region investigating spatial variation in the rates below the provincial level. One such study, carried out by Statistics South Africa (2010), only described the district level observed spatial rates in fertility, which, with all things being equal, is linked to timing of childbirth and marriage (Manda and Meyer 2005; Palamuleni 2011). However, the Statistics South Africa study did not undertake any modelling of dependence of the observed rates between districts. Thus, the lack of studies investigating childbearing and marriage rates for lower levels than provinces has adversely affected local government health-policy planning regarding maternal and reproductive health.

To the best of our knowledge, this is the first attempt to employ the recent methodological advances in spatial modelling that accounts for multiple outcomes (see, for example Chap. 8). We use joint spatial models to investigate dependence structures between and within rates of timing of childbearing and marriage. In the context of substantive issues within maternal and child health, we investigate the spatial distributions of hazard of early childbearing and marriage using spatially dependent models to account for the spatial correlation of the two maternal health events. We are not aware of any previous work that uses joint spatial hazards models to estimate geographical distribution of hazard rates for multiple maternal health outcomes, at least within the sub-Saharan African region.

9.4.1 Application Data

We use data from South African Demographic and Health Survey (SADHS) of 1998, which was a nationally representative probability sample of nearly 12,000 women between the ages of 15 and 49 years (Department of Health 2002). The women were selected using a two-stage sampling design; using enumeration areas (EAs) as primary sampling units and households as secondary sampling units. We extracted the following women-level explanatory variables for use in the models: *urban or rural residence*, used to capture effects of urbanisation and modernisation of timing of childbearing and marriage; *birth cohort*, used to capture effects of changing generations and behaviour on early childbearing and marriage; and *education level* of woman, to capture the effects of social status and modernisation of women. In addition, we model the health district spatial random effect to account for unmeasured and unobserved district-level risk factors, such as differences in social and material deprivation (this was not available for the study time) and cultural influences, both of which have been shown to contribute to differences in the timing of childbearing and marriage. Some of the observed characteristics of the sample women are shown in Table 9.1.

9.4.2 Results

In a preliminary analysis, we used the Kaplan-Meier product limit method to calculate proportion of the women that were mothers and proportion of women have been married by various ages across the different population groups. These are shown in Fig. 9.1a, b, for timing of childbearing and timing of marriage, respectively. There are ethnic differences in the timing of both childbearing and marriage. However, the ethnic effects are not systematic: while Black African and Coloured women start childbearing at younger ages than White and Indian women, Black African women enter marriage much later than White and Indian women.

We then fitted three models to the data: two separate univariate spatially correlated survival model for timing of first childbirth and first marriage, and a four-way random frailty model for the bivariate time-to-event data outcome (timing of first childbirth and first marriage). The fit of the models was implemented in WinBUGS simulation-based Bayesian estimation software (Lunn et al. 2000). For each model, we ran three parallel MCMC chains for 20,000 iterations from over-dispersed starting positions. All models had rapid mixing and convergence to the stationary distribution within 5,000 iterations. Posterior summaries were obtained using the remaining $3 \times 15{,}000 = 45{,}000$ iterations. The effects of birth cohort, type of residence, ethnicity and education on the risks of timing of first childbirth and first marriage, from fitting the various spatial models, are shown in Table 9.2, together with the various random effects parameter estimates. Since, in all three models, all the predictor effects are similar and are significant at the 5%-level, we concentrate on the hazard ratios from the multivariate frailty model.

Table 9.1 Distributions of characteristics of women aged 15–49 years, South Africa Demographic and Health Survey, 1998

Characteristic	Frequency	Percent
Birth cohort		
1948–1959	2,746	23.40
1960–1969	3,331	28.39
1970–1979	4,037	34.40
1980–1983	1,621	13.81
Place of residence		
Urban	6,518	55.54
Rural	5,217	44.46
Region of residence		
Western Cape	919	7.83
Eastern Cape	2,756	23.49
Northern Cape	1,041	8.87
Free State	936	7.98
Kwazulu-Natal	1,826	15.56
North West	931	7.96
Gauteng	1,057	9.01
Mpumalanga	1,131	9.64
Limpopo	1,138	9.70
Ethnicity of woman		
Black/African	8,993	77.03
Coloured	1,533	13.13
White	755	6.47
Asian/Indian	393	3.37
Education level of woman		
No education	810	6.90
Grade 1–7	3,134	26.71
Grade 8–11	5,175	44.10
Grade 12	1,754	14.95
Higher	862	7.35
Total	11,753	100

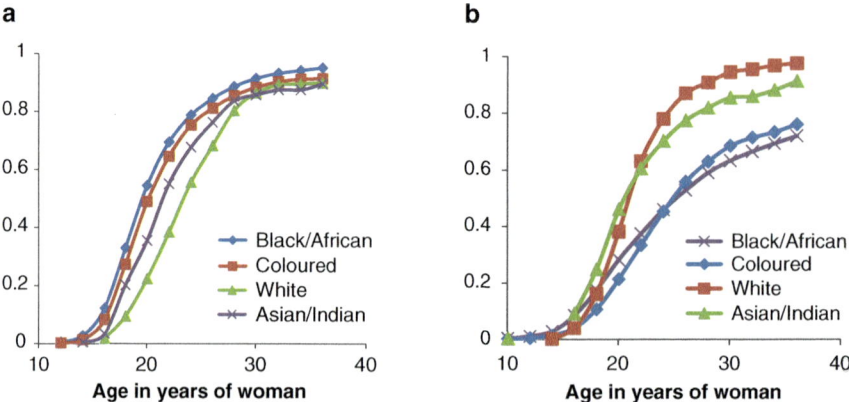

Fig. 9.1 (a) Proportion of women who are already mothers by population group. (b) Proportion of women who have been married before by population group

Overall, women born in the earlier decades before the 1980s have significantly higher rates of early childbearing and marriage. For instance, women born in the 1960s had rates of first childbirths and first marriage that are about 7 and 10 times the rates of the women born in the 1980s. Compared to women with more than 12 years of schooling years, women with lower years of education have significantly higher rates of early motherhood and marriage. In addition, women residing in the rural areas have significantly higher rates of first childbirth and marriage. Racial differences among the sampled women in the age at first childbirth and marriage are observed, with Black African and Coloured women being more likely than White and Indian women to be early mothers. On the other hand, Black African and Coloured women have rates of marriage about half that of White women. Indian and White women have similar rates for both timing of childbearing and marriage.

In all the models, the condition structured variation is larger than that for the structured variation. This is also reflected in the larger contribution of the structured random effect to the total variation. The hazard rates for timing of first marriage are more variable than those of timing of first childbirth. As the variations and contributions could not be taken as negligible, especially of the structured random effects, it indicates there are still missing important covariates that are causing spatial correlation in the observed data. The estimated fitted hazards on the log-scale for various spatial models of the risk of timing of first childbirth and timing of first marriage are shown in Fig. 9.2a–d. These figures show that both rates are highest in the north-eastern provinces of Limpopo, Mpumalanga, Kwazulu-Natal, and parts of Eastern Cape province. Districts in the most urbanised and economically advanced provinces of Gauteng and Western Cape, and metropolitan districts have lower rates of early childbearing. Most metropolitan districts, and those districts that are in the more economically developed provinces, have higher rates of early marriage than those districts that are more rural (results not shown).

9.5 Discussion

We have used recent methodological and estimation techniques in spatial epidemiology to model multiple time-to-event data that are spatially correlated. We have extended the spatially correlated survival model to enable similarities in putative risk factors to be identified by appropriate statistical modelling and estimation of the timing to first childbirth and timing to first marriage in South Africa. This has been achieved within a multiple membership multiple classification construction in modelling spatially dependent outcomes (Browne et al. 2001). The computations of the model parameters were carried out within a Bayesian hierarchical multivariate survival frailty model. In using Bayesian methods, as implemented using MCMC computational algorithms, we were able to fit and estimate a more realistic model that captures various sources of variation. We avoided the need to adopt model simplifications or approximations.

Table 9.2 Median (95% CI) hazards ratios of various background characteristics for first childbirth and first marriage by various spatially correlated survival models

Parameter	Univariate spatial models		A multivariate spatial model	
	Timing of first childbirth	Timing of first marriage	Timing of first childbirth	Timing of first marriage
Birth cohort				
1948–1959	6.502 (5.420, 8.091)	11.290 (8.617, 16.510)	6.324 (5.374, 7.831)	11.690 (8.805, 17.840)
1960–1969	6.949 (5.786, 8.625)	10.080 (7.719, 16.780)	6.743 (5.754, 8.352)	10.500 (7.849, 15.990)
1970–1979	5.357 (4.468, 6.660)	5.416 (4,125, 7.899)	5.200 (4.442, 6.434)	5.622 (4.196, 8.597)
1980–1983	1.000	1.000	1.000	1.000
Ethnicity of woman				
Black/African	1.154 (1.046, 1.271)	0.400 (0.357, 0.443)	1.151 (1.038, 1.268)	0.392 (0.353, 0.444)
Coloured	1.106 (0.983, 1.243)	0.497 (0.432, 0.570)	1.116 (0.78, 1.247)	0.503 (0.437, 0.581)
White	1.000	1.000	1.000	1.000
Asian	0.992 (0.839, 1.169)	0.919 (1.118, 1.285)	1.002 (0.851, 1.162)	0.918 (0.770, 1.081)
Place of residence				
Urban	1.000	1.000	1.000	1.000
Rural	1.119 (1.061, 1.178)	1.200 (1.118, 1.285)	1.114 (1.060, 1.177)	1.190 (1.108, 1.278)
Education of woman				
None	1.677 (1.481, 1.883)	1.900 (1.652, 2.196)	1.672 (1.483, 1.869)	1.909 (1.669, 2.181)
Grade 1–7	1.748 (1.582, 1.927)	1.779 (1.569, 2.019)	1.739 (1.577, 1.922)	1.792 (1.602, 2.019)
Grade 8–11	1.583 (1.434, 1.741)	1.401 (1.244, 1.577)	1.572 (1.424, 1.732)	1.408 (1.266, 1.571)
Grade 12	1.162 (1.049, 1.288)	1.068 (0.945, 1.206)	1.158 (1.048, 1.281)	1.074 (0.968, 1.204)
Higher	1.000	1.000	1.000	1.000
Random effects				
Unstructured standard deviation	0.029 (0.014, 0.066)	0.174 (0.107, 0.267)	0.062 (0.015, 0.098)	0.150 (0.074, 0.217)
Structured standard deviation	0.136 (0.077, 0.214)	0.372 (0.150, 0.6001)	0.102 (0.042, 0.155)	0.537 (0.350, 0.719)
Proportion structured variation	0.865 (0.397, 0.977)	0.566 (0.101, 0.830)	0.436 (0.063, 0.933)	0.730 (0.534, 0.907)
Correlation unstructured effects	–	–	0.532 (−0.331, 0.884)	
Correlation structured effects	–	–	0.887 (−0.145, 0.991)	

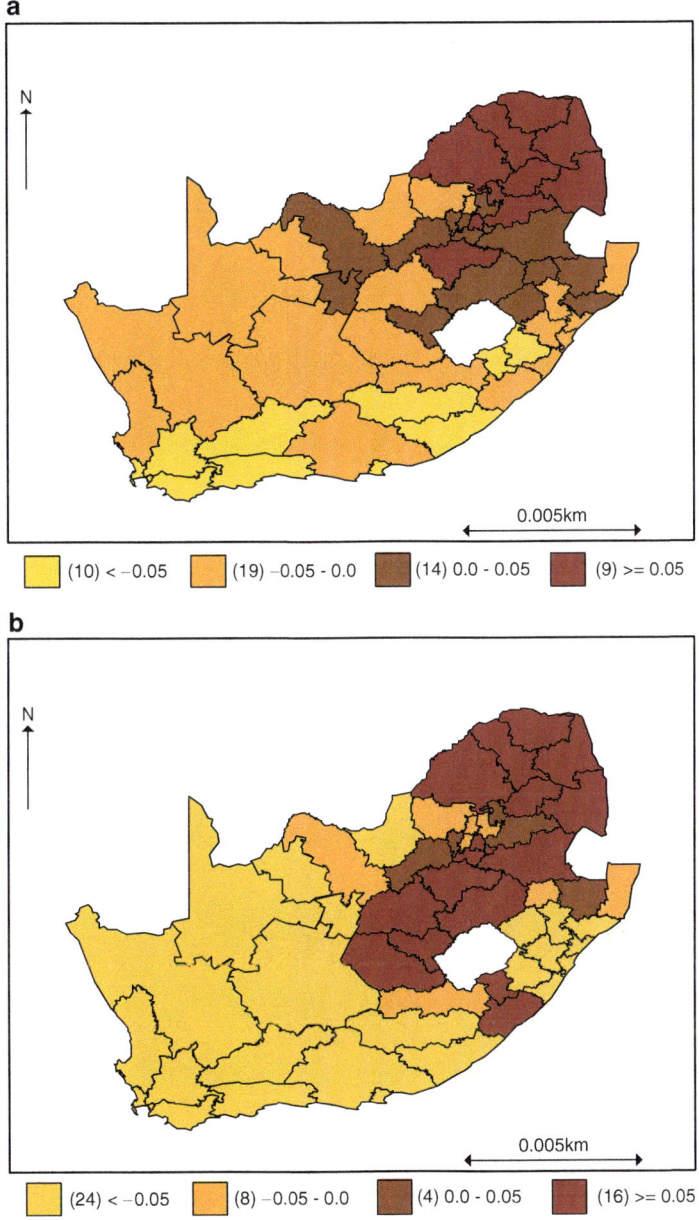

Fig. 9.2 (**a**) Estimated district level first childbirth log-hazards for the univariate spatial survival model of timing of first childbirth. (**b**) Estimated district level first marriage log-hazards for the univariate spatial survival model of timing of first marriage. (**c**) Estimated district level first childbirth log-hazards for the multivariate spatial survival model. (**d**) Estimated district level first marriage log-hazards for the multivariate spatial survival model

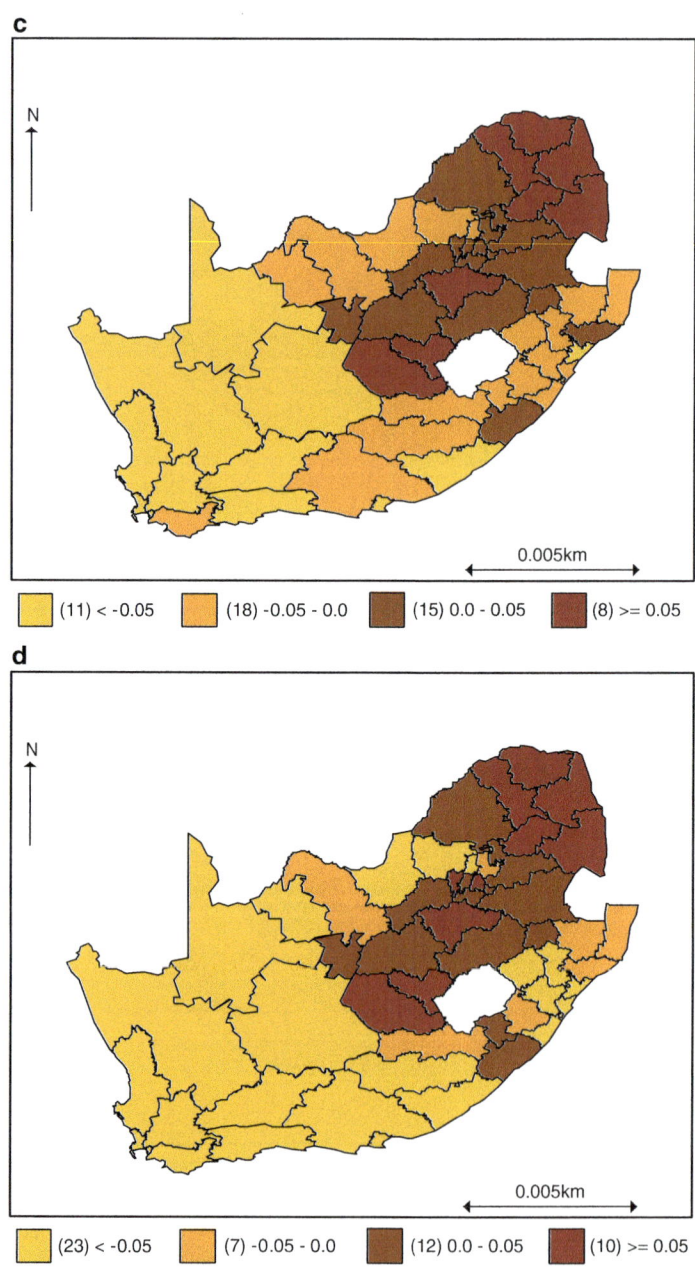

Fig. 9.2 (continued)

We investigated the effects of birth cohort, ethnicity, education and type of residence in the timing of first childbirth and marriage. This investigation is paramount in the context of public health policy; more so in measuring progress towards meeting some of the Millennium Development Goals (Human Sciences Research Council (HSRC) 2009). The fitted results of the fixed effects confirm previous findings regarding women's age, education, place of residence, and ethnic differences in the timing of first childbirth and first marriage (Palamuleni et al. 2007; Upchurch et al. 1998). These differences operate through various avenues, such as socioeconomic status and cultural differences (Jewkes et al. 2009; South 1993). The added benefits of our modelling approach has been in the generation of maps of the smoothed frailties. Such maps have the potential to reveal districts that could be targeted for further investigations, or where effective use of limited resources could optimally target maternal and child health outcomes at local government levels (Statistics South Africa 2010).

We could also have used *exceedance* maps which, rather than plotting the fitted hazard rates, show probabilities that the hazard rates exceed a certain threshold. In modelling the baseline hazards for each event, we opted for simplicity in using piecewise constant hazards for each event averaged across the districts. We could have allowed the baseline hazards to vary from district to district, as in Carlin and Hodges (1999). Under this scenario, the district-specific baseline hazard could then be modelled with an independent and identically distributed or a spatially correlated random variable, as suggested by Banerjee et al. (2003). Other extensions could be considered where the baseline hazards are modelled non-parametrically using mixture distributions (Cai and Meyer 2011).

9.6 Conclusions

We have demonstrated the utility of recent developments in the modelling of multiple events data that are spatially dependent over many small areas. These methods allow simultaneous modelling and estimation of multiple survival outcomes, where estimates of similarities and differences in the risk effects are possible, in addition to estimating within and cross spatial correlation effects. In terms of substantive issues, the methods can be applied to produce robust covariate-adjusted maps that may indicate underlying latent risk profiles. Such maps may help the search for possible persistent spatial correlations, which may suggest links with district-specific covariates and thus help policy-making bodies and stakeholders to prioritise the available resources to places and sub-groups that are in greater need. It is hoped that this work will encourage a greater uptake of these methods by researchers and practitioners in maternal and child health, especially in the developing countries where such data are routinely collected but not always appropriately analysed.

9.7 Further Reading

The concept of frailty was developed by Vaupel et al. (1979) for univariate survival data, and it was subsequently developed by Clayton (1978), Oakes (1982), Clayton (1991), Clayton and Cuzick (1985) for bivariate model based on a gamma frailty effect; the later also extending to account for covariates. Hougaard (2000) present an excellent introduction into the concepts of frailty and important different frailty model specification estimation procedures. In particular, the shared frailty models for various forms of bivariate and multivariate survival distributions are presented and exemplified with typical data sets. Most of these earlier developments have been on independent and identically distributed frailty effects. Recently, extensions to modelling spatially structured shared frailty effects have been developed and can be found in Banerjee and Carlin (2003a); Banerjee et al. (2003b); and Banerjee et al. (2004) using the CAR model. We proposed a MMMC model which was based on the concept of a multivariate spatial model outlined by Leyland et al. (2000) and Browne and colleagues (2001), which accounts for both unstructured heterogeneity and spatially structured random effects. These closely adhere to applications of previous spatial modelling carried out by Feltbower et al. (2005) and Manda et al. (2009).

References

Abrahantes, J. C., Legrand, C., Burzykowski, T., Janssen, P., Ducrocq, V., & Duchateau, L. (2007). Comparison of different estimation procedures for proportional hazards model with random effects. *Computational Statistics and Data Analysis, 51*, 3913–3930.

Andersen, P. K., & Gill, R. D. (1982). Cox's regression models for counting processes. *The Annals of Statistics, 10*, 1100–1120.

Banerjee, S., & Carlin, B. P. (2003). Semiparametric spatio-temporal frailty modeling. *Environmetrics, 14*, 523–535.

Banerjee, S., Wall, M. M., & Carlin, B. P. (2003). Frailty modeling for spatially correlated survival data, with application to infant mortality in Minnesota. *Biostatistics, 4*, 123–142.

Banerjee, S., Carlin, B. P., Alan, E., & Gelfand, A. E. (2004). *Hierarchical modeling and analysis for spatial data*. Boca Raton: Chapman & Hall.

Besag, J., York, J., & Mollie, A. (1991). Bayesian image restoration, with two applications in spatial statistics (with discussion). *Annals of the Institute of Statistical Mathematics, 43*, 1–59.

Browne, W. J., Goldstein, H., & Rasbash, J. (2001). Multiple membership multiple classification (MMMC). *Statistical Modelling, 1*, 103–124.

Cai, B., & Meyer, R. (2011). Bayesian semiparametric modeling of survival data based on mixtures of B-spline distributions. *Computational Statistics and Data Analysis, 55*, 1260–1272.

Carlin, B. P., & Hodges, J. S. (1999). Hierarchical proportional hazards regression models for highly stratified data. *Biometrics, 55*, 1162–1170.

Clayton, D. G. (1978). A model for association in bivariate life tables and its application in epidemiological studies of familial tendency in chronic disease incidence. *Biometrika, 65*, 141–152.

Clayton, D. G. (1991). A Monte Carlo method for Bayesian inference in frailty models. *Biometrics, 47*, 467–485.

Clayton, D. G., & Cuzick, J. (1985). Multivariate generalizations of the proportional hazards model (with discussion). *Journal of the Royal Statistical Society A, 148*, 82–117.

Department of Health, Medical Research Council, Measure DHS+. (2002). *South Africa Demographic and Health Survey 1998*. Pretoria: Department of Health.

Feltbower, R. G., Manda, S. O. M., Gilthorpe, M. S., Greaves, M. F., Parslow, R. C., Kinsey, S. E., Bodansky, H. J., Patricia, A., & McKinney, P. A. (2005). Detecting small area similarities in the epidemiology of childhood acute lymphoblastic leukaemia and type 1 diabetes: A Bayesian approach. *American Journal of Epidemiology, 161*, 1168–1180.

Gupta, N., & Mahy, M. (2003). Adolescent childbearing in sub-Saharan Africa: Can increased schooling alone raise ages at first birth? *Demographic Research, 8*, 93–106.

Hougaard, P. (2000). *Analysis of multivariate survival data*. New York: Springer.

Human Sciences Research Council. (2009) *Teeange pregnancy in South Africa-with specific focus on school-going children* (Full report). Pretoria: Human Sciences Research Council.

Jewkes, R., Morrell, R., & Christofides, N. (2009). Empowering teen ages to prevent pregnancy: Lessons from South Africa. *Culture, Health and Sexuality, 11*, 675–688.

Kalule-Sabiti, I., Palamuleni, M., Makiwane, M., & Amoateng, A. Y. (2007). Family formation and dissolution patterns. In A. Y. Amoateng & T. B. Heaton (Eds.), *Families and households in post-apartheid South Africa: Socio-demographic perspectives* (pp. 89–112). Cape Town: HSRC Press.

Leyland, A. H., Langford, I. H., Rasbash, J., & Goldstein, H. (2000). Multivariate spatial models for event data. *Statistics in Medicine, 19*, 2469–2478.

Lloyd, C. B., & Mensch, B. S. (2006). *Marriage and childbirth as factors in school exit: An analysis of DHS data from sub-Saharan Africa*. New York: Population Council.

Lunn, D. J., Thomas, A., Best, N., & Spiegelhalter, D. (2000). WinBUGS: A Bayesian modelling framework: concepts, structure, and extensibility. *Statistics and Computing, 10*, 325–337.

Magadi, M. (2004). Poor pregnancy outcomes among adolescents in South Nyansa region of Kenya. Working paper: A04/04 Statistical Sciences Research Institute. University of Southampton.

Manda, S. O. M. (2011). A nonparametric frailty model for clustered survival data. *Communications in Statistics – Theory and Methods, 40*(5), 863–875.

Manda, S. O. M., & Leyland, A. (2007). An empirical comparison of maximum likelihood and Bayesian estimation methods for multivariate spatial disease model. *South African Statistical Journal, 41*, 1–21.

Manda, S. O. M., & Meyer, R. (2005). Age at first marriage in Malawi: A Bayesian multilevel analysis using a discrete time-to-event model. *Journal of the Royal Statistical Society A, 168*, 439–455.

Manda, S. O. M., Feltbower, R. G., & Gilthorpe, M. S. (2009). Investigating spatio-temporal similarities in the epidemiology of childhood leukaemia and diabetes. *European Journal of Epidemiology, 24*, 743–752.

Oakes, D. (1982). A concordance test for independence in the presence of censoring. *Biometrics, 38*, 451–455.

Palamuleni, M. E. (2011). Socioeconomic determinant of age at first marriage in Malawi. *International Journal of Sociology and Anthropology, 3*, 224–235.

Palamuleni, M. E., Kalule-Sabiti, I., Makiwane, M. (2007). Fertility and child bearing in South Africa. In A. Y. Amoateng & T. B. Heaton (Eds.), *Families and households in post-apartheid South Africa: Sociol-demographics perspectives* (pp. 113–134). Cape Town: HSRC Press.

Sargent, D. J. (1998). A general framework for random effects survival analysis in the Cox proportional hazards setting. *Biometrics, 54*, 1486–1497.

Sastry, N. (1997). A nested frailty model for survival data, with an application to the study of child survival in northeast Brazil. *Journal of the American Statistical Association, 92*, 426–435.

Sharma, A. K., Verma, K., & KhatriS, K. A. T. (2003). Determinants of pregnancy in adolescents in Nepal. *Indian Journal of Paediatrics, 69*, 19–22.

South, S. J. (1993). Racial and ethnic differences in the desire to marry. *Journal of Marriage and Family, 55*, 357–370.

Statistics South Africa. (2010). *Estimation of fertility from the 2007 Community Survey of South Africa/Statistics South Africa*. Pretoria: Statistics South Africa.

Upchurch, D. M., Levy-Storms, L., Sucoff, C. A., & Aneshensel, C. S. (1998). Gender and ethnic differences in the timing of first sexual intercourse. *Family Planning Perspectives, 30*, 121–127.

Vaupel, J. W., Manton, K. G., & Stallard, E. (1979). The impact of heterogeneity in individual frailty on the dynamics of mortality. *Demography, 16*, 439–454.

Chapter 10
Meta-analysis of Observational Studies

Darren C. Greenwood

10.1 Introduction

Meta-analysis has become a popular means of pooling estimates from a number or randomised controlled trials (RCTs) where there remains uncertainty over the benefit of particular interventions. Similar uncertainty can exist in observational epidemiology when a number of studies provide contradictory results. However, observational studies such as those used to investigate lifecourse epidemiology present particular challenges for meta-analysis (Sutton et al. 2000). Results are often prone to large heterogeneity because of different populations sampled, different designs, different outcome or exposure definitions, adjustment for different covariates, and vulnerability to biases that randomised controlled trials are largely immune from.

Even if the studies are conducted and analysed in identical fashion, results may be presented in a number of different ways in the different publications. Relative risks may have been presented for a unit increment of a continuous exposure, giving the linear trend. Alternatively, the exposure may have been categorised into groups containing equal numbers of individuals, or some other categorisation, with relative risks for each category compared with a reference category. This categorisation could be into any number of groups.

The potential bias introduced by such categorisation is a form of measurement error, and is discussed in Chap. 2. Alternatively the data may have been presented as mean exposure for cases compared to controls. In this chapter methods for meta-analysis of observational studies are illustrated using a real example from a meta-analysis in the field of diet and cancer.

D.C. Greenwood (✉)
Division of Biostatistics, Centre for Epidemiology and Biostatistics,
Leeds Institute of Genetics, Health & Therapeutics, University of Leeds, Leeds, UK
e-mail: D.C.Greenwood@leeds.ac.uk

10.2 General Principles

For meta-analysis to be possible, all the differently presented results from the observational studies need to be converted to one metric. Combining studies with entirely different designs, e.g. cohort and case-control studies, is often unreasonable, and so analyses should be stratified by design and separate estimates presented (Sutton et al. 2000). Even so, substantial heterogeneity is common between studies of the same design, due to different population structures and adjustment for confounding. It is important to characterise these differences in tables and to explore any heterogeneity using standard tools such as stratified forest plots and meta-regression techniques.

Epidemiologists sometimes like to compare extreme categories of exposure, such as the highest versus lowest categories. Although this allows most studies to be combined, this is often unwise for the following reasons: categorisation often differs between studies, definition of quantiles depends on the population exposure distribution, and categorisation loses information by introducing measurement error (see Chap. 2). These issues introduce unwanted heterogeneity that often render the combined estimates useless. The common metric that reduces these problems is to present results as a linear dose-response trend.

10.3 Statistical Methods for Deriving Dose-Response

To allow these different studies to be included in the same meta-analysis, all results need to be converted to a relative risk for a unit increase of exposure, giving a linear dose-response trend. This is done using the methods attributable to Greenland and Longnecker (1992) (the "pool last" approach) and Chêne and Thompson (1996). The method of Greenland and Longnecker is particularly useful in that it (i) provides dose-response estimates that take account of the correlation between the estimates for each category induced by using the same reference group (Berlin et al. 1993; Greenland and Longnecker 1992), and (ii) enables derivation of dose-response relative risk estimates that are adjusted for whatever confounding factors were considered in the particular study.

Using the notation given in Greenland and Longnecker (1992), these methods are applied in the following steps:

Step 1. Use an iterative algorithm to estimate the cell counts A_x and B_x, where A_x is the fitted number of cases at exposure level x and B_x is the number of non-cases.

Step 2. Let L_x be the adjusted log relative risk for exposure level x when $x \neq 0$ compared to the reference level (assumed to be $x = 0$). For $x \neq z$, estimate the correlation r_{xz} between L_x and L_z by $r_{xz} = (1/A_0 + 1/B_0)/s_x s_z$ for case-control studies, $r_{xz} = (1/A_0 - 1/B_0)/s_x s_z$ for cohort studies without person-time, and $r_{xz} = 1/(A_0 s_x s_z)$ for cohorts involving person-time, where s_x^2 is the crude variance estimate. Calculating s_x^2 depends on the study type too: $s_x^2 = (1/A_x + 1/B_x + 1/A_0 + 1/B_0)$ for case-control studies, $s_x^2 = (M_1/A_xA_0 - 1/N_0 - 1/N_x)$ for cohort studies without person-time, and $s_x^2 = M_1/A_xA_0$ for cohort studies with person-time data, where N_x is the total number of subjects at exposure level x, and M_1 is the total number of cases.

Step 3. Estimate the covariance c_{xz} of L_x and L_z by $c_{xz} = r_{xz}\sqrt{v_x v_z}$ where v_x is the estimated variance of L_x.

Step 4. Estimate the dose-response slope b^* (and the variance of its estimate, v_b^*) by weighted least squares for correlated outcomes as follows: $b^* = v_b^* \mathbf{x}'C^{-1}\mathbf{L}$ and $v_b^* = (\mathbf{x}'C^{-1}\mathbf{x})^{-1}$ where $\mathbf{x}$ is the vector of exposure levels excluding the reference level, and C is the estimated covariance matrix of $\mathbf{L}$, and has diagonal element v_x and off-diagonal element c_{xz}. When the mean exposure in the reference category is non-zero, appropriate subtraction from the remaining category means is required. For linear trends this is simply subtracting the mean for the reference category from all category means.

The information required to derive a dose-response is not presented in the majority of papers and a number of approaches should taken in order to derive the information required. These need to be applied in the following order of priority:

1. Where the exposure is measured as a continuous variable, and the dose-response slope given, then this should be used directly. This does not allow extension to nonlinear trends. Where nonlinear trends need to be modelled, results based on three or more categories are required.
2. Where the slope (and its standard error or confidence interval) is not given in the text, these should be estimated using the methods of Greenland and Longnecker (1992) using the mean exposure in each category given in the paper. No additional assumptions are required.
3. Greenland and Longnecker's method requires the total numbers of cases and controls to be known, and starting estimates for the number of cases in each category. Where these are not presented, values should be estimated based on the ratio of cases to controls, the basis for any categorisation using quantiles (whether based on the whole population or just controls), or on the information contained in each category estimated from the width of the confidence intervals.
4. The mean exposure for each category is rarely given, so the methods of Chêne and Thompson(1996) can be used to estimate the means for use in the Greenland and Longnecker technique. This approach makes the assumption of a normally distributed exposure, or a distribution that could be transformed to normality. Many environmental or dietary exposures will follow a lognormal distribution adequately enough for these purposes. This is not necessarily the case for exposures where a large group of unexposed individuals may reasonably be assumed to come from a separate distribution, i.e. zero-inflated, or a mixture of two distributions. Episodically consumed foods such as alcohol or meat are two examples where this approach may not

be appropriate. Where an unexposed group can be treated separately, this may still allow the remainder of category means to be modelled, providing enough categories exist.
5. Where it is not possible to derive mean exposures for each category, the midpoints can be used instead as a basis for the Greenland and Longnecker technique.
6. Where no confidence intervals for estimates (RR or OR) are given in the paper, but approximate standard errors can be obtained from the cell counts, these can be used to derive approximate confidence intervals for the adjusted estimates. Greenland and Longnecker's method can then be applied using means or midpoints, as described above.
7. Using the methods of Chêne and Thompson, one can also derive an estimate of the dose-response slope through a weighted logistic regression if the mean exposure for cases and controls is known. This method also requires the numbers of cases and controls to be known, and a measure of variability such as standard deviation for each group. Unless the means presented were adjusted means, this would yield an unadjusted estimate.
8. Where the above methods cannot be used, the methods of Chêne and Thompson can still be applied to derive a dose-response curve directly from cell counts, if individual cell counts are provided. This estimate would unfortunately be unadjusted for any confounding, even if the relative risks presented in the study were adjusted, because it is only based on the cell counts.
9. Where these fail, a comparison based on the extreme categories can be used to estimate the dose-response trend, ignoring the information from categories in-between. This still requires information to quantify the exposure so the mean exposure in each category can be estimated. This does not allow extension to nonlinear curves.

Alternative methods to those of Greenland and Longnecker are possible, so long as the correlation structure is properly modelled, e.g. using a Bayesian framework.

10.4 Information Required for Meta-analysis

The quality of presentation of results of observational studies lags behind randomised controlled trials (Elm et al. 2007). It is therefore common to find insufficient information for the dose-response to be estimated from one of the above approaches. To be included, they need one of the following combinations of pieces of information to be derivable or at least approximately estimable:

- Dose-response slope and measure of uncertainty, i.e. standard error or confidence interval.
- Mean exposure in each category, the total number of cases and controls, estimated relative risks for each category, a way of quantifying uncertainty around these estimates, e.g. confidence intervals.

- Range of exposure for each category, the total number of cases and controls, estimated relative risks for each category, a way of quantifying uncertainty around these estimates, e.g. confidence intervals.
- Mean exposure for cases and controls separately, number of cases and controls, along with a measure of uncertainty in the mean, e.g. standard deviation or standard error.

The method of Greenland and Longnecker should be applied using standard errors that depend on the study type (cohort) and the form of the relative risk estimate (relative risk or odds ratio). For these cohort studies, relative risks derived from person-years of exposure should also be taken into account if presented. For the purpose of meta-analysis, it may be possible for estimates of relative risk to be treated as good approximations because of the outcome, i.e. odds ratios may be considered as a good approximation to the relative risk in some situations (Greenland et al. 1986; Greenland and Thomas 1982).

10.5 Excluding Studies

Where the information required for meta-analysis is not available, studies cannot be included in that meta-analysis. As discussed above, whilst allowing wider inclusion of studies, comparison of extreme categories introduces heterogeneity.

For example, as part of the World Cancer Research Fund and American Institute for Cancer Research series of systematic literature reviews of *"Food, Nutrition, Physical Activity and the Prevention of Cancer"*, a systematic review was conducted of the association between processed meat intake and gastric cancer (World Cancer Research Fund/American Institute for Cancer Research 2007). All original, aetiological, peer-reviewed studies were considered with no exclusions on the basis of study quality or publication date, or language. Data were extracted from 29 studies, but of these, only 17 studies (59%) contained sufficient information to contribute to the dose-response meta-analysis. Of these, 9 were case-control studies prone to substantial recall and selection biases, leaving just 8 cohort studies, 28% of the initial number of studies extracted. It is typical for the more recent studies to provide better quality information. Similarly a greater proportion of cohort studies tend to contain more information useable for meta-analysis than the case-control studies, although in some fields cohort studies are rare.

10.6 Selecting Results to Include

Cohort studies sometimes publish more than one paper from the same study, separated by a number of years' follow-up. In this situation the paper containing the larger number of cases should usually be used, which is often the most recent paper. In the even more common situation where the same exposure is analysed in several ways, with different levels of adjustment, a decision needs to be made regarding which model is the one with the "most appropriate" adjustment for confounding. The most appropriate adjustment is often the maximally adjusted analysis given in the paper, or the one with the narrower confidence intervals. However, the best model is not always the maximally adjusted one and sometimes a model with less adjustment is more appropriate because it avoids collinearity and over-adjustment (see Chap. 1). Where estimates are presented only by subgroup, e.g. men and women, then the subgroups can be included in the meta-analysis separately and give valid overall pooled estimates. However, this leads to underestimation of the heterogeneity by including the same study as an apparently independent observation, and incorrect degrees of freedom in the test for heterogeneity, so it is better to first pool these subgroup results and include this pooled estimate as the single result from that study.

10.7 Separate Zero Exposure Groups

Where there was a category representing a zero exposure, i.e. non-consumers, then this presents a situation similar to that discussed in Chap. 6. For the purposes of estimating the category means required for Greenland and Longnecker's method, this zero category may be treated separately for the purposes of estimating means in each category. For example, for processed meat intake, this would include vegetarians. Such "never" categories often lead to a peak in the distribution at zero, which means that the data follow neither a normal nor a lognormal distribution. By using a mean of zero for the "never" category and estimating means for the other categories separately, this allows distributional assumptions to be made for the remaining exposure categories, and therefore more studies can be included in a meta-analysis.

10.8 Presentation

Because of the large potential for heterogeneity in meta-analysis of observational studies, it is often appropriate to present both fixed and random effects estimates. It is also helpful to view the trends in relative risk estimates across each study visually, and to present scatter plots with the area of the circles plotted for each estimate being proportional to the precision associated with that estimate. These plots aid assessment of linearity of response.

When assessing whether estimates from smaller studies differ from larger studies, either visually using funnel plots, or using Begg's test or Egger's test, it is important to consider this assessment as investigating "small study bias" rather than "publication bias". That is because there are other possible causes for this effect other than differential probability of publication. In observational studies it is possible that smaller studies are less biased, if they are carried out in more detail, whereas large studies may contain poorer exposure measures.

Finally, a checklist has been developed that summarizes recommendations for reporting meta-analyses of observational studies, known as the Meta-analysis Of Observational Studies in Epidemiology (MOOSE) guidelines. (Stroup et al. 2000) The checklist covers reporting of the relevant background, search strategies, methods, presentation and discussion of results, and how conclusions are reported.

10.9 Practical Example

10.9.1 Introduction and Methods

The World Cancer Research Fund and American Institute for Cancer Research series of systematic literature reviews of *"Food, Nutrition, Physical Activity and the Prevention of Cancer"* form a seminal series of meta-analyses of observational studies (World Cancer Research Fund/American Institute for Cancer Research 2007). All original, aetiological, peer-reviewed studies were considered with no exclusions on the basis of study quality or publication date, or language. Studies were identified through a comprehensive literature search (Butrum et al. 2006). One of the reviews conducted was of the association between processed meat intake and gastric cancer. Data were extracted from eight cohort studies (Galanis et al. 1998; Gonzalez et al. 2006; Khan et al. 2004; McCullough et al. 2001; Ngoan et al. 2002; Nomura et al. 1990; van den Brandt et al. 2003; Zheng et al. 1995).

In order to combine studies presenting results as portions of processed meat with those presenting results as grams of intake, a standard portion size was used to convert portions to grams, based on standard food tables (Ministry of Agriculture 1988).

10.9.2 Results

Study characteristics are given in Table 10.1 with category definitions and relative risk estimates given in Table 10.2. It is sometimes helpful to also to show these results graphically for each study, converted into standard portion sizes. The forest plot shows results for both the fixed effects with inverse-variance weighting ("I-V overall") and DerSimonian and Laird random effects ("D+L overall") analyses (DerSimonian and Laird 1986) (Fig. 10.1). The fixed effects estimate of relative risk was 1.02 (95% CI: 1.00–1.05) per 20 g/day of processed meat. There was hardly any excess heterogeneity within the cohort studies ($I^2 = 1\%$). The random effects estimate of relative risk was almost the same as the fixed effects estimate because there was very little excess heterogeneity (relative risk = 1.03, 95% CI: 1.00–1.05).

Table 10.1 Study characteristics

Author (Year)	Country and subject characteristics	Age (mean)	Subjects' gender	N cases	Size of cohort	Case ascertainment	Follow up, loss to follow up	Dietary method	Covariate adjustment						
									Age	Sex	SES	Other nutrients	Smoking	Energy intake
Nomura et al. (1990)	USA, Japanese residents of Hawaii	45+	M	150	7,990	Hospital records	19 years, 1.3% lost	FFQ	Y					
Zheng et al. (1995)	USA, mostly white, post-menopausal	55–69	F	26	34,691	Cancer registry	7 years, <1% lost per year	FFQ	Y		Y		Y	
Galanis et al. (1998)	USA, Japanese residents of Hawaii	18+ (46)	M/F	108	11,907	Cancer registry	14.8 years, 10.7% lost	FFQ	Y	Y	Y			
McCullough et al. (2001)	USA, multi-ethnic	30+	M	910	435,744	Death register	14 years, 1.2% lost	FFQ	Y		Y	Y	Y	
McCullough et al. (2001)	USA, multi-ethnic	30+	F	439	532,952	Death register	14 years, 1.2% lost	FFQ	Y		Y	Y	Y	
Ngoan et al. (2002)	Japan	15–96 (60)	M/F	62	13,250	Resident registry	13 years, <1% lost	FFQ	Y	Y		Y	Y	
van den Brandt et al. (2003)	Netherlands	55–69	M/F	282	120,852	Cancer registry	6.3 years, none lost	FFQ	Y	Y	Y		Y	
Khan et al. (2004)	Japan	40+ (58)	M	36	1,488	Multiple methods	14 years, 8.5% lost	FFQ	Y				Y	
Khan et al. (2004)	Japan	40+ (58)	F	15	1,619	Multiple methods	14 years, 8.5% lost	FFQ	Y				Y	
Gonzalez et al. (2006)	Europe, multi-ethnic	35–70 (52)	M/F	330	521,457	Cancer registry	6.5 years, % lost not reported	FFQ + 24 h-recall	Y	Y	Y	Y	Y	Y

10 Meta-analysis of Observational Studies

Table 10.2 Category definitions and relative risks. 95% confidence intervals are given in parentheses

Author (Year)	Subjects' gender	Reference category	Category 2	Category 3
Nomura et al. (1990)	M	0–1 times/week RR = 1.0	2–4 times/week RR = 1.0 (0.7, 1.4)	5+ times/week RR = 1.3 (0.9, 2.0)
Zheng et al. (1995)	F	0–4.4 times/month RR = 1.0	4.4–12 times/month RR = 0.9 (0.3, 2.9)	13+ times/month RR = 2.2 (0.8, 6.0)
Galanis et al. (1998)	M/F	0 times/week RR = 1.0	1–2 times/week RR = 0.9 (0.6, 1.4)	3+ times/week RR = (0.6, 1.7)
McCullough et al. (2001)	M	0–0.9 days/week RR = 1.00	1–4.4 days/week RR = 1.03 (0.86, 1.23)	4.5+ days/week RR = 1.08 (0.87, 1.33)
McCullough et al. (2001)	F	0–1.4 days/week RR = 1.0	1.5–2.9 days/week RR = 0.99 (0.79, 1.24)	3+ days/week RR = 1.11 (0.88, 1.39)
Ngoan et al. (2002)	M/F	2–4 times/month RR = 1.0	2–4 times/week RR = 0.7 (0.3, 1.3)	1+ times/day RR = (0.8, 5.4)
van den Brandt et al. (2003)	M/F	0 g/day RR = 1.00	0.1–3.0 g/day RR = 0.86 (0.63, 1.17)	3.1+ g/day RR = 0.95 (0.67, 1.35)
Khan et al. (2004)	M	0–3 times/month RR = 1.0	2–7 times/week RR = 1.0 (0.5, 2.1)	
Khan et al. (2004)	F	0–3 times/month RR = 1.0	2–7 times/week RR = 0.7 (0.2, 2.6)	
Gonzalez et al. (2006)	M/F	RR = 2.11 (1.08, 4.14) per 50 g/day increment		

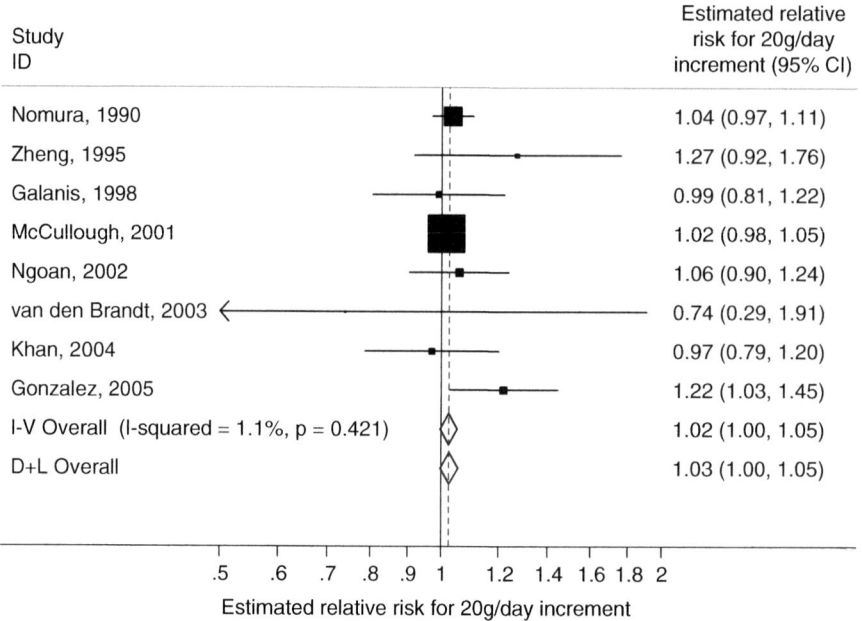

Fig. 10.1 Forest plot for fixed-effects meta-analysis ignoring measurement error

What little heterogeneity existed was explored by meta-regression on each of the following factors specified *a priori*: year of publication, mean age, gender, ethnicity and nationality of study participants, dietary assessment method used, number of categories used to define the exposure, statistical method used to derive dose-response slope, unit of exposure measurement, adjustment for age, sex, smoking, *helicobacter pylori* status, socio-economic status, alcohol consumption, anthropometric measures, total energy intake, ethnicity, family history of gastric cancer, nutrient intake, non-nutrient intake, physical activity, other concomitant diseases, and presence of infection, either by matching or through modelling. There was no strong evidence that any of these factors were associated with variation in the estimates.

Egger's test suggested no evidence of any small-study bias, though power for this test would be low. The possibly more informative funnel plot showed no evidence of asymmetry.

In addition to the sensitivity analyses outlined previously, each individual study was omitted in turn to investigate the sensitivity of the pooled estimates to inclusion or exclusion of particular studies. No single study had any great influence on the pooled estimate; exclusion of no one study caused the pooled estimates to change substantially.

10.10 Correcting for Measurement Error in Pooled Estimates

Substantial work has been done by others on correction for the effects of missing data in the context of meta-analysis, allowing for the uncertainty that it introduces using Bayesian methods (Sutton et al. 2000; White et al. 2008a, b). In simple situations it is possible to apply the methods described in Chap. 2 to the estimates from each study before pooling, to correct for the effects of measurement error on pooled estimates in meta-analysis. A particular problem for meta-analysis of published data is that the exposure is often presented in categorized form, thus suffering from loss of information and associated bias introduced by this form of measurement error. Bayesian methods can be used to address these issues, with the benefit of taking into account the uncertainty in the measurement error variance, and flexibility for use with non-additive or non-classical measurement error mechanisms.

10.11 Nonlinear Trends and Meta-Analysis

10.11.1 Methods

So far the methods described have assumed that there is a linear dose-response curve. It is possible that the curve is nonlinear, and for some exposures, particularly dietary components such as alcohol intake, this is likely. Considering a non-linear dose-response curve is not possible using Greenland and Longnecker's "pool last" approach outlined in Sect. 10.3, i.e. slopes derived before pooling, but is possible if means and covariance matrices from individual studies are pooled *before* estimating the slopes, known as the "pool first" approach (Greenland and Longnecker 1992).

One way to fit a nonlinear curve, using the "pool first" approach within Stata, is to select the best fitting nonlinear dose-response curve from a limited but flexible family of fractional polynomials (Bagnardi et al. 2004; Royston et al. 1999; Royston and Altman 1994, 2000). For the example in this chapter, the family of second-order fractional polynomials were used with $\ln(RR|x) = \beta_1 x^p + \beta_2 x^q$, with p and q taking values of $-2, -1, -0.5, 0, 0.5, 1, 2, 3$. When p or q are zero, x^p or x^q are taken to be $\ln(x)$. When p = q, the model is taken as $\ln(RR|x) = \beta_1 x^p + \beta_2 x^q \ln(x)$. These provided simple models but still with a good range of possible curves, including a range of commonly observed tick-shaped (J-shaped) and U-shaped curves. The best model was the one that gave the most improvement (decrease) in deviance compared to the linear model.

The "pool-first" approach is similar to the "pool-last" approach outlined in Sect. 10.3 but more flexible for including covariates. Using the same notation as

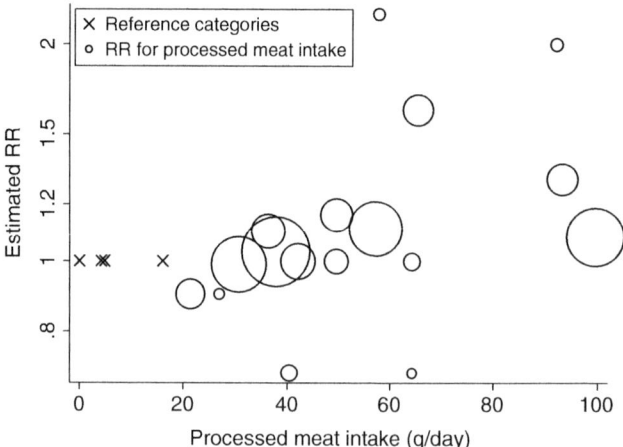

Fig. 10.2 Scatterplot of ln(RR) vs. processed meat. The area of the circle representing each estimate is proportional to the precision associated with that estimate. Reference categories are indicated by points with ln(RR) = 0

before, let $\mathbf{x}_k$, and $\mathbf{L}_k$ be vectors of exposure levels for study k excluding the reference levels, C_k be the estimated covariance matrix for $\mathbf{L}_k$, G be a block-diagonal matrix whose kth diagonal block is C_k^{-1}. The pooled estimate of the coefficients $\hat{\beta}$ is $VX'G\mathbf{L}$, with estimated covariance matrix $V = (X'GX)^{-1}$. The model fit can be assessed by comparing $\mathbf{e}'G\mathbf{e}$ to a chi-squared distribution on degrees of freedom equal to the number of elements in $\mathbf{e} - 2$, where $\mathbf{e}$ is the vector of residuals $\mathbf{e} = \mathbf{L} - X\hat{\beta}$.

When the mean exposure in the reference category is non-zero, the value of the fractional polynomial function evaluated at the mean of the reference category needs to be subtracted first.

10.11.2 Results

A scatterplot of log relative risk of gastric cancer against level of processed meat intake was plotted with the area of the plotting symbol proportional to the precision of the relative risk associated with it. This represents the raw data extracted in a way that summarises the observations clearly on one graph (Fig. 10.2).

The best fitting fractional polynomial (based on the deviance) was $\ln(RR|x) = \beta_1 x^3 + \beta_2 x^3 \ln(x)$ with $\beta_1 = 6.17 \times 10^{-6}$ (s.e. $= 3.35 \times 10^{-6}$) and $\beta_2 = {}^-1.31 \times 10^{-6}$ (s.e. $= 7.30 \times 10^{-7}$).

The coefficients appear small because of the size of x^3 and $x^3 \ln x$. This model had the lowest deviance (Chi-squared goodness of fit test $= 9.0$, on 13 df, $p = 0.78$) but

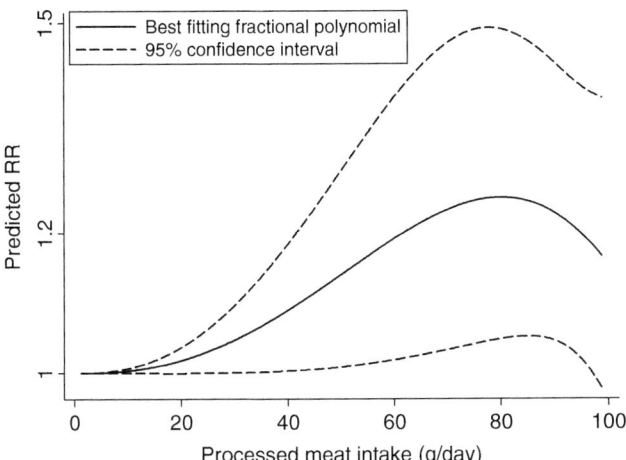

Fig. 10.3 Predicted relative risk vs. processed meat intake from fractional polynomial model. Shaded area represents 95% confidence interval around fitted curve

was not significantly better than the linear model (decrease in deviance = 2.0, on 1 df, p = 0.16). This curve is plotted in Fig. 10.3 with 95% confidence bands. The curve shows very little excess risk for the first 30–40 g/day of processed meat rising more steeply to a peak risk with 80 g/day intake before dropping slightly with higher intakes. For higher intakes, the confidence intervals are very wide, so this curve could also indicate a threshold effect beyond which additional processed meat intake does not confer any further harm. The risks associated with intakes of processed meat above 20 g/day were statistically significant, though 95% confidence intervals include negligible effects for intakes up to 40–50 g/day.

10.11.3 Potential Alternative Approaches

Eilers (2007) has also viewed the problem of nonlinear dose-response curves in meta-analysis as a latent trait on which the categorised exposure is based. Eilers considers a non-parametric smooth latent distribution of event probabilities, and uses an EM algorithm to do it. Further work could extend this to allow for measurement error. Extensions of established multilevel methods for meta-analysis (Higgins et al. 2001; The Fibrinogen Studies Collaboration 2006) (see also Chap. 5) and latent variable methods within a Bayesian framework (Higgins et al. 2001; Salanti et al. 2006; Spiegelhalter et al. 2007; Sutton et al. 2000, 2008) (see also Chaps. 8 and 9) may also be successfully applied.

10.12 Software

The methods of Greenland and Longnecker have been implemented in the Stata function "glst.ado". This implementation includes both fixed and random effects meta-analysis, and both the "pool last" or "pool first" methods. This allows exploration of heterogeneity as well as modelling linear and nonlinear dose-response curves. However, substantial work can sometimes be required to extract and derive the appropriate information from the included studies, and some additional programming is required to select an appropriate fractional polynomial and plot the curves. A package such as WinBUGS or JAGS is required for work within the Bayesian framework (Spiegelhalter et al. 2007; Plummer 2003).

10.13 Individual Patient Data

Most statistical techniques to correct for confounding (other than design-based methods such as matching or stratification), incomplete data and measurement error require access to individual patient data. Rather than pooling estimates from each study, a better approach to reaching overall combined estimates is to access the individual patient data, and analyse these. With this approach, confounding in each study is handled consistently, because the same covariates can be included in the model for each study, provided the data has been collected. This provides a solution to heterogeneity from adjustment for covariates. Similarly, imputation for incomplete data and correction for measurement error (see Chap. 2) can be achieved, using standard methods that can take full account of uncertainty involved in the process. However, although adjustment for confounding can use the same covariates, not all studies will have recorded the same information, so analysis often defaults to the lowest common denominator.

Where some published results do not present the information required to include the study in meta-analysis, with access to the individual patient data this is no longer a problem. However, gaining access to individual patient data often is a problem, and so combined analyses may still contain an unrepresentative sample of studies. It is less likely that data from older studies will be available. Current studies may not wish to give access to data from ongoing research. Datasets will be in differing formats, with different definitions, interpretations and categorisation of similar important items.

Examples of successful pooling of individual patient data from observational studies include for the investigation of birth size and breast cancer risk where 32 observational studies were successfully pooled (Collaborative Group on Pre-Natal Risk Factors and Subsequent Risk of Breast Cancer 2008), and the MRC Centre for Nutritional Epidemiology in Cancer Prevention and Survival (CNC), a collaboration of eight universities in the United Kingdom to pool cohorts investigating diet and cancer using similar methodology (Bingham and Day 2006).

10.14 Conclusions

Ultimately, the amount of information presented in observational studies on which meta-analyses are based appears to be inadequate for the task. In addition, substantial heterogeneity if often found, introduced by adjustment for different covariates, differing exclusion criteria and categorisation of exposures. This adds further argument for the use of individual patient meta-analysis in these situations. Further discussion and an extensive bibliography can be found in Sutton et al. (2000).

References

Bagnardi, V., Zambon, A., Quatto, P., & Corrao, G. (2004). Flexible meta-regression functions for modeling aggregate dose-response data, with an application to alcohol and mortality. *American Journal of Epidemiology, 159*(11), 1077–1086.

Berlin, J. A., Longnecker, M. P., & Greenland, S. (1993). Meta-analysis of epidemiologic dose-response data. *Epidemiology, 4*(3), 218–228.

Bingham, S. A., & Day, N. (2006). Commentary: Fat and breast cancer: Time to re-evaluate both methods and results? *International Journal of Epidemiology, 35*(4), 1022–1024.

Butrum, R., Cannon, G., Heggie, S., Kroke, A., Miles, L., Norman, H., El Sherbini, N., James, C., Stone, E., Thompson, R., & Wiseman, M. (2006). *Food, Nutrition, Physical Activity and the Prevention of Cancer: a Global Perspective. Systematic Literature Review Specification Manual* (Second expert report), Washington DC: World Cancer Research Fund/American Institute for Cancer Research. http://www.wcrf.org/research/research_pdfs/slr_manual_15.doc.

Chene, G., & Thompson, S. G. (1996). Methods for summarizing the risk associations of quantitative variables in epidemiologic studies in a consistent form. *American Journal of Epidemiology, 144*(6), 610–621.

Collaborative Group on Pre-Natal Risk Factors and Subsequent Risk of Breast Cancer. (2008). Birth size and breast cancer risk: Re-analysis of individual participant data from 32 studies. *PLoS Medicine, 5*(9), 1372–1386.

DerSimonian, R., & Laird, N. (1986). Meta-analysis in clinical trials. *Controlled Clinical Trials, 7*, 177–188.

Eilers, P. H. C. (2007). Data exploration in meta-analysis with smooth latent distributions. *Statistics in Medicine, 26*(17), 3358–3368.

Elm, E. V., Altman, D. G., Egger, M., Pocock, S. J., Gotzsche, P. C., Vandenbroucke, J. P., & STROBE, I. (2007). Strengthening the reporting of observational studies in epidemiology (STROBE) statement: Guidelines for reporting observational studies. *British Medical Journal, 335*(7624), 806–808.

Galanis, D. J., Kolonel, L. N., Lee, J., & Nomura, A. (1998). Intakes of selected foods and beverages and the incidence of gastric cancer among the Japanese residents of Hawaii: A prospective study. *International Journal of Epidemiology, 27*(2), 173–180.

Gonzalez, C. A., Jakszyn, P., Pera, G., Agudo, A., Bingham, S., Palli, D., Ferrari, P., Boeing, H., Del Giudice, G., Plebani, M., Carneiro, F., Nesi, G., Berrino, F., Sacerdote, C., Tumino, R., Panico, S., Berglund, G., Siman, H., Nyren, O., Hallmans, G., Martinez, C., Dorronsoro, M., Barricarte, A., Navarro, C., Quiros, J. R., Allen, N., Key, T. J., Day, N. E., Linseisen, J., Nagel, G., Bergmann, M. M., Overvad, K., Jensen, M. K., Tjonneland, A., Olsen, A., Bueno-de-Mesquita, H. B., Ocke, M., Peeters, P. H., Numans, M. E., Clavel-Chapelon, F., Boutron-Ruault, M. C., Trichopoulou, A., Psaltopoulou, T., Roukos, D., Lund, E., Hemon, B., Kaaks, R., Norat, T., & Riboli, E. (2006). Meat intake and risk of stomach and esophageal adenocarcinoma within the European Prospective Investigation into Cancer and Nutrition (EPIC). *Journal of the National Cancer Institute, 98*(5), 345–354.

Greenland, S., & Longnecker, M. P. (1992). Methods for trend estimation from summarized dose-response data, with applications to meta-analysis. *American Journal of Epidemiology, 135*(11), 1301–1309.

Greenland, S., & Thomas, D. C. (1982). On the need for the rare disease assumption in case-control studies. *American Journal of Epidemiology, 116*(3), 547–553.

Greenland, S., Thomas, D. C., & Morgenstern, H. (1986). The rare-disease assumption revisited. *American Journal of Epidemiology, 124*(6), 869–883.

Higgins, J. P., Whitehead, A., Turner, R. M., Omar, R. Z., & Thompson, S. G. (2001). Meta-analysis of continuous outcome data from individual patients. *Statistics in Medicine, 20*(15), 2219–2241.

Khan, M. M., Goto, R., Kobayashi, K., Suzumura, S., Nagata, Y., Sonoda, T., Sakauchi, F., Washio, M., & Mori, M. (2004). Dietary habits and cancer mortality among middle aged and older Japanese living in Hokkaido, Japan by cancer site and sex. *Asian Pacific Journal of Cancer Prevention, 5*(1), 58–65.

McCullough, M. L., Robertson, A. S., Jacobs, E. J., Chao, A., Calle, E. E., & Thun, M. J. (2001). A prospective study of diet and stomach cancer mortality in United States men and women. *Cancer Epidemiology, Biomarkers & Prevention, 10*(11), 1201–1205.

Ministry of Agriculture, F. a. F. (1988). *Food portion sizes* (2nd ed.). London: HMSO.

Ngoan, L. T., Mizoue, T., Fujino, Y., Tokui, N., & Yoshimura, T. (2002). Dietary factors and stomach cancer mortality. *British Journal of Cancer, 87*(1), 37–42.

Nomura, A., Grove, J. S., Stemmermann, G. N., & Severson, R. K. (1990). A prospective study of stomach cancer and its relation to diet, cigarettes, and alcohol consumption [see comment]. *Cancer Research, 50*(3), 627–631.

Plummer, M. (2003). JAGS: A program for analysis of bayesian graphical models using gibbs sampling. *Proceedings of the 3rd International Workshop on Distributed Statistical Computing (DSC 2003)*, March 20–22, Vienna, Austria.

Royston, P., & Altman, D. G. (1994). Regression using fractional polynomials of continuous covariates: Parsimonious parametric modelling. *Applied Statistics, 43*, 429–467.

Royston, P., & Altman, D. G. (2000). A strategy for modelling the effect of a continuous covariate in medicine and epidemiology. *Statistics in Medicine, 19*, 1831–1847.

Royston, P., Ambler, G., & Sauerbrei, W. (1999). The use of fractional polynomials to model continuous risk variables in epidemiology. *International Journal of Epidemiology, 28*, 964–974.

Salanti, G., Higgins, J. P., & White, I. R. (2006). Bayesian synthesis of epidemiological evidence with different combinations of exposure groups: Application to a gene-gene-environment interaction. *Statistics in Medicine, 25*(24), 4147–4163.

Spiegelhalter, D. J., Thomas, A., Best, N. G., & Lunn, D. (2007). *WinBUGS user manual: Version 1.4.3.* Cambridge: MRC Biostatistics Unit.

Stroup, D. F., Berlin, J. A., Morton, S. C., Olkin, I., Williamson, G. D., Rennie, D., Moher, D., Becker, B. J., Sipe, T. A., Thacker, S. B., & for the Meta-analysis of Observational Studies in Epidemiology Group. (2000). Meta-analysis of observational studies in epidemiology: A proposal for reporting. *Journal of the American Medical Association, 283*(15), 2008–2012.

Sutton, A. J., Abrams, K. R., Jones, D. R., Sheldon, T. A., & Song, F. (2000). *Methods for meta-analysis in medical research.* Chichester: Wiley.

Sutton, A. J., Kendrick, D., & Coupland, C. A. C. (2008). Meta-analysis of individual- and aggregate-level data. *Statistics in Medicine, 27*(5), 651–669.

The Fibrinogen Studies Collaboration. (2006). Regression dilution methods for meta-analysis: Assessing long-term variability in plasma fibrinogen among 27 247 adults in 15 prospective studies. *International Journal of Epidemiology, 35*(6), 1570–1578.

van den Brandt, P. A., Botterweck, A. A., & Goldbohm, R. A. (2003). Salt intake, cured meat consumption, refrigerator use and stomach cancer incidence: A prospective cohort study (Netherlands). *Cancer Causes & Control, 14*(5), 427–438.

White, I. R., Higgins, J. P., & Wood, A. M. (2008a). Allowing for uncertainty due to missing data in meta-analysis – Part 1: Two-stage methods. *Statistics in Medicine, 27*(5), 711–727.

White, I. R., Welton, N. J., Wood, A. M., Ades, A. E., & Higgins, J. P. (2008b). Allowing for uncertainty due to missing data in meta-analysis – Part 2: Hierarchical models. *Statistics in Medicine, 27*(5), 728–745.

World Cancer Research Fund/American Institute for Cancer Research. (2007). *Food, nutrition, physical activity and the prevention of cancer: A global perspective*. Washington DC: World Cancer Research Fund/American Institute for Cancer Research.

Zheng, W., Sellers, T. A., Doyle, T. J., Kushi, L. H., Potter, J. D., & Folsom, A. R. (1995). Retinol, antioxidant vitamins, and cancers of the upper digestive tract in a prospective cohort study of postmenopausal women. *American Journal of Epidemiology, 142*(9), 955–960.

Chapter 11
Directed Acyclic Graphs and Structural Equation Modelling

Yu-Kang Tu

11.1 Introduction

One of the major challenges for epidemiologists is to understand and infer causal relationships between risk factors and health outcomes in the population by analysing data from observational studies. For many risk factors, it is either unethical or impractical to conduct randomised controlled trials to test their health effects. It would therefore be very desirable if there is a methodology for observational studies to discover causes and effects amongst variables or at least confirm or refute the proposed causal relationships. Epidemiologists need a methodology which is sort of a combination of the directed acyclic graphs (DAGs, see Chap. 1) for conceptual construction of causal models and regression analysis for testing those models. It is therefore surprising that structural equation modelling (SEM) has not been so frequently used in epidemiology as in the social sciences, given that both epidemiologists and social scientists want to delineate causes and effects from observational data. The difference between DAGs and path diagrams in SEM is trivial: the path between two variables can only have one direction in DAGs (Greenland and Brumback 2002; Iacobucci 2008), whilst in SEM the paths can be in both directions at once. An individual path in SEM is tested in the same way as the regression coefficient is in regression analysis, and model fit indices provided by SEM software packages help the analysts to assess the adequacy of the proposed causal model compared to the observed associations in the sample data (Pearl 2000; Kline 2011).

Why then is SEM still under-utilised in epidemiology? This is a question posed by Der (2002) a few years ago. The answers cited included that SEM used unfamiliar terminology, because mathematical models in SEM are formulated in

Y.-K. Tu (✉)
Division of Biostatistics, Centre for Epidemiology and Biostatistics, Leeds Institute of Genetics, Health & Therapeutics, Faculty of Medicine and Health, University of Leeds, Leeds, UK
e-mail: Y.K.Tu@leeds.ac.uk

matrix algebra, and the first SEM software, LISREL, uses eight matrices in Greek letters; the restriction in the assumptions of variables requires that the outcome variables need to be continuous and follow multivariate normality; it is quite tedious to set up SEM models to test interaction amongst variables and non-linear relationship. More importantly, two different causal models may imply the same covariance structure and consequently, it is impossible to tell which is better, known as the equivalent models problem. Recent advances in SEM theory and software development has nevertheless resolved some of these issues. We now known that the maximum likelihood estimator is quite robust to the violation of multivariate normality, and new estimation methods do not require the strict assumption of multivariate normality (Shipley 2000). Software packages can now estimate non-continuous outcome variables (Skrondal and Rabe-Hesketh 2004; Muthen and Muthen 2006; Hancock and Samuelson 2007). From a statistical viewpoint, all general and generalised linear models (such as linear regression, analysis of variance, and logistic regression), and multivariate statistics (such as path analysis, multivariate analysis of variance, canonical correlation, and factor analysis) are part of SEM family. As a result, almost all epidemiologists are 'doing' SEM every day, though most of them are not aware of this.

Since Karl Jöreskog first proposed his famous LISREL model in 1970s, SEM has become a very important research tool for quantitative social scientists, because it provides a very powerful and versatile framework for formulating research hypotheses and testing them. SEM is a vast and rapidly evolving field, and there are more than a dozen of textbooks and monographs dedicated entirely to SEM. Chapter-length introduction can be found in many statistics textbooks covering multivariate methods. Therefore, the aim of this Chapter is not to explain the mathematical theory of SEM or to demonstrate how to use SEM software. Instead, the aim of this Chapter is to discuss the relation between DAGs and SEM, rationale behind SEM, and the limitation of SEM philosophy. Readers who are interested in applying this methodology can consult the textbooks and software manuals for further details. The structure of this Chapter is as follows: we first explain the path diagrams used by SEM and the similarity between them and DAGs (Sects. 11.2 and 11.3). Then, we explain how SEM may be useful for the identifications of causal relationships (Sects. 11.4 and 11.5). Finally, we explain the philosophy behind SEM testing and its limitations (Sect. 11.6).

11.2 Path Diagrams

Path diagram is a graphical presentation of linear models. Both observed and unobserved variables can be included in the diagram. When we become familiar with the rules of path diagrams, they can be used to visualise the causal relationships amongst the variables in the model. Observed variables are usually in squares and unobserved (latent) variables in circles. For instance, in a bivariate Pearson product-moment correlation between variable X and Y, both are observed

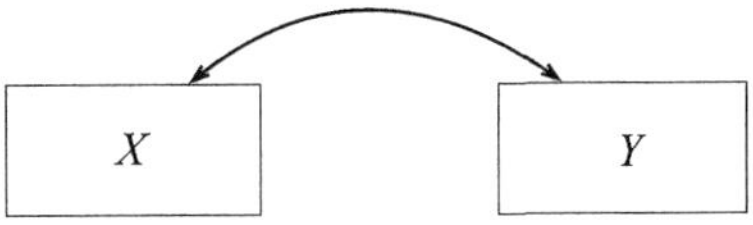

11 Directed Acyclic Graphs and Structural Equation Modelling

Fig. 11.1 Path diagram for correlation between X and Y

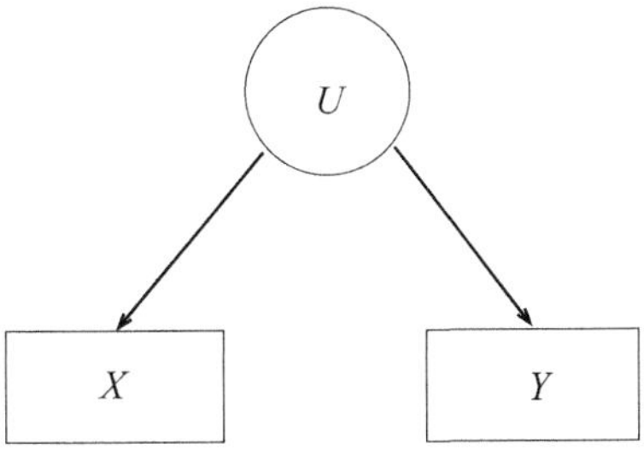

Fig. 11.2 Path diagram for observed correlation between X and Y caused an unobserved common ancestor of U

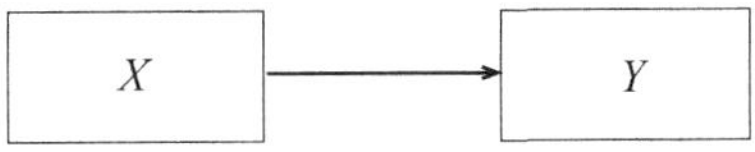

Fig. 11.3 Path diagram for regressing Y on X

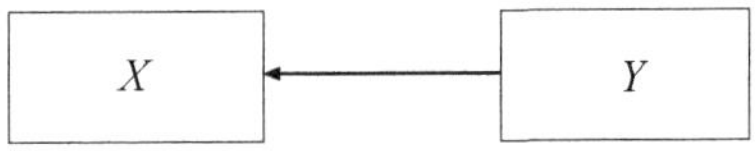

Fig. 11.4 Path diagram for regressing X on Y

variables and there is no direction in their relationship. As a result, X and Y are connected by a double arrow (Fig. 11.1). We may think of the correlation without causal direction as a manifestation of an unobserved causal variable, i.e. the observed correlation between X and Y is due to a latent variable U which is the cause of both X and Y (Fig. 11.2). Therefore, if we can identify U and measure it, X and Y would become independent conditional on U. In mathematical notations, this relationship amongst the three variables is noted as $Y \perp X | U$ following the notations introduced in Chaps. 1 and 4. From a statistical viewpoint, this means that the partial correlation between X and Y is zero after the adjustment of U, and regression coefficient for X is zero when Y is regressed on both X and U together.

When substantive theory suggests that X is a cause of Y, i.e. when X changes, Y will change accordingly, we draw a single arrow from X to Y (Fig. 11.3). In contrast, if we believe Y is a cause of X, the arrow should be drawn from Y to X (Fig. 11.4). Note that from a pure statistical viewpoint, these four models in Figs. 11.1, 11.2, 11.3 and 11.4 are not distinguishable, i.e. without knowledge external to the system, it is impossible to tell which model is true, because all the four models make the same prediction in the observed relationship between X and Y in a non-experimental setting. All the four models imply an observed correlation between X and Y, although the causal relationships between X and Y are different.

Passive observation such as measuring X and Y in a sample from a population is insufficient to identify which model is true. In other words, testing the statistical relationship between X and Y alone is not able to discriminate between the variety of possible models. We need to test the causal relationship using active observation, i.e. we need to intervene into the system, observe the consequences, and compare them to the predictions made by the models.

For instance, the causal models in Figs. 11.1, 11.2 and 11.4 suggests that if we change X, Y will not change because X is not a cause of Y. Therefore if change in Y does occur when we increase X by one unit in a selected sample by conducting an experiment, the three causal models in Figs. 11.1, 11.2 and 11.4 are rejected because their predictions are refuted by the experiment. On the other hand, if change in Y does not occur when we increase X by a unit, the three causal models are tentatively accepted because their predictions pass the experiment, but further experiments are required to tell which of the three models is the best. For instance, we can increase Y by a unit and see if X will change. If X changes, this means that the causal models in Figs. 11.1 and 11.2 are rejected, because according to their predictions, Y is not a cause of X and should not change (Tu et al. 2008).

Suppose we do not observed any change in X when Y is increased by one unit, and this will reject the prediction by the model in Fig. 11.4. But what about the models in Figs. 11.1 and 11.2? How can we know which one is the best? In fact, there is no genuinely causal relationship in the model in Fig. 11.1, and as a result, no experiment can be undertaken to test its truthfulness. This is why in DAGs, double arrows are not allowed. For the causal model in Fig. 11.2, although there is no double arrow, conducting experiments to test it will not be easy. First, we need to identify the unobserved variable U and measure it. When U increases, we expect to see changes in both X and Y. The problem is if we observe no change in X and Y, this is not sufficient to reject the model, because we might identify an incorrect U. Therefore, the model in Fig. 11.2 needs to pass three tests: (1) when X changes, Y does not change; (2) when Y changes, X does not change; (3) U is identified and when U changes both X and Y change. Then we may tentatively accept this model as the most plausible one amongst the three causal models.

The discussion so far may look recognisable for readers who are familiar with the writings of Sir Karl Popper, an influential philosopher of science in the last century. His famous slogan: conjectures and refutations, has once been considered as the demarcation criteria between science and pseudo-science. A good scientific theory clearly specifies the conditions where it may be rejected, i.e. to make predictions which have not been but can be observed, and then experiments are designed to test the predictions. If the scientific theory passes the test, its truth-content has increased; if it fails the test, it may need to be modified or in extreme circumstances rejected. Of course, in real research, the process is quite complex, as we need to take into account the accuracy of our measurements and to decide the extent of deviations between predictions and observations that suffice to falsify our theory. Note that according to Popperian philosophy, we cannot 'prove' a theory true by undertaking an experiment or observation, because the theory may fail in the next test. This is an asymmetry in the acceptance and refutation of a scientific theory: one experiment or observation may refute a theory forever but only corroborate it (Popper 2002).

Popperian philosophy was once very popular amongst natural and social scientists, and there have been many discussions about its application in epidemiology. In SEM literature, Popper's philosophy has been used to defend the values of SEM in finding causal relationships in data from passive observations (Bollen 1989). In the following sections, we will discuss why it is not always easy to practice (so-called naïve) Popperian conjectures and refutations in SEM.

11.3 Directed Acyclic Graphs

One limitation of classical SEM analysis is that the manifest (observed) variables for the outcomes have to be continuous variables such as Y in Fig. 11.3 and X in Fig. 11.4 (there is no such limitation for X in Fig. 11.3 and Y in Fig. 11.4). Recent advances in SEM theory and software development have overcome this by implementing new estimation procedures (Little et al. 2007; Muthén 2001). These new developments make SEM a useful tool for causal modelling in epidemiology, because many outcome variables in epidemiology are binary or counts. DAGs, which have been known to epidemiologists for nearly two decades, have received greater attention in the last few years (see Chaps. 1 and 4 for more details). They have mainly been used by epidemiologists to identify confounders and potential biases in the estimation of causal relationships, and DAGs are a particular type of path diagrams.

11.3.1 Identification of Confounders

The question of which variables are confounders and should be adjusted for in statistical analysis has been a controversial issue within epidemiology (Weinberg 2005; Kirkwood and Sterne 2003; Jewell 2004). Only with the consideration of DAGs can the relevant issue be resolved. According to DAGs theory, confounders are variables which are causally associated with both the outcome *and* exposure but are *not* on the causal pathway from the exposure to the outcome variable (Greenland et al. 1999; Pearl 2000; Tu et al. 2005; Glymour 2006; Glymour and Greenland 2008). For instance, variable Z is a confounder for the relation between the exposure X and the outcome Y in Fig. 11.5a, because there are arrows from Z to X and Y (i.e. they are causally associated), and Z is *not* on the causal path from X to Y. In contrast, Z is not a confounder for the relation between the exposure X and the outcome Y in Fig. 11.5b, because although there are arrows from Z to Y and from X to Z (i.e. they are causally associated), Z *is* on the causal path from X to Y. Therefore, if we want to estimate the impact of X on Y, Z is a confounder and should be adjusted for according to Fig. 11.5a, but Z is not a confounder according to 11.5b. From the viewpoint of path diagram, the adjustment of Z in Fig. 11.5b is the partition of direct and indirect effect, and this is very common in SEM literature.

Fig. 11.5 Path diagram for confounding: (**a**) Z is a confounder for the relationship between X and Y; (**b**) Z is a not confounder for the relationship between X and Y, because Z is on the causal pathway from X to Y

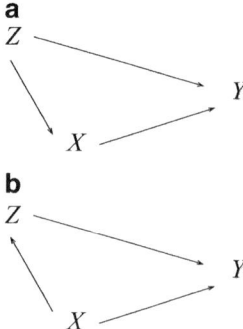

11.3.2 Direct and Indirect Effects

Most SEM software can produce the results of direct and indirect effects upon request. The path from X to Y in Fig. 11.5b is interpreted as the direct effect of X on Y, and the path from X to Z and Y is the indirect effect of X on Y. To estimate the former, we need to adjust for an intermediate variable between X and Y. This practice is also known as 'mediation' analysis in social sciences (MacKinnon 2008). The total effects are just the sum of direct and indirect effects. Therefore, although the adjustment of Z in a regression model will change the estimate of regression coefficient for X, it matters little in SEM because both unadjusted and adjusted regression coefficients are reported: the former is the total effects and the latter the direct effects.

11.3.3 Backdoor Paths and Colliders

We may ask why Z is a confounder and should be adjusted for in Fig. 11.5a and what would happen if Z is not adjusted for. Before we answer this question, we first look at Fig. 11.2 again. Suppose the arrows from U to X and Y represent positive associations. When U increases, we will observe that both X and Y increase. If we do not know that there is U behind the observed increases in X and Y, we may therefore conclude that either X influences Y or vice versa, but actually if we change the values of X (or Y), nothing would happen to Y (or X). U is therefore a confounder for the relation between X and Y, and this can be identified by tracing the path from X to Y or Y to X known as a backdoor path (see Chap. 1). When there are backdoor paths from the exposure to the outcome, the estimate of their causal relation is contaminated (in statistical jargon, biased). To block the backdoor paths, variables such as U need to be adjusted for, and in epidemiological terminology, these variables are confounders.

A related issue is to identify colliders in DAG (see Chap. 1 for the definition of a collider). Consider Fig. 11.6. There are paths from X to Z and Y to Z, i.e. changing

Fig. 11.6 Path diagram for Z regressed on X and Y, and X and Y are uncorrelated

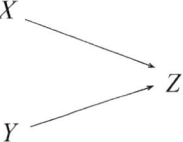

either X or Y will give rise to change in Z, but changes in X will not cause changes in Y, and vice versa. However, if we adjust for Z when we regress Y on X (or X on Y), we will find a spurious association between Y and X. The non-mathematical explanation for this phenomenon is as follows: we know both X and Y can influence X, say, positively; if we observe a positive change in Z, we know either X or Y is the cause but we are uncertain of which is the cause. However, if we then know X had changed, that Y had also changed becomes less probable than that Y had not, so a negative relation between X and Y would be observed. Mathematically speaking, X and Y are independent unconditionally, but they are dependent, conditional on Z. In this scenario, Z acts as a collider, because two arrows (one from X and the other from Y) go toward it, so Z blocks the pathway from X to Y (and Y to X). However, statistical adjustment of Z will open this path, and X and Y will become correlated.

In path diagram, X and Y are assumed to independent, i.e. when their relationships with Z are estimated, the correlation between X and Y will be constrained to be zero, even though their observed correlation may not be zero.

11.3.4 Example of a Complex DAG

Suppose we want to estimate the "true effect" of X on Y in Fig. 11.7, which variables should be measured and adjusted for (Greenland and Brumback 2002)? As discussed before, variables to be adjusted for are confounders, i.e. the adjustment of these variables can block the backdoor paths from X to Y. The most obvious confounder in Fig. 11.7 is Z, as there is a backdoor path: $X \leftarrow Z \rightarrow Y$. Following the same principle, U and V are also confounders for the estimation of the causal effects of X on Y. The question is do we need to adjust for all three variables? For instance, suppose that it would take a lot of efforts and resources to measure either U or V, so the question is to determine the minimum set of confounders for statistical adjustment (see Chap. 1 for the definition of minimum set of confounders). We then note that when Z is blocked (i.e. statistically adjusted for), the backdoor path from X to U, Z and Y is also blocked. As a result, blocking Z will block two backdoor paths from X to Y. The same applies to V. When Z is blocked, the backdoor path from X to Z, V and Y is also blocked. However, does this mean that the adjustment of Z would be sufficient to block *all* the backdoor paths? The answer is no, because Z is also a collider for U and V. When Z is adjusted for, a new backdoor path from X to U, V and Y is opened, and therefore, the minimum set of confounders is either Z and U or Z and V.

Fig. 11.7 Path diagram for a complex scenario, where the aim of investigation is to estimate an unbiased relation between X and Y

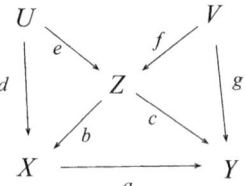

11.4 Implied Correlation Matrix in SEM

Structural equation modelling (SEM) looks at the model in Fig. 11.7 from a slightly difference perspective. To simplify our discussion, we standardise all the variables used in Fig. 11.7, so that their means are zero and their variances are one. The lower case letters accompanying each path represent the standardised path coefficients which can be interpreted as standardised regression coefficients from multiple regression analysis. From Fig. 11.7 it is possible to work the estimated correlations between each pair of variables in the model using Sewell Wright's Rules of Tracing (Loehlin 2004). Wright was a geneticist and invented path analysis in 1920s. His path analysis was largely ignored by statisticians but adopted by econometricians in 1950s. In 1960s and 1970s, path analysis and factor analysis were incorporated into one single general statistical framework, SEM, by Karl Jöreskog and others.

Wright's rules can be summarised as follows:

1. No loops are allowed. In tracing from one variable to another, the same variable cannot be passed through twice.
2. No going forward and then backward. Once following a path forward, e.g. following the path from X to Y ($X \rightarrow Y$) in Fig. 11.7, it is not allowed to follow backward across the path, e.g. following the path backward from Y to Z ($Y \leftarrow Z$) in Fig. 11.7 not allowed. However, going backward and then forward is possible, e.g. flowing the path backward from Y to Z ($Y \leftarrow Z$) and then from Z to X ($X \rightarrow Y$) in Fig. 11.7 is allowed.
3. Only one double arrow is allowed in tracing from the first variable to the last variable, e.g. tracing from X to Y is allowed in Fig. 11.1.

Note that we will not need rule No.3 for DAGs for reasons explained previously, and the rule No.2 is equivalent to how we identify backdoor paths and colliders in the previous section. It is better to use examples to explain how to apply these rules. For instance, the correlation between U and V in Fig. 11.7 is zero according to the rule No.2. The correlation between X and Z is $(b + d*e)$. The former is a direct effect from Z to X and the latter the confounding effect due to U, i.e. the estimated correlation between X and Z is the sum of the genuine effect and the spurious confounding effects. If the model is correct, this will also be the observed correlation between X and Z in the population. The correlation between X and Y is

$(a + b*c + d*e*c + b*f*g)$ of which a is the genuine (unconfounded) effect of X on Y. We can write down all the mathematical relationships between observed (on the left hand side of the equations) and estimated (the the right hand side of the equations) correlations as:

$$r_{U,V} = 0; \tag{11.1}$$

$$r_{X,Z} = b + d*e; \tag{11.2}$$

$$r_{X,Y} = a + b*c + d*e*c + b*f*g; \tag{11.3}$$

$$r_{X,V} = b*f; \tag{11.4}$$

$$r_{X,U} = d + b*e; \tag{11.5}$$

$$r_{U,Z} = e; \tag{11.6}$$

$$r_{U,Y} = e*c + e*b*a + d*a; \tag{11.7}$$

$$r_{V,Y} = g + f*c + f*b*a; \tag{11.8}$$

$$r_{V,Z} = f; \tag{11.9}$$

$$r_{Z,Y} = c + b*a + e*d*a + f*g; \tag{11.10}$$

There are seven standardised regression coefficients in Eqs. 11.1–11.10: the seven lower case letters, and there are ten known correlation coefficients on the left hand side of the equations. Some standardised regression coefficients have already been given from the equations, e.g. $e = r_{U,Z}$ and $f = r_{V,Z}$, but the other five remain to be estimated. As there are more correlations than unknown parameters, there is no unique solution, and SEM in general uses maximum likelihood method to minimise the differences between the observed and estimated correlations. If the proposed model is correct, the estimated correlations amongst the five variables would be exactly observed correlations in the population, and the unconfounded effect of X on Y is therefore a.

Suppose we mistakenly believe that Fig. 11.8 is the correct model for the relationships amongst X, Y and Z instead of Fig. 11.7. The relationships between the observed and estimated correlations become:

$$r_{Z,X} = b'; \tag{11.11}$$

$$r_{Z,Y} = b' + a'*c'; \tag{11.12}$$

$$r_{X,Y} = a' + b'*c'; \tag{11.13}$$

Fig. 11.8 The same research question as the one in Fig. 11.7, but here variables U and V are not included in the model, yielding biased estimate for the relation between X and Y

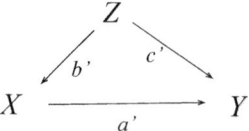

It becomes apparent that $a' \neq a$, i.e. the estimated effect of X on Y in Fig. 11.8 is biased.

11.5 Model Testing in SEM

The basic rationale behind the model testing in SEM is straightforward: multiple linear equations are used to specify causal relationship between variables some of which are manifest variables (observed and collected by the researchers), while others are latent variables derived from the observed variables by specifying their relations using equations, such as those in factor analysis. The multiple equations in each causal model describe particular correlation structure between the observed variables which is usually presented as a correlation (or covariance) matrix Σ. The estimation procedure is to minimise the difference between Σ and the observed correlation or covariance matrix $\mathbf{S}$ formulated by a likelihood function:

$$F_{ML} = \log\left|\sum\right| - \log|\mathbf{S}| + trace\left(\mathbf{S}\sum{}^{-1}\right) - (p+q),$$

where p and q is the number of independent and dependent variables, respectively.

A χ^2 test is then used to evaluate the difference between these two matrices by taking into account the number of the estimated parameters in the proposed model. When the χ^2 value is large (i.e. the difference between the two matrices is large) relative to the model's degree of freedom, the proposed model is rejected, i.e. the causal relationships in the proposed model might be mis-specified. When the χ^2 value is small, we do not reject the model or even tentatively accept the model as adequate.

Why do we only tentatively accept the proposed model as adequate when the χ^2 value is small? This is because of the possibility of equivalent models. In other words, our model may actually be wrong in terms of the causal relations amongst variables but happen to estimate the same correlation structure (the same $\mathbf{S}$) of the 'true' model. For example, suppose the true relationship is $Y \rightarrow X \rightarrow Z$, but we wrongly specify their relationships as $Z \rightarrow X \rightarrow Y$. Both models imply that the three variables are correlated and Y and Z are independent conditional on X. Therefore, both models will obtain the same χ^2 value with the same one degree of freedom.

One controversy in the SEM model testing is whether a large χ^2 value relative to the model degree of freedom necessarily means that the proposed model is wrong and should be modified or even rejected, because the statistical power of the χ^2 test to reject a model increases with the sample size. As a result, a causal model whose model fit deems acceptable in a small sample is considered unacceptable when the sample size increases. The problem is inherent in hypothesis testing (Gardner and Altman 1986; Altman and Bland 1995). Therefore, many alternative model fit indices have been proposed that take into account the sample size and model degrees of freedom. Many software packages also provide modification indices to help researchers identify possible ways to modify the models to reduce the χ^2 value. Model modification should be guided by more than just the reduction in the χ^2 value, because this may be entirely caused by chance, and the modified model may make little sense from a theoretical point of view.

A more fundamental issue in SEM model testing is why the aim of SEM is to produce a model that has the same correlation/covariance structure in the sample as that in the population. The rationale is that if a model faithfully represents the "true" causal relationships amongst variables, the estimated relationships should correspond to the observed ones in the data. In reality, there may be biases in the data collection that cause the observed correlation/covariance structure to deviate from the true one in the population. Furthermore, reality is often complex, and many of the causes and effects may be subtle and intricate; we may never be able to capture a full picture. Even if we do, the model may be too complex to be useful, and a simpler model with a simplified version of theory may be more useful for our understanding of reality. According to the popular version of Popperian philosophy (we call it popular version, because Popper himself recognised the process of conjectures and refutations is far more complex in the practice of science), a model may survive many attempts to refute it, but if it fails just one test, we should modify or even reject it. Is it always a good approach that we give up our carefully formulated model and modify our theory because it does not fit one data set? Or should we try to identify the reasons for the poor fit, such as random sampling errors?

11.6 No Causes In No Causes Out

Nancy Cartwright, a prominent philosopher of science, argued "no causes in, no causes out" (Cartwright 1989), and epidemiologists will never prove or refute a causal relationship from observational studies, if causes and effects are not part of their statistical models. Causality has to be incorporated into statistical analysis, if we want to make causal inference from the results. DAGs have been used widely by many studies in justifying the adjustments of confounders and corrections for biases. We agree that both DAGs and path diagrams are very useful tools for explicitly formulating the causal relationships amongst variables in the models. However, DAGs and path diagrams cannot turn passive observations into active ones, i.e. the conditional relationships and covariance structure in the proposed DAGs and path diagrams may be very close to the ones in the sample data, but this alone may not be able to prove the proposed causal relationships. Ideally, we would like to conduct experiments to make changes to the system in the model and observed whether the consequence follows the prediction made by the model. This may not always be feasible and does not mean no causal inference can be made without experiments. For example, we could never take Moon away from our galaxy and then see what change this might cause to how the Earth moves around the sun; but we still believe Newton's law is correct. Causal thinking can still be incorporated in the statistical analysis and causal inference can still be made using data from careful observations (Arah 2008, Tu 2009).

11.7 Further Reading

Two book chapters (Glymour 2006, and Glymour and Greenland 2008) provide a comprehensive but accessible coverage of DAGs for epidemiologists. Judea Pearl's book (Pearl 2000) discusses both DAGs and SEM in much deeper depth, but people without strong statistical background may find it difficult. Kline (2011) and Loehlin (2004) are both good introductory textbooks on SEM without relying too much on linear algebra for explaining the concepts.

References

Altman, D. G., & Bland, J. M. (1995). Absence of evidence is not evidence of absence. *BMJ, 311*, 485.
Arah, O. A. (2008). The role of causal reasoning in understanding Simpson's paradox, Lord's paradox, and the suppression effect: Covariate selection in the analysis of observational studies. *Emerging Themes in Epidemiology, 5*, 5.
Bollen, K (1989). Structural equations with latent variables. Hoboken, NJ: Wiley.
Cartwright, N. (1989). *Nature's capacities and their measurement*. Oxford: Oxford University Press.
Der, G. (2002). Commentary: Structural equation modelling in epidemiology: Some problems and prospects. *International Journal of Epidemiology, 31*, 1199–1200.
Gardner, M. J., & Altman, D. G. (1986). Confidence intervals rather than P values: estimation rather than hypothesis testing. *BMJ, 292*, 846–850.
Glymour, M. M. (2006). Using causal diagrams to understand common problems in social epidemiology. In J. M. Oakes & J. S. Kaufman (Eds.), *Methods in social epidemiology* (pp. 393–428). San Francisco: Jossey-Bass.
Glymour, M. M., & Greenland, S. (2008). Causal diagrams. In K. J. Rothman, S. Greenland, & T. L. Lash (Eds.), *Modern epidemiology* (3rd ed., pp. 183–209). Philadelphia: Lippincott Williams & Wilkins.
Greenland, S., & Brumback, B. (2002). An overview of relations among causal modelling methods. *International Journal of Epidemiology, 31*, 1030–1037.

Greenland, S., Pearl, J., & Robins, J. M. (1999). *Causal Diagrams for epidemiologic research.* Epidemiology, 10, 37–48.

Hancock, G., & Samuelson, K. M. (Eds.). (2007). *Advances in latent variable mixture models.* Charlotte: IAP.

Iacobucci, D. (2008). *Mediation analysis.* Thousand Oaks: Sage.

Jewell, N. P. (2004). *Statistics for Epidemiology.* Boca Raton, Florida: Chapman & Hall.

Kirkwood, B., & Sterne, J. A. C. (2003). *Essential medical statistics* (2nd ed.). London: Blackwell.

Kline, R. B. (2011). *Principles and practice of structural equation modeling* (3rd ed.). New York: Guilford press.

Little, T. D., Preacher, K. J., Selig, J. P., & Card, N. A. (2007). New developments in latent variable panel analyses of longitudinal data. *International Journal of Behavioral Development, 31*, 357–365.

Loehlin, J. C. (2004). *Latent variable models* (4th ed.). Mahwah: Lawrence Erlbaum Associates.

MacKinnon, D. P. (2008). *Introduction to statistical mediation analysis.* Mahwah: Lawrence Erlbaum Associates.

Muthén, B. (2001). Second-generation structural equation modelling with a combination of categorical and continuous latent variables: New opportunities for latent class/latent growth modeling. In L. M. Collins & A. Sayer (Eds.), *New methods for the analysis of change* (pp. 291–322). Washington, DC: American Psychological Association.

Muthén, L. K., & Muthén, B. (2006). *Mplus user's guide* (4th ed.). Los Angeles: Muthén & Muthén.

Pearl, J. (2000). *Causality: Models, reasoning, and inference.* Cambridge: Cambridge University Press.

Popper, K. R. (2002). *Conjectures and refutations.* London: Routledge.

Shipley, B. (2000). *Cause and correlation in biology.* Cambridge: Cambridge University Press.

Skrondal, A., & Rabe-Hesketh, S. (2004). *Generalized latent variable modelling: Multilevel, longitudinal and structural equation models.* Boca Raton: Chapman & Hall/CRC.

Tu, Y. K., West, R., Ellison, G. T. H., et al. (2005). Why evidence for the fetal origins of adult disease might be a statistical artifact: The "reversal paradox" for the relation between birth weight and blood pressure in later life. *American Journal of Epidemiology, 161*, 27–32.

Tu, Y. K., Gunnell, D. J., & Gilthorpe, M. S. (2008). Simpson's paradox, Lord's paradox, and suppression effects are the same phenomenon – The reversal paradox. *Emerging Themes in Epidemiology, 5*, 2.

Tu, Y. K. (2009) Commentary: Is structural equation modelling a step forward for epidemiologists? *International Journal of Epidemiology, 38*, 249–251.

Weinberg, C. R. (2005). Invited commentary: Barker meets Simpson. *American Journal of Epidemiology, 161*, 33–35.

Chapter 12
Latent Growth Curve Models

Yu-Kang Tu and Francesco D'Auito

12.1 Introduction

Many clinical and epidemiological studies make repeated measurements of continuous variables during the period of observation. Statistical analysis of longitudinal data often requires advanced, sophisticated methods to explore the complexity of information within the data. Standard statistical methodologies include the use of summary statistics (Senn et al. 2000), multilevel modelling (MLM) (Goldstein 1995; Hox 2002; Raudenbush and Bryk 2002; Gilthorpe et al. 2003; Singer and Willett 2003; Twisk 2003; Twisk 2006) and generalized estimating equations (GEE) (Liang and Zeger 1986; also see Chap. 15 on Generalised Additive Models).

During the development of MLM in the social sciences (also known as random effects modelling in biostatistics), another statistical methodology, latent growth curve modelling (LGCM), has been developed (Byrne and Crombie 2003; Bollen and Curran 2006; Duncan et al. 2006) within the framework of structural equation modelling (SEM) (Bollen 1989; Loehlin 2004; Kline 2011; see also Chap. 11). Theoretical development in the last decade has shown that MLM yields the same answers as those of SEM with regards to longitudinal data analysis (Curran 2003; Bauer 2003; Steele 2008), and therefore SEM software can be used to analyze multilevel or random effects models. This discovery has a potential to have a great

Y.-K. Tu (✉)
Division of Biostatistics, Centre for Epidemiology and Biostatistics, Leeds Institute of Genetics, Health & Therapeutics, Faculty of Medicine and Health, University of Leeds, Leeds, UK
e-mail: Y.K.Tu@leeds.ac.uk

F. D'Auito
Department of Periodontology, Eastman Dental Institute, University College London, London, UK

impact on practical data analysis, especially in clinical and epidemiological research, because the SEM framework offers greater flexibility than MLM in statistical modelling with the incorporation of latent variables (Curran 2003). The aim of this chapter is to present a concise introduction to LGCM for epidemiologists showing the possible benefits they might gain from using this methodology for some study designs compared to MLM or GEE when modelling longitudinal data. The structure of this chapter is as follows. In Sect. 12.2, we explain how commonly used statistical methods such as simple and multiple linear regression can be visualized using path diagrams. In Sect. 12.3, we use an example from a clinical trial to explain how to employ LGCM to test a two-level growth curve model. In Sect. 12.4, we show how LGCM can provide greater flexibility in modelling non-linear growth curves and changing processes of multiple outcomes. Finally, we conclude in Sect. 12.5 by discussing the advantages and limitations of LGCM. We use statistical software Mplus (version 5.2, Muthén and Muthén 2006) for LGCM analysis throughout this chapter.

12.2 Path Diagram for Linear Regression

As discussed in Chap. 11, structural equation modelling (SEM) can be considered as a general theoretical framework for all univariate and multivariate linear statistical models, i.e. correlation, linear regression, analysis of variance, multivariate analysis of variance, canonical correlation, and factor analysis. Whilst SEM can be expressed using linear algebra, a sometimes clearer way to appreciate the concepts of SEM is through understanding the path diagrams of these statistical models. As shown in Chap. 11, path diagrams are a graphical way of presenting the relationships amongst variables in statistical models. Some SEM software provides a graphical interface for users to draw path diagrams for their models on the computer, and the software then performs the analyses specified in the path diagrams.

12.2.1 The Path Diagram for Simple Linear Regression

To illustrate how to draw path diagrams for growth models, we begin with a simple example of linear regression with one outcome variable (known as the dependent variable) and one explanatory variable (known as the independent variable or covariate). Figure 12.1 is the path diagram for a simple linear regression model given as:

$$y = b_0 + b_1 x + e; \tag{12.1}$$

12 Latent Growth Curve Models

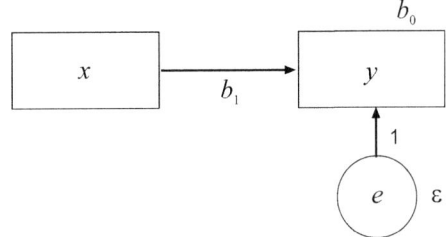

Fig. 12.1 Path diagram for simple linear regression in Eq. 12.1. The factor loading b_1 in the path diagram is equivalent to the regression coefficient b_1 in Eq. 12.1

where y is the outcome variable, x the explanatory variable, e the residual error term, b_0 the intercept, and b_1 the regression coefficient for x.

From Eq. 12.1, we see that when x is zero, y is b_0, and when x increases by one unit, y is expected to increase by the amount of b_1. The residual error term is the difference between the observed values of the outcome and the predicted values of the outcome. In path diagrams, observed variables such as x and y are within squares, and latent (unobserved) variables such as residual errors (e in Eq. 12.1) are within circles. An arrow from variable x to variable y in a path diagram means that x affects y in the specified statistical model, but y does not affect x. In contrast, a double arrow connecting x and y means that these two variables are correlated without specific causal direction. When there is no arrowed line (single or double) between x and y, this means that x and y are assumed to be causally independent, i.e. the underlying population correlation between them is assumed to be zero in the specified model. For instance, x and e are assumed to be uncorrelated, and this is one of the assumptions behind regression analysis: explanatory variables and residual errors are independent.

The arrow from one variable to another is called a *path* in the diagram. In Fig. 12.1, there are two paths that specify the relationships between variables in the model: one from x to y, and another from e to y. As a result, two parameters associated with those two paths may need to be estimated. The parameter for the path from x to y is b_1, which is unknown and needs to be estimated, but another parameter for the path from e to y is fixed to be unity. Only one free parameter for the relationship between x and y requires estimation, though other free parameters also require estimation, for example, the variances of x and e.

12.2.1.1 Regression Weights, Path Coefficients, and Factor Loadings

In linear regression, b_1 is usually known as the regression coefficient, but in SEM, the parameters for the paths are sometimes called path coefficients or factor loadings. Despite the confusing jargon, all these terms can be interpreted as regression coefficients, and in this Chapter, we simply call them regression coefficients. One exception is where double arrow are used between two variables: the estimated path coefficient with a double arrow is the covariance between the two variables.

12.2.1.2 Exogenous and Endogenous Variables

In a path diagram such as Fig. 12.1, variables like x are known as exogenous variables because there is no arrow from another variable in the model directed towards them. In contrast, variables like y are known as endogenous variables, because there is at least one arrow from other variables (x in this model) directed toward it. Endogenous variables are accompanied by residual errors, such as e in our model, because it is unlikely that the variations in y can be completely explained by x. SEM estimates the means and variances for exogenous variables whilst estimating the intercepts for the endogenous variables. This is because the variance of an endogenous variable is derived from exogenous variables as well as residual errors associated with the endogenous variable. For example, in the linear regression given in Eq. 12.1, the intercept for y will be estimated by b_0. Both the mean and variance of x will be estimated, although they are not explicitly expressed in Eq. 12.1. The mean of the residual errors is fixed to zero and the path from it to the associated endogenous variable is fixed to be unity (reflected by the regression coefficient for e in Eq. 12.1 being 1). Therefore, the only parameter to be estimated is its variance. The mean and variance of y can then be derived from Eq. 12.1. Note that observed and unobserved variables can be exogenous or endogenous variables.

12.2.2 The Path Diagram for Multiple Linear Regression

Multiple linear regression tests the relationship between one outcome variable and more than one explanatory variable. Fig. 12.2 is the path diagram for a multiple linear regression with three explanatory variables denoted:

$$y = b_0 + b_1 x_1 + b_2 x_2 + b_3 x_3 + e; \qquad (12.2)$$

where y is the outcome variable, x_1 to x_3 the explanatory variables, e the residual error term, b_0 the intercept, and b_1 to b_3 the regression coefficients for x_1 to x_3, respectively.

In Fig. 12.2, the three paths from each of the three explanatory variables to y are equivalent to the regression coefficients given by Eq. 12.2, and the interpretations of these paths are the same as that for the regression coefficients. Note that there are three double arrows in Fig. 12.2 that connect x_1, x_2 and x_3, representing the covariances amongst the three explanatory variables (their means and variances will also be estimated). This indicates the relationship between y and each x is determined whilst also taking into account the correlations amongst the three explanatory variables. Note that when multiple regression analysis is undertaken using standard software packages, the explanatory variables are always assumed to be correlated, whether or not subsequent interpretation of the regression coefficients recognizes this.

Fig. 12.2 The path diagram for multiple regression

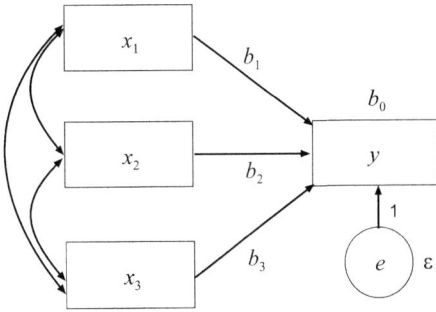

12.3 Univariate Latent Growth Curve Models

12.3.1 Data

For illustration, we use data from a randomized controlled trial (RCT) on the effects of periodontal treatments on clinical outcomes and laboratory biomarkers for systematic inflammation (Tonetti et al. 2007). In general, the treatments of gum (periodontal) diseases aim to control infection and inflammation by eradicating the periodontal pathogens within the dental plaque on the tooth or root surfaces. The periodontal pocket is the small space between a tooth and the surrounding gum (gingivae), and its healthy depth is usually about 1–3 mm. As periodontal disease progresses, the depth of periodontal pocket increases due to both the swollen gum (caused by inflammation) and the loss of attachment between the tooth and the surrounding supporting structure (such as periodontal ligament and bone). Pocket depth is measured by a periodontal probe with markings, and it is the most commonly used clinical variable for measuring periodontal diseases and treatment effects. Many recent studies have shown an association between periodontal infection and an increased risk of cardiovascular diseases. The aim of the original study was to test whether changes in clinical outcomes were associated with the changes in inflammatory biomarkers and vascular function.

The details of the RCT have been reported elsewhere (Tonetti et al. 2007). To summarise, 120 patients with chronic periodontal diseases were randomized into two groups: the control group (59 patients) received conventional periodontal treatment (CPT), i.e. professional cleaning of teeth without removal of dental plaque and calculus in the periodontal pockets. This is the treatment what patients would receive from their general dentist. The test group (61 patients) received intensive periodontal treatment (IPT), i.e. specialist periodontal treatments to remove dental plaque and calculus within periodontal pockets within a single appointment. It is called intensive, because traditionally the specialist treatment was usually given in several appointments over a few weeks. Previous studies have shown that intensive periodontal treatment may induce short-term sharp rise in the level of inflammatory biomarkers.

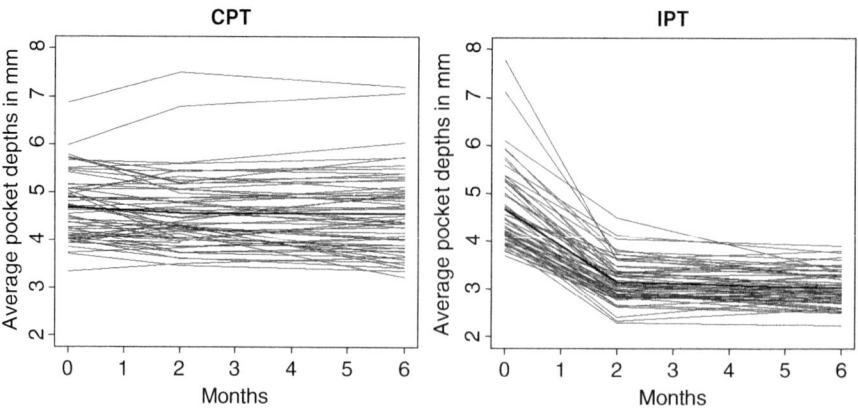

Fig. 12.3 Profile plots for pocket depths at baseline, 2 and 6 months

Full mouth pocket depths have been measured three times over this 6-month study: baseline, 2 months and 6 months. Blood tests for inflammatory biomarkers were undertaken at baseline, 1 day, 7 days, 1 month, 2 month and 6 months. In this section, we first look at the difference in the changes in pocket depths, and Fig. 12.3 shows the individual trajectories of pocket depths for the two groups.

12.3.2 Multilevel Model

A two-level multilevel model for the analysis of change in the pocket depths for these patients can be written as:

$$PD_{ij} = \pi_{0ij} + \pi_{1j} Month_{ij}; \qquad (12.3)$$

$$\pi_{0ij} = \beta_0 + \beta_2 Tx_j + e_{0ij} + u_{0j}; \qquad (12.4)$$

and

$$\pi_{1j} = \beta_1 + \beta_3 Tx_j + u_{1j}; \qquad (12.5)$$

Expanding by substituting π_{0ij} and π_{1j}, the new multilevel model becomes:

$$PD_{ij} = \beta_0 + \beta_1 Month_{ij} + \beta_2 Tx_j + \beta_3 Tx^* Month_{ij} + u_{1j} Month_{ij} + u_{0j} + e_{0ij} \quad (12.6)$$

where PD is the average full mouth pocket depth in millimeters on the ith occasion (level-1, $i = 1, 2, 3$) for the jth subject (level-2, $j = 1, \ldots, 120$), $Month$ is time in months since baseline (i.e. 0, 2, 6), Tx_j is a binary variable (IPT coded 1 and CPT code 0), and $Tx*Month_{ij}$ is a product interaction term between Tx and *Month* (i.e. *Months* multiplied by Tx).

The two-level multilevel model given by Eqs. 12.3–12.5 is a linear growth model, i.e. a straight line was fitted to the distance measured on three occasions between baseline and 6 month for each of the 120 patients. The baseline pocket depths and their changes varied across patients, so there were variations in the intercepts and slopes of the fitted straight lines. These variations were modelled as normally distributed random effects in MLM, and as we shall explain later, modelled as latent variables in LGCM.

The intercept β_0 is the average baseline pocket depth for the CPT group, and β_2 (the regression coefficient for Tx_j) is the additional baseline pocket depth for the IPT group, i.e. the average baseline distance for boys is $\beta_0 + \beta_2$. The regression coefficient for $Month_{ij}$ is β_1, which is the estimated average change in pocket depth per month for CPT; and β_3 (the regression coefficient for the interaction term $Tx*Month_{ij}$) is the difference in the slopes between the CPT and IPT groups. The slope, β_1, is the predicted amount of changes in the pocket depth *per month* for the CPT group, and the total amount of growth is therefore $\beta_1 * 6$. The slope for the IPT group is $\beta_1 + \beta_3$, and the total amount of predicted growth in the depth is $(\beta_1 + \beta_3) * 6$. As a result, the difference in the growth between the two groups is $\beta_3 * 6$.

12.3.3 Latent Growth Curve Model (LGCM)

The multilevel model in Sect. 12.3.2 can be specified using LGCM, and the path diagram in Fig. 12.4 shows the general concept of LGCM. As explained previously, observed and measured variables are represented by squares. In this model, the observed variables are the three measurements of pocket depths made at baseline (*PD0M*), 2 months (*PD2M*), and 6 months (*PD6M*). Note that software for MLM usually requires the data in long format, for example, the variable PD_{ij} in Eqs. 12.3 and 12.6 is created by stacking the three measurements of pocket depth into one column. In contrast, software for LGCM requires the data in wide format, i.e. the outcome measured on different occasions is treated as three separate variables. Another observed variable in the model is Tx, which is a binary variable (CPT is coded 0 and IPT coded 1). The parameters $m3$ and $v3$ are the mean and variance of Tx.

The latent variables are represented by circles: $F1$ and $F2$ are two latent variables which model the growth trajectories (i.e. the change patterns) for the pocket depth. The parameters $m1$ and $m2$ are the intercepts for $F1$ and $F2$; the $D1$ and $D2$ are residual error terms for $F1$ and $F2$. Recall that for endogenous variables (i.e. $F1$, $F2$, and the three measurements of pocket depth in this model) only the intercepts are estimated, because they are affected and 'explained' by exogenous variables (i.e. Tx in this model) and their associated residual errors (D and E). Like residual error terms in regression analysis, the means of $D1$ and $D2$ are fixed to

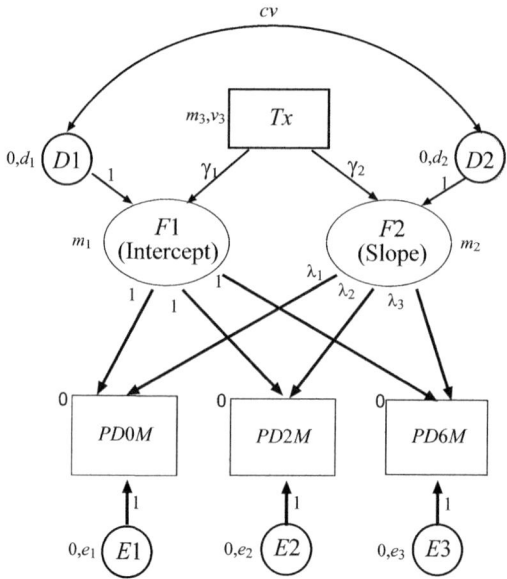

Fig. 12.4 Path diagram for univariate latent growth curve models. Observed variables such as *Tx* and *PD* are in squares and latent variables such as *F1* and *F2* are in circles. *D1* and *D2* are residual errors for *F1* and *F2*, respectively. *E1*, *E2*, and *E3* are residual errors for *PD0M*, *PD2M* and *PD6M*, respectively

be zero, and $d1$ and $d2$ are their variances, respectively. $E1$ to $E3$ are the error terms for each observed variable; $E1$ to $E3$ are assumed to be uncorrelated and to have a mean of zero. By contrast, the two latent variables $F1$ and $F2$ are assumed to be correlated (there is a double arrow between them indicating that their covariance is estimated in Fig. 12.4).

Note that $F1$ and $F2$ are unobserved (latent) variables or factors, which means that unlike PD, they are not directly measured but are estimated by extracting information from the observed variables. Therefore, the meaning of $F1$ and $F2$ depends upon how this information is extracted, i.e. it depends upon how the relationships between them and PD are defined in the model by specifying the parameters for the arrows from $F1$ and $F2$ to PD. The regression coefficients for the arrows from $F1$ to the three measurements of PD are fixed to be unity, and those for the arrows from the residual errors (D and E) are also fixed to be unity. So a latent growth curve model or structural equation model can be viewed as an attempt to use multiple equations to define the relationships amongst observed and unobserved variables in the model.

For instance, the equation for the relationship between $PD0M$ and other variables in Fig. 12.4 is given as:

$$PD0M = 1^*F1 + \lambda_1^*F2 + 1^*E1. \qquad (12.7)$$

Similarly, the equation for $PD2M$ and $PD6M$ in Fig. 12.5 are given as:

$$PD2M = 1^*F1 + \lambda_2^*F2 + 1^*E2. \qquad (12.8)$$

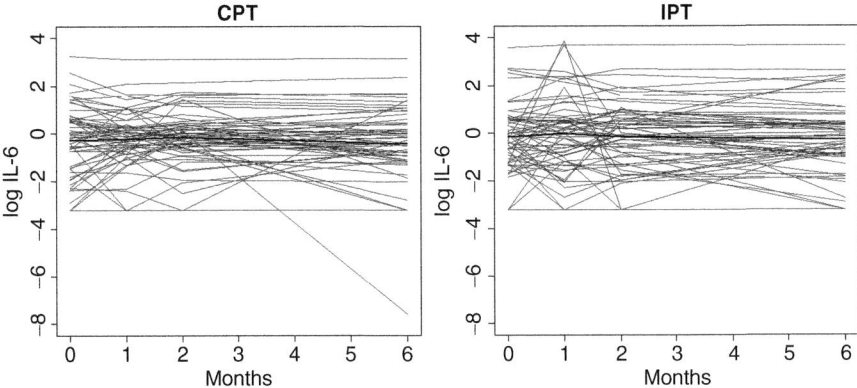

Fig. 12.5 Profile plots for log transformed IL-6 levels in blood samples at baseline, 1, 2 and 6 months

$$PD6M = 1^*F1 + \lambda_3{}^*F2 + 1^*E3. \qquad (12.9)$$

$$F1 = m1 + \gamma_1{}^*Tx + 1^*D1. \qquad (12.10)$$

$$F2 = m2 + \gamma_2{}^*Tx + 1^*D2; \qquad (12.11)$$

where $m1$ an $m2$ are the intercepts in Eqs. 12.10 and 12.11 for $F1$ and $F2$, respectively; and $\lambda 1, \lambda 2, \lambda 3, \lambda 4, \gamma 1, \gamma 2$ are regression coefficients. Recall the simple linear regression given by Eq. 12.1: $y = b_0 + b_1 x + e$, where b_0 and b_1 are two unknown parameter which need to be estimated. The regression coefficient for e is actually fixed to be unity just like those for $E1$ to $D2$ in Eqs. 12.7–12.11. Therefore, we can view LGCM (or SEM in general) as a system of multiple equations for the relationships amongst the observed and latent variables and to identify their relationships by solving these equations simultaneously. In Eqs. 12.7–12.11, some of the parameters have been given (such as the factor loadings fixed to be unity), and the unknown parameters, such as γ and λ, need to be estimated. In Fig. 12.4, all the means of residual errors are fixed to be zero, just like the means of residual errors in the ordinary regression models. It is noted that the intercepts of observed outcome variables *PD0M, PD2M and PD6M* in Eqs. 12.7–12.9 are also fixed to be zero, because the expected means of these variables will be estimated via the latent variables $F1$ and $F2$.

12.3.3.1 Equivalence Between MLM and LGCM

To specify a LGCM model (given by Eqs. 12.7–12.11) equivalent to MLM given by Eqs. 12.3–12.5, we fix the regression weights for the paths from $F2$ to *PD0, PD2M and PD6M*, i.e. $\lambda 1, \lambda 2$ and $\lambda 3$, to be 0, 2 and 6, respectively, to match the time when they are measured. The latent variables $F1$ and $F2$ are then equivalent to the estimated baseline pocket depths and the estimated changes in pocket depths over 6 months, respectively. Recall that Eq. 12.7 is written as: $PD0M = 1^*F1 + \lambda_1^*F2 + 1^*E1$. When $\lambda_1 = 0$, $PD0M = 1^*F1 + 1^*E1$, i.e. $PD0M$ is decomposed into a latent variable $F1$ and residual errors variable $E1$. On the other hand, $F1$ can be viewed as the unobserved true $PD0M$ by removing the measurement errors and random variations. Therefore, $F2$, which is estimated from the differences between $PD0M$, $PD2M$ and $PD6M$, is the estimated change from $F1$.

The variances of $D1$ and $D2$ ($d1$ and $d2$), i.e. the variations in the estimated baseline pocket depths and changes in pocket depths, are equivalent to the random effects of the intercept (u_{0j}) and slope (u_{1j}) in Eqs. 12.4 and 12.5, respectively. By constraining the variances of $E1$, $E2$, and $E3$, i.e. $e1$, $e2$, and $e3$, to be equal, they are equivalent to e_{0ij} in Eq. 12.4. In Eqs. 12.5 and 12.6, β_3 is the difference in the change in average pocket depth per month between CPT and IPT groups over the 6-month observation, and its equivalent in LGCM is γ_2. The equivalents of β_0, β_1, and β_2 in LGCM are $m1$, $m2$ and γ_1.

In summary, for longitudinal data analysis, both MLM and LGCM estimate a linear growth trajectory (i.e. a change pattern) for each patient. Variations in the intercepts and slopes of these trajectories, regarded as random effects in MLM, are explicitly specified in LGCM as latent variables, because unlike PD, which is directly observed and measured, these trajectories and their variations (random effects) are unknown and need to be estimated.

12.3.4 Analysis Using LGCM

The results from Mplus using maximum likelihood estimation are shown in Table 12.1. Mplus (and other SEM software) provides many additional indices for accessing model fit. Two most commonly used are the Chi-square test and Root Mean Square Error of Approximation (RMSEA). The Chi-square value for the model is 250.5 with 4 degrees of freedom ($P < 0.001$), and RMSEA is 0.717. In SEM, the null hypothesis for the Chi-square test is that there is no difference in the covariance structures between the proposed model and the data, and a P-value greater than 0.05 means that we cannot reject the null hypothesis. This is different from the usual null hypothesis testing where researchers seek to reject the null hypothesis. In contrast, a small RMSEA means that the proposed model fits the data relatively well (0.06 is usually used as the cut-off value) (Kline 2011). Apparently, this linear latent curve model is not acceptable and requires modification. Moreover, the estimated variance of $D2$ is -0.013, which is not acceptable, because the variance is the square of the standard deviation and should always be a positive value. The case of negative variance is known as a Heywood Case in SEM literature (Loehlin 2004; Kline 2011), i.e. an offending estimate which indicates serious flaws in the model specifications. This should not be surprising, as Fig. 12.3 clearly shows

Table 12.1 Results of univariate latent growth curve models for pocket depths following the SEM outlined in Fig. 12.4

Linear model					Nonlinear model					Nonlinear model with additional path				
Regression coefficients					**Regression coefficients**					**Regression coefficients**				
		Estimate	SE	P			Estimate	SE	P			Estimate	SE	P
F1	→ Tx	−0.392	0.124	0.002	F1	→ Tx	−0.009	0.135	0.948	F1	→ Tx	−0.007	0.135	0.959
F2	→ Tx	−0.218	0.017	<0.001	F2	→ Tx	−0.253	0.017	<0.001	F2	→ Tx	−0.249	0.018	<0.001
PD0	→ F1	1			PD0	→ F1	1			PD0	→ F1	1		
PD0	→ F2	0			PD0	→ F2	0			PD0	→ F2	0		
PD2M	→ F1	1			PD2M	→ F1	1			PD2M	→ F1	1		
PD2M	→ F2	2			PD2M	→ F2	5.448	0.12	<0.001	PD2M	→ F2	4.717	0.296	<0.001
PD6M	→ F1	1			PD6M	→ F1	1			PD6M	→ F1	1		
PD6M	→ F2	6			PD6M	→ F2	6			PD6M	→ F2	6		
										PD2M	→ Tx	−0.231	0.088	0.009
Intercepts					**Intercepts**					**Intercepts**				
		Estimate	SE	P			Estimate	SE	P			Estimate	SE	P
F1		4.652	0.088	<0.001	F1		4.682	0.097	<0.001	F1		4.681	0.096	<0.001
F2		−0.023	0.012	0.058	F2		−0.024	0.012	0.041	F2		−0.026	0.013	0.039
Covariances					**Covariances**					**Covariances**				
		Estimate	SE	P			Estimate	SE	P			Estimate	SE	P
D1	↔ D2	0.028	0.009	0.003	D1	↔ D2	−0.032	0.007	<0.001	D1	↔ D2	−0.034	0.008	<0.001
Correlations					**Correlations**					**Correlations**				
		Estimate					Estimate					Estimate		
D1	↔ D2	*			D1	↔ D2	−0.562			D1	↔ D2	−0.555		
Variances					**Variances**					**Variances**				
		Estimate	SE	P			Estimate	SE	P			Estimate	SE	P
E1		0.387	0.05	<0.001	E1		0.041	0.005	<0.001	E1		0.038	0.005	<0.001
E2		0.387	0.05	<0.001	E2		0.041	0.005	<0.001	E2		0.038	0.005	<0.001
E3		0.387	0.05	<0.001	E3		0.041	0.005	<0.001	E3		0.038	0.005	<0.001
D1		0.184	0.07	<0.001	D1		0.51	0.071	<0.001	D1		0.507	0.071	<0.001
D2		−0.013	0.003	0.058	D2		0.006	0.001	<0.001	D2		0.007	0.001	<0.001
Model fit indices					**Model fit indices**					**Model fit indices**				
Chi-square	df = 4	250.508		<0.001	Chi-square	df = 3	7.642		0.054	Chi-square	df = 3	1.629		0.443
RMSEA		0.717			RMSEA		0.114			RMSEA		0		

*Because the variance of D2 is negative, it is impossible to calculate the correlation coefficient that the change in pocket depths did not appear to be linear. Traditional approach would be to add a quadratic term for *Month* in order to fit a curve-linear model. However, as there are only three measurements of pocket depths, quadratic curve fitting is not the best approach. Although results seem to suggest that patients in IPT group had lower average pocket depth at baseline (-0.392 mm, $P < 0.001$) and greater pocket depth reduction (-0.218 mm, $P < 0.001$), the validity of these results is highly questionable.

12.3.5 Non-linear Latent Growth Curve Model

The observed trajectories shown in Fig. 12.3 suggest a non-linear growth curve, and there are many simple and advanced approaches to model non-linear curves in the statistical literature (see Chap. 15). Because there are only three measurements of pocket depths over the 6-month period, most advanced methods, such as fractional polynomials and splines (see Chap. 15), are not suitable.

LGCM provides an elegant way to model the non-linear growth curve. Recall that in the linear growth curve model, the paths from *F2* to *PD0M, PD2M and PD6M* ($\lambda 1, \lambda 2,$ and $\lambda 3$) are fixed to be 0, 2 and 6, respectively. To capture the non-linearity, we can fixed the first path ($\lambda 1$) to be 0 and the final path ($\lambda 3$) to be 6 but allow $\lambda 2$ to be a free parameter for estimation (Bollen and Curran 2006; Duncan et al. 2006; Tu et al. 2008). If the estimated values for $\lambda 2$ are close to 2, this indicates that the growth curves are approximately linear. The results from this approach using Mplus (Table 12.2) show that $\lambda 2$ is 5.45, indicating that most of the change in pocket depths occurred during the first 2 months. The Chi-square value for the model is 7.64 with 3 degrees of freedom ($P = 0.054$) and RMSEA $= 0.114$. In contrast to the results from the previous model, patients in the IPT group did not have a significantly lower average pocket depth at baseline (-0.009 mm, $P = 0.948$), but they did show greater pocket depth reduction (-0.253 mm, $P < 0.001$) at 6 months.

The large difference in the Chi-square values between the linear and nonlinear models indicates a substantial improvement in the model fit. However, the Chi-square value and RMSEA are still not ideal. The *P*-value for the Chi-square test is just greater than 0.05, whereas the statistical power of the Chi-square test to reject a structural equation model is related to sample size. As our sample size is moderate, we should not feel complacent about the result of the Chi-square test. Also note that when the degree of freedom becomes zero, the model will get a perfect fit, i.e. the Chi-square value will certainly become zero. This is known as a saturated model. The aim of statistical model building is therefore to seek models that approximate the relationships between variables in a parsimonious way. A good model is one with a small Chi-square value relative to the model's degree of freedom. In this nonlinear model, it is assumed that changes in pocket depth within both the CPT and IPT groups followed similar patterns, but the profile plots in Fig. 12.3 showed that there was a steeper change in pocket depth for the IPT group between baseline

Table 12.2 Results of univariate latent growth curve models for IL-6 following the SEM outlined in Fig. 12.4

Linear model					
Regression coefficients					
			Estimate	SE	P
F1	←	Tx	0.121	0.240	0.614
F2	←	Tx	0.001	0.044	0.982
tIL6_0	←	F1	1		
tIL6_0	←	F2	0		
tIL6_1	←	F1	1		
tIL6_1	←	F2	1		
tIL6_2	←	F1	1		
tIL6_2	←	F2	2		
tIL6_6	←	F1	1		
tIL6_6	←	F2	6		
Intercepts					
			Estimate	SE	P
F1			−0.220	0.171	0.199
F2			−0.032	0.032	0.316
Covariances					
			Estimate	SE	P
D1	↔	D2	−0.046	0.031	0.141
Correlations					
			Estimate		
D1	↔	D2	−0.234		
Variances					
			Estimate	SE	P
E1			0.632	0.058	<0.001
E2			0.632	0.058	<0.001
E3			0.632	0.058	<0.001
E4			0.632	0.058	<0.001
D1			0.412	0.224	<0.001
D2			0.027	0.008	0.001
Model fit indices					
Chi-square		df = 10	11.49		0.32
RMSEA			0.035		

and 2 months. This may be the cause of misfit, and to accommodate this subtle difference in the trends, we add an additional path from *Tx* to *PD2M* in Fig. 12.4. This additional path is to capture the additional change in pocket depth between baseline and 2 months in the IPT group. After adding the additional path, the Chi-square value becomes 1.63 with 2 degrees of freedom ($P = 0.44$) and RMSEA is zero, indicating a further improvement in model fit. This final model shows both groups had similar average pocket depths at baseline, but the IPT group achieved greater pocket depth reduction (−0.249 mm, $P < 0.001$) at 6 months.

12.4 Multivariate LGCM

One advantage of LGCM over other approaches is that it provides a flexible framework to test the relationships for multiple outcomes, i.e. we can test the growth curve models of different outcomes and their associations. In this section, we use LGCM to test the relationships between change in pocket depth and the level of interleukin-6 (IL-6), an inflammatory biomarker.

Four measurements of IL-6 made at baseline, 1, 2 and 6 months are used for our analysis. Like many blood tests results, the distributions of IL-6 are severely positively skewed, so a natural log transformation of the original variables are undertaken to make their distribution symmetrical before LGCM analysis is conducted. The profile plots in Fig. 12.5 shows the trends in the levels of log transformed IL-6 during the 6-month observations. We first fit a linear latent curve model, and the results show a very good model fit (Table 12.2). IL-6 levels slightly decreased after 6 months and there is no statistically significant difference in the baseline IL-6 levels or change in IL-6 between the two treatment groups.

Figure 12.6 shows the conceptual path diagram of the multivariate latent curve model for pocket depths and IL-6 after periodontal treatments. We hypothesize that patients with greater baseline pocket depths would have higher levels of IL-6 at baseline, and patients with greater reduction in pocket depths would also have greater reduction in IL-6 levels. Table 12.3 shows that the Chi-square value of the multivariate model is 21.43 with 21 degrees of freedom ($P = 0.43$) and RMSEA is 0.013, and both tests indicate an acceptable model fit. The results from Mplus show that patients with 1 mm greater baseline pocket depths had 0.29 unit greater log transformed IL-6 at baseline (0.29, $P = 0.291$), and patients with 1 mm greater reduction in pocket depths had 0.394 unit greater reduction in IL-6 levels ($P = 0.21$). Patients with greater average pocket depths at baseline also showed greater reduction in IL-6 levels (0.065, $P = 0.078$). Nevertheless, none of these associations are statistically significant. Patients in the IPT group showed greater reduction in pocket depths (0.249 mm, $P < 0.001$) than the CPT group, but there is no statistically significant difference in the reduction of IL-6 levels between the two groups. Therefore, though the directions of relationships between the changes in pocket depths and IL-6 levels follow what have been hypothesized, the effect sizes are not sufficiently large to reject the null hypothesis. A larger study with greater statistical power is therefore required to test the complex relationships between these two outcomes.

12.5 Conclusion

In this article, we demonstrate how to apply LGCM to analyze longitudinal data. These methods, if applied properly, can be very useful and powerful statistical tools for epidemiological researchers. Any statistical method has its limitations, and LGCM is no exception. In our examples, the intervals between the measurements

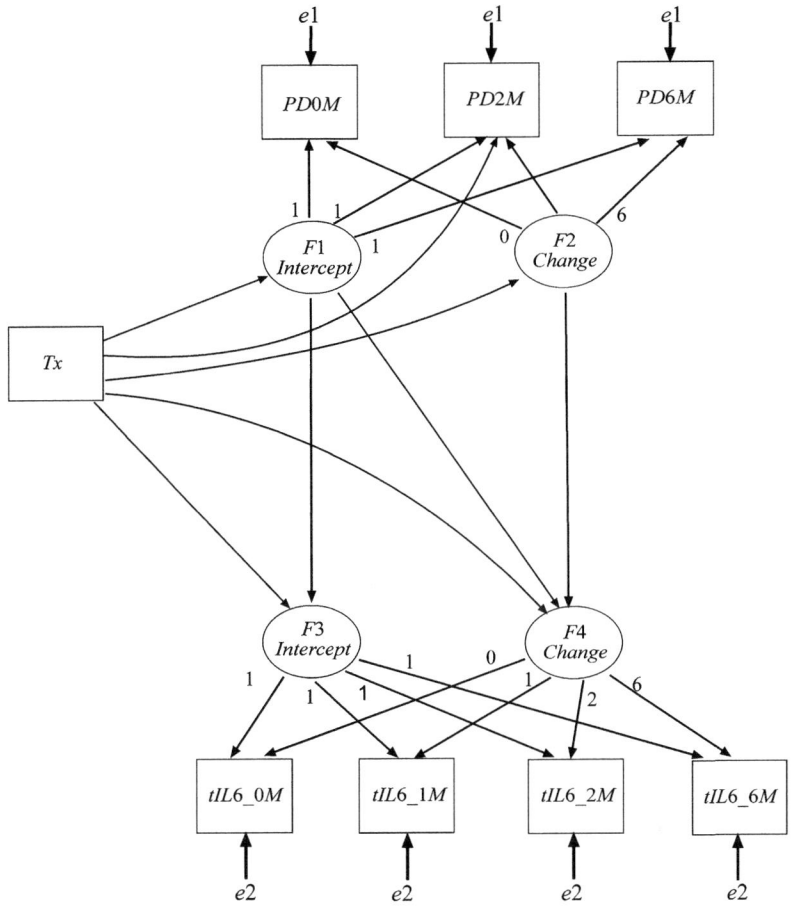

Fig. 12.6 Path diagram for multivariate latent growth curve model. To simplify the presentation, the residual errors for $F1$ to $F4$ ($D1$ to $D4$) are omitted. The variances ($e1$) of residual error terms ($E1$) for the three pocket depths are fixed to be equal, and the variances ($e2$) of four residual errors ($E2$) for log transformed IL-6 measured at baseline ($tIL6\_0M$), 1 month ($tIL6\_1M$), 2 months ($tIL6\_2M$) and 6 months ($tIL6\_6M$), respectively, were also fixed to be equal

of outcomes were approximately identical for all subjects. If, for example, PD was measured at baseline, 2 and 6 months after interventions for some patients but at baseline, 4 and 7 months for others, this will not pose any problem in the analyses employing multilevel modeling, but this is currently a problem when undertaking LGCM for some SEM software packages (though not a problem for Mplus). This reflects the limitations of current statistical software rather than the method itself. Therefore, researchers should choose the methods (and software) best suited for their research questions and study design. We strongly encourage epidemiologists to consult professional statisticians when they plan to use these methods to analyze their longitudinal data.

Table 12.3 Results of multivariate latent growth curve models following the SEM outlined in Fig. 12.6

Regression coefficients:					
			Estimate	S.E.	P
F1 (PD)	←	Tx	−0.007	0.135	0.959
F2 (PD)	←	Tx	−0.248	0.018	<0.001
F3 (tIL-6)	←	Tx	0.123	0.237	0.604
F4 (tIL-6)	←	Tx	0.100	0.090	0.265
F3	←	F1	0.290	0.172	0.091
F4	←	F2	0.394	0.314	0.290
F4	←	F1	0.065	0.037	0.078
PD2M	←	Tx	4.714	0.296	<0.001
Intercepts					
			Estimate	S.E.	P
F1			4.681	0.096	<0.001
F2			−0.026	0.013	0.039
F3			−1.578	0.822	0.055
F4			−0.324	0.170	0.057
Covariances					
			Estimate	S.E.	P
D1	↔	D2	−0.034	0.008	<0.001
D3	↔	D4	−0.050	0.031	0.103
Correlations					
			Estimate		
D1	↔	D2	−0.555		
D3	↔	D4	−0.268		
Variances					
			Estimate	S.E.	P
D1			0.507	0.071	<0.001
D2			0.007	0.001	<0.001
D3			1.369	0.219	<0.001
D4			0.026	0.008	<0.001
E1			0.038	0.005	<0.001
E2			0.632	0.058	<0.001
Model fit indices					
Chi-square		df = 21	21.43		0.43
RMSEA			0.013		

12.6 Further Reading

For readers with knowledge of linear algebra, Bauer (2003) and Curran (2003) explain why MLM and LGCM yield the same results. Bollen and Curran (2006) and Duncan et al. (2006) are two textbooks dedicated to LGCM. The former is more mathematical. Many examples for the applications of LGCM can be found in psychological journals. Tu et al. (2008) provides an example for applying LGCM to biomedical data with multiple outcomes.

References

Bauer, D. J. (2003). Estimating multilevel linear models as structural equation models. *Journal of Educational and Behavioral Statistics, 28*, 135–167.

Bollen, K. A. (1989). *Structural equations with latent variables*. New York: Wiley.

Bollen, K. A., & Curran, P. J. (2006). *Latent curve models*. Hoboken: Wiley.

Byrne, B. M., & Crombie, G. (2003). Modeling and testing change: An introduction to the latent growth curve model. *Understanding Statistics, 2*, 177–203.

Curran, P. (2003). Have multilevel models been structural equation models all along? *Multivariate Behavioral Research, 38*, 529–569.

Duncan, T. E., Duncan, S. C., & Strycker, L. A. (2006). *An introduction to latent variable growth curve modeling* (2nd ed.). Mahwah: Laurence Erlbaum Associates.

Gilthorpe, M. S., Zamzuri, A. T., Griffiths, G. S., et al. (2003). Unification of the "burst" and "linear" theories of periodontal disease progression: A multilevel manifestation of the same phenomenon. *Journal of Dental Research, 82*, 200–205.

Goldstein, H. (1995). *Multilevel statistical models* (2nd ed.). New York: Wiley.

Hox, J. (2002). *Multilevel analysis*. Mahwah: Laurence Erlbaum Associates.

Kline, R. B. (2011). *Principles and practice of structural equation modeling* (3rd ed.). New York: Guilford Press.

Liang, K. Y., & Zeger, S. L. (1986). Longitudinal data analysis using generalized linear models. *Biometrika, 73*, 13–22.

Loehlin, J. C. (2004). *Latent variable models: An introduction to factor, path, and structural equation analysis* (4th ed.). Mahwah: Laurence Erlbaum Associates.

Muthén, L. K., & Muthén, B. (2006). *Mplus user's guide* (4th ed.). Los Angeles: Muthén & Muthén.

Raudenbush, S. W., & Bryk, A. S. (2002). *Hierarchical linear model* (2nd ed.). Thousand Oaks: Sage Publication.

Senn, S., Stevens, L., & Chaturvedi, N. (2000). Repeated measures in clinical trials: Simple strategies for analysis using summary measures. *Statistics in Medicine, 19*, 861–877.

Singer, J. B., & Willett, J. D. (2003). *Applied longitudinal data analysis*. New York: Oxford University Press.

Steele, F. (2008). Multilevel models for longitudinal data. *Journal of the Royal Statistical Society Series A, 171*, 1–15.

Tonetti M. S., D'Aiuto F., Nibali L., Donald A., Storry C., Parkar M., Suvan J., Hingorani A. D., Vallance P., Deanfield J. (2007) Treatment of periodontitis and endothelial function. New Engl J Med, *356*(9), 911–920.

Tu, Y. K., Jackson, M., Kellett, M., & Clerehugh, V. (2008). Direct and indirect effects of interdental hygiene in a clinical trial. *Journal of Dental Research, 87*, 1037–1042.

Twisk, J. W. R. (2003). *Applied longitudinal data analysis for epidemiology*. Cambridge, UK: Cambridge University Press.

Twisk, J. W. R. (2006). *Applied multilevel analysis*. Cambridge, UK: Cambridge University Press.

Chapter 13
Growth Mixture Modelling for Life Course Epidemiology

Darren L. Dahly

13.1 Introduction

Life course epidemiology is the study of how physical and social exposures occurring across the entire life course, or even inter-generationally, can impact chronic disease risk later in life (Ben-Shlomo and Kuh 2002). The life course approach to chronic disease epidemiology is not a new one, though it was overshadowed during much of the twentieth century by research on the importance of adulthood lifestyle risk factors such as smoking and diet (Kuh and Ben-Shlomo 2004). Recently, however, the life course approach to epidemiology has been given more attention by researchers, funding agencies, and policy makers (Ben-Shlomo and Kuh 2002; De Stavola et al. 2006; Kuh and Ben-Shlomo 2004; Kuh et al. 2003; Pickles et al. 2007).

A key life course theme is the Developmental Origins of Health and Disease (DOHaD) paradigm. In its most basic formulation, it hypothesises that environmental influences during critical periods of development can impact physiology in a manner that increases disease risk later in life (Gillman 2005; Gluckman and Hanson 2004; Barker 2004). While early DOHaD research focused on nutritional and other influences during foetal development (Barker 2001), there is a growing interest in post-natal influences, particularly in the role that post-natal growth may play in the aetiology of later obesity, diabetes, and cardiovascular disease (Ong and Loos 2006; Baird et al. 2005; Monteiro and Victora 2005; Stein et al. 2005; Stettler 2007).

Not surprisingly, reviews of published research paint a complex picture. Some evidence suggests rapid growth in early infancy is associated with obesity later in life (Baird et al. 2005; Monteiro and Victora 2005; Ong and Loos 2006), while other research suggests that poor growth in early life is associated with diabetes and heart disease (Eriksson et al. 2001; Eriksson et al. 2003). Existing evidence largely

---

D.L. Dahly (✉)
Division of Biostatistics, Centre for Epidemiology and Biostatistics,
Leeds Institute of Genetics, Health & Therapeutics, University of Leeds, Leeds, UK
e-mail: d.l.dahly@leeds.ac.uk

consists of observed associations between the rate of weight change over a specific period in infancy or childhood (e.g. birth to 6 months) and later disease. Building upon this research, more sophisticated approaches such two stage least squares (Healy 1974; Gale et al. 2006; Keijzer-Veen et al. 2005; Adair et al. 2009), multi-level spline models (Ben-Shlomo et al. 2008), and partial least squares regression (Tu et al. 2010) have been employed to try and identify critical periods where growth is associated with later disease, independent of final attained size and growth in other periods. One important limitation of these methods is that they fail to consider that growth may be more important than the sum of its parts, i.e. they do not consider possible interactions between varying rates of growth over different periods of time. Recognising this, some have suggested that later disease is associated with overall patterns of pre- and postnatal growth (Victora and Barros 2001). To investigate this possibility, we need a way to identify mutually exclusive groups of people who share a similar growth trajectory, and then relate those groups to later disease and other covariates. This chapter aims to illustrate the utility of growth mixture models for just this purpose.

13.2 Mixture Models

Epidemiologists often aim to detect meaningful differences in groups of people (e.g. by treatment group, gender, or social class). We typically group people based on the hypothesis being tested, and then relate group membership to other covariates through a statistical model (e.g. a linear regression of systolic blood pressure on treatment arm in a randomized controlled trial). In some cases we might expect the association to vary across levels of another observed variable, such as gender, which could be tested by including the appropriate product interaction term in the model (see Chap. 17). However, there could also be unmeasured characteristics that modify the impact of treatment. This concept is referred to as *unobserved heterogeneity*.

Mixture modelling, broadly speaking, is a clustering method that aims to detect unobserved heterogeneity by allowing model parameters to vary across a multinomial latent class variable. The complexity of the model can range from a simple mean to very complex structural equation models. When the underlying model is a latent growth curve (see Chap. 12), the addition of a latent class variable results in a *Growth Mixture Model* (Jung and Wickrama 2008; Muthén and Muthén 2000). While must be specified in advance (a point we will come back to shortly), and the prior probabilities of membership in each class are estimated.

By allowing the parameters describing the latent growth curve to vary across classes, growth mixture models can be used to identify mutually exclusive subgroups of individuals who share a similar growth curve. Growth mixture modelling has been illustrated in studies of alcohol use (Li et al. 2001; Muthén and Muthén 2000; Muthén 2001), criminology (Kreuter and Muthén 2008), and educational attainment (Muthén 2001). To date, this method has been largely overlooked in life course epidemiology (a rare examples include Li et al. 2007; Østbye et al. 2011).

To illustrate the method for an audience of applied life course researchers, we used growth mixture modelling to group individuals based on their body mass index (BMI) trajectories from birth to 2 years, and then related subgroup membership to later systolic blood pressure and waist circumference, while controlling for socio-economic status (SES). We recommend that the reader become familiar with Chapters. 6 (which includes an overview of mixture models), 11 (structural equation models) and 12 (latent growth curve models), before continuing here.

13.3 Data

Data are from 1,620 young adult males enrolled in the Cebu Longitudinal Health and Nutrition Survey (CLHNS), a community based study of a 1-year birth cohort living in Metropolitan Cebu, Philippines. Detailed information on the study design is given by Adair et al. (2010), and data are available to download at http://www.cpc.unc.edu/projects/cebu.

Surveys were conducted during the third trimester of pregnancy; birth; bimonthly to 24 months; and at 8.5, 11.5, 16, 19, and 21.5 years (mean ages). The estimated trajectories are based on 13 measures of BMI from birth to 24 months, calculated as kg/m^2 from measured lengths and weights using standard techniques (Lohman et al. 1988). BMI is a measure of body mass that is relatively independent of height/length across the life course and is most often used as a proxy for adiposity in population based studies. While it is correlated with percent body fat, there are limitations to it use (Hall and Cole 2006), though these concerns go beyond the scope of this chapter.

We focused on systolic blood pressure and waist circumference as the distal health outcomes, measured in young adulthood. The former was calculated as the mean of three repeat measures using a mercury sphygmomanometer taken after a 10 min seated rest; the latter was measured in cm at the midpoint between the bottom of the ribs and the top of the iliac crest. We also included SES scores, measured at birth and young adulthood, as key covariates. These were derived from a principal components analysis of interviewer observed household goods and housing materials (Vyas and Kumaranayake 2006; Victora et al. 2008).

13.4 Statistical Modelling

We estimated a variety of statistical models for this analysis, all of which are described in detail below. We started with a latent growth curve model that only included the repeated BMI measures from the first 2 years of life. We then extended this to a growth mixture model though the inclusion of a categorical latent class variable. We then modeled class membership as a predictor of the two distal health outcomes, systolic blood pressure and waist circumference, while controlling for SES at birth and young adulthood. While we are not able to cover every detail for each estimated model, all models were estimated using Mplus 5.2 (Muthén & Muthén, Los Angeles, USA), and the code used is included in the appendices.

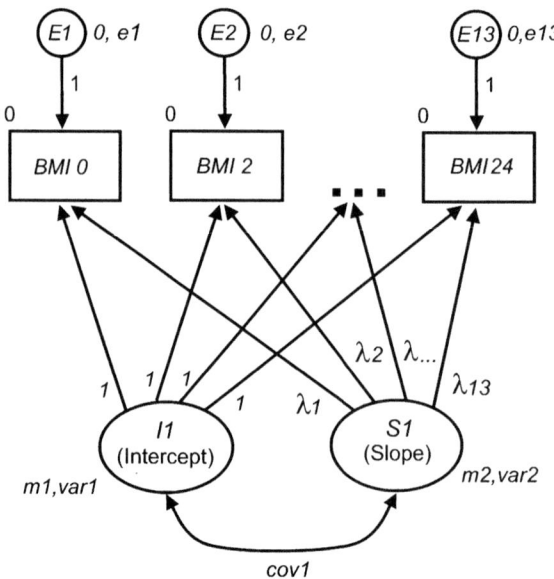

Fig. 13.1 Graphical representation of a latent growth curve model (13.4.1) for body mass index (BMI) from zero (birth) to 24 months. The model hypothesizes that the observed value of a person's BMI at any time point is a function of random intercept and slope factors and time specific random error

13.4.1 Latent Growth Curve Model

First we estimated a latent growth curve model which will serve as the base of our later mixture modelling. The model is presented graphically in Fig. 13.1. It includes the following variables: the 13 observed measures of BMI (abbreviated by the ellipsis ...), the corresponding time specific latent error terms (E), and the latent intercept and slope growth factors ($I1$ and $S1$). Freely estimated parameters include the error variances ($e1$-$e13$), the intercept and slope variances ($var1$, $var2$) and means ($m1$, $m2$), and the covariance of the slope and intercept ($cov1$). The error means and the intercepts of the measured BMI variables are set at zero, and the factor loadings for $I1$ are set at one. The factor loadings $\lambda 1$ and $\lambda 2$ are set at zero and one, respectively. The remaining factor loadings are freely estimated ($\lambda 3$-$\lambda 13$), resulting in a freed-loading model (Bollen and Curran 2006; Meredith and Tisak 1990). While this complicates the interpretation of the slope factor, freeing these factor loadings helps us avoid making any a priori assumptions regarding the functional form of the BMI trajectory. This seems particularly advantageous given our eventual goal of identifying unobserved heterogeneity in the BMI trajectories.

The estimated parameters, standard errors, and multiple indices of model fit are given in Table 13.1. Mean BMI at birth, $m1$, was 12.40 kg/m^2 (SE 0.036); mean change in BMI from birth to month 2, $m2$, was 3.27 kg/m^2 (SE 0.045). Both growth factors had a non-zero variance ($var1$ and $var2$), and their covariance, $cov1$, was negative.

Table 13.1 Results from the latent growth curve model (13.4.1)

	Estimate	SE	R^2		Estimate	SE
Means				Covariance		
I1 *(m1)*	12.401	0.036	–	I1 and S1 *(cov1)*	−0.217	0.066
S2 *(m2)*	3.274	0.045	–			
				Factor loadings		
Variances				$\lambda 1$ (BMI$_0$)	0.000	–
I1 *(var1)*	0.642	0.073	–	$\lambda 2$ (BMI$_2$)	1.000	–
S1 *(var2)*	0.930	0.077	–	$\lambda 3$ (BMI$_4$)	1.326	0.019
				$\lambda 4$ (BMI$_6$)	1.382	0.019
e1 (BMI$_0$)	1.425	0.076	0.26	$\lambda 5$ (BMI$_8$)	1.311	0.017
e2 (BMI$_2$)	2.240	0.084	0.14	$\lambda 6$ (BMI$_{10}$)	1.225	0.016
e3 (BMI$_4$)	1.765	0.069	0.36	$\lambda 7$ (BMI$_{12}$)	1.158	0.015
e4 (BMI$_6$)	1.205	0.050	0.53	$\lambda 8$ (BMI$_{14}$)	1.105	0.014
e5 (BMI$_8$)	0.841	0.036	0.64	$\lambda 9$ (BMI$_{16}$)	1.072	0.014
e6 (BMI$_{10}$)	0.640	0.028	0.70	$\lambda 10$ (BMI$_{18}$)	1.047	0.014
e7 (BMI$_{12}$)	0.495	0.022	0.75	$\lambda 11$ (BMI$_{20}$)	1.032	0.013
e8 (BMI$_{14}$)	0.439	0.019	0.76	$\lambda 12$ (BMI$_{22}$)	1.037	0.014
e9 (BMI$_{16}$)	0.414	0.018	0.74	$\lambda 13$ (BMI$_{24}$)	1.034	0.014
e10 (BMI$_{18}$)	0.362	0.017	0.76			
e11 (BMI$_{20}$)	0.393	0.018	0.73			
e12 (BMI$_{22}$)	0.529	0.023	0.63			
e13 (BMI$_{24}$)	0.661	0.028	0.56			

MODEL FIT: χ^2 3,998.352, 75df, p < 0.0001 (where adequate model fit is often indicated when p > 0.05); Comparative Fit Index 0.757; Tucker Lewis Index 0.747; Log Likelihood −23,771.442; Akaike Information Criterion 51,599.237; Bayesian Information Criterion 51,755.552; Root Mean Square Error of Approximation 0.180 (90% CI 0.175–0.184); Standardized Root Mean Square Residual 0.207

Using the time specific error variances (*e1-e13*) estimated by the model, and the observed variances of the BMI measures, we can calculate R^2 values. They show that the model explains much of the variation in BMI from 6 to 24 months (~50–75%), but considerably less of the variation from birth to 4 months.

The freely estimated factor loadings ($\lambda 3$- $\lambda 13$) can be interpreted as the change in BMI from birth, relative to the change in BMI from birth to 2 months (accomplished by setting their respective λ at zero and one, respectively). In other words, the scale of the slope factor is the change in BMI (kg/m^2) from birth to 2 months. For example, the estimate of $\lambda 3$ indicates that BMI increased 1.33 times more from birth to 4 months than it did from birth to month 2. According to the model, BMI increased rapidly from birth to 6 months, and then slowly declined to month 24.

Figure 13.2 displays the model estimated mean BMI trajectory, along with the observed trajectories of 20 randomly selected individuals. While the mean curve is what we would expect, given what we know about BMI in infancy (e.g. Cole et al. 2000), there is clearly a great deal of variation around the curve. In a latent growth curve model, deviations from the mean trajectory are explained by individual variation in the growth factors and time specific errors. However, a cursory inspection of Fig. 13.2 suggests that this explanation may be inadequate,

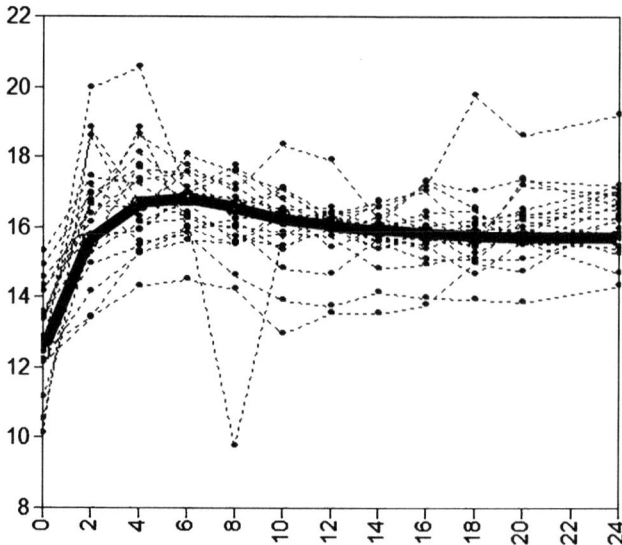

Fig. 13.2 Estimated mean BMI curve in infancy (*heavy solid line*) from the latent growth curve model (13.4.1), and observed curves for 20 randomly selected individuals (*dashed lines*)

particularly as there there are apparent differences between individuals in the timing of peaks and troughs in the curve. This phase variation (Hermanussen and Meigen 2007), while potentially very important, cannot be captured by the latent growth curve model since the estimated factor loadings (λ) that describe the functional form of the BMI curve are fixed effects (i.e. assumed to be the same for every individual in the sample). The poor model fit, indicated by the various criteria given in Table 13.1, further suggests that this parameterization of BMI changes in infancy is not a very good one. Next we set out to determine whether the variation in BMI trajectories is better explained by the idea that our overall sample contains subgroups characterized by BMI curves with different functional forms.

13.4.2 Growth Mixture Modelling

To test this idea, we added a categorical latent variable to the latent growth curve model we just described. Each parameter that was freely estimated in the latent growth curve model was allowed to vary across latent classes (including any estimated factor loadings) with the following exception: the variances of the growth factors, *var1* and *var2*, were constrained as zero in all classes. These constraints to the growth mixture model result in a specific form that is referred to as *latent class growth analysis* (Jung and Wickrama 2008) or *semi-parametric group-based longitudinal models* (Nagin 1999), and was largely popularized by the SAS procedure TRAJ (Jones et al. 2001).

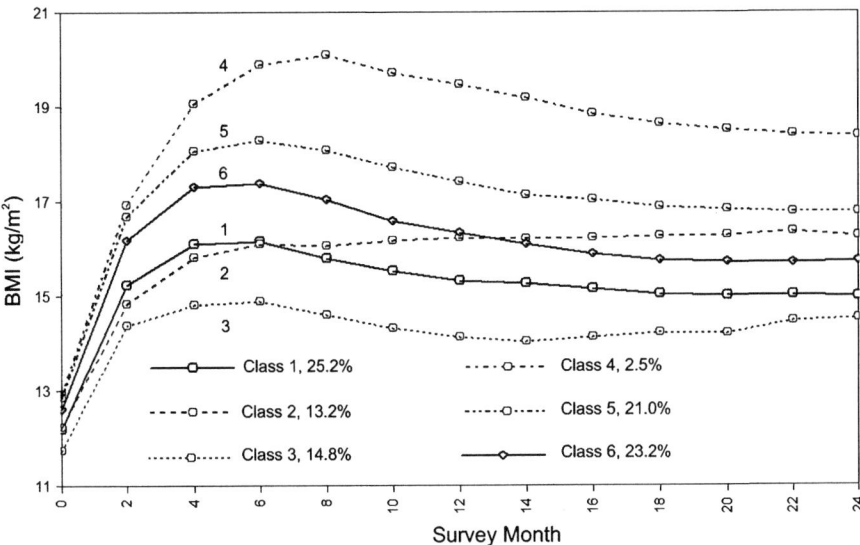

Fig. 13.3 Latent class growth analysis (13.4.2): BMI trajectories for the 6-class solution

The model makes the following theoretical statement: individual variation around the mean BMI trajectory exists because our population is composed of subgroups, each with their own distinct curve. In other words, the mean population BMI curve we are trying to parameterize is in reality a mixture of different subgroup BMI curves, each described by their own distinct set of parameters. Furthermore, this model says that within latent classes there is no individual variation in the growth factors that make up the trajectory, only time specific error variances.

Ideally, the researcher will have an a priori hypothesis about the number of latent classes they expect to find. However, these models are more often used in an exploratory manner, asking the question, "How many latent classes are needed to best describe the data." A key challenge to mixture modelling is that the "ideal" number of classes is not something that is estimated. Instead, the number of latent classes to include in the model must be specified in advance. Thus, in practice, multiple models are estimated, each specifying a different number of latent classes, and a "best" model is chosen. While there are no concrete rules for determining the optimum number of classes, the standard criteria are the degree to which the latent classes can be meaningfully interpreted, the fit to the observed data, and the quality with which it classifies individuals into latent classes. Each of these criteria should be evaluated across all estimated models, but for brevity, we will focus on a 6-class model from the outset.

13.4.2.1 Substantive Interpretation

The estimated mean BMI trajectories for each class are given in Fig. 13.3. Class 1 contains 25.5% of the sample and has a similar functional form to the latent growth curve model estimated in Sect. 13.4.1. With the exception of classes 2 and 4, the other class trajectories have a functional form similar to the class 1 trajectory. Conversely, the class 2 curve is characterized by a low birth BMI, followed by a slow but steady gain in BMI that doesn't peak until the 22nd month, while Class 4, which only contains 2.5% of the sample, is characterized by rapid early increase in BMI that continues to 8 months (vs. 6 months in the other classes).

13.4.2.2 Model Fit

While the 6-class solution results in interesting groups with potentially important differences between them, does it fit the data better than other solutions? Unlike most structural equation models, Pearson χ^2 tests (comparing the observed covariance matrix to the model estimated matrix) cannot be used to distinguish mixture models with different numbers of specified latent classes (Garrett and Zeger 2000). We must instead rely on likelihood based statistics, such as the log likelihood, the Akaike Information Criterion, and the Bayesian Information Criterion (Nylund et al. 2007). There is no definitive answer as to which fit index is best, though there is some suggestion that BIC out-performs the other two (Nylund et al. 2007).

Table 13.2 includes information on model fit for a series of models specifying between one and nine latent classes. Typically we are looking for the model that gives the largest log likelihood and the smallest Akaike Information Criterion and Bayesian Information Criterion, though failure to arrive at these extrema is common in practice. The values can be plotted to help the researcher weigh improvements in model fit versus parsimony (similar to the scree plots often used in factor analysis; see Jackson 1993). For example, Fig. 13.4 indicates large improvements in the Bayesian Information Criterion moving from one to three latent classes, and then more moderate improvements with additional classes. Other tests of model fit possible in Mplus include the Lo-Mendel-Rubin likelihood ratio test (Lo et al. 2001) and parametric bootstrapped likelihood ratio test (McLachlan and Peel 2000), though their properties under various scenarios are not as well understood, and they require more time and computing power to estimate.

13.4.2.3 Classification Quality

For each individual, we can estimate the posterior probabilities of membership in each latent class (using Bayes' theorem, Dolan et al. 2005). High classification quality occurs when individuals have a high probability of being placed in one class, and low probabilities of being placed in other classes. Mplus output includes the average probability of latent class membership for individuals assigned to their most likely latent class. These averages for the 6-class LCGM are given in Table 13.3. For example, among people assigned to class 1 (row 1), the mean probability of being in class 1 is 81%. When these data are arranged as they are in Table 13.3, a high classification quality is indicated by higher values along the diagonal. This information is also summarized by the entropy value (Table 13.2), with values closer to 1 indicating better classification quality (Celeux and Soromenho 1996).

Table 13.2 Model characteristics, including indicators of model fit, for the latent class growth analysis, comparing solutions with one to nine latent classes specified (13.4.2)

Number of latent classes	1	2[a]	3	4	5	6	7	8	9
Number of parameters	26	53	80	107	134	161	188	215	242
Log Likelihood	−31,816.1	–	−27,162.2	−26,487.4	−26,035.3	−25,754.7	−25,486.9	−25,288.6	−25,109.8
AIC	63,684.19	–	54,484.4	53,188.8	52,338.5	51,831.3	51,349.9	51,007.2	50,703.6
BIC	63,824.33	–	54,915.6	53,765.6	53,060.8	52,699.1	52,363.2	52,166.1	52,008.1
aBIC	63,741.74	–	54,661.5	53,425.6	52,635.1	52,187.7	51,766.0	51,483.1	51,239.3
Entropy	NA	–	0.33	0.85	0.83	0.81	0.81	0.80	0.80

NA not applicable

[a] The 2 class model did not converge

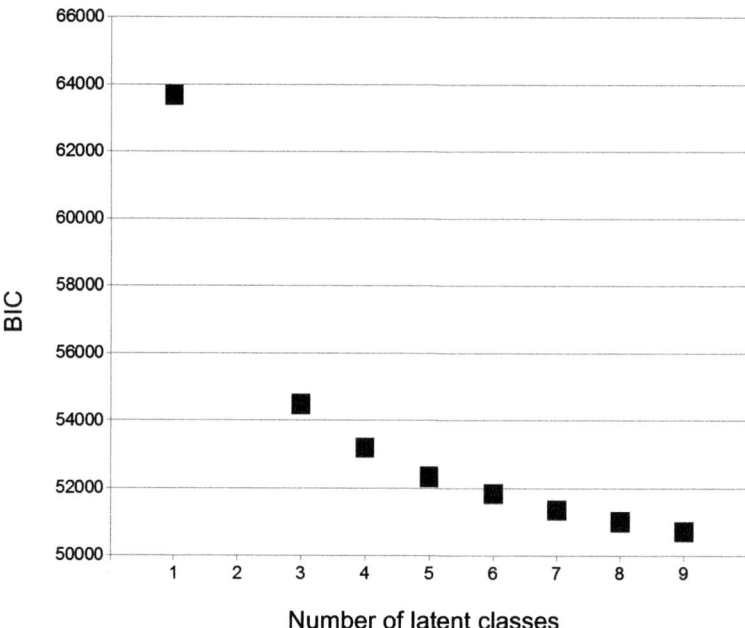

Fig. 13.4 Bayesian Information Criteria values for the latent class growth analysis (13.4.2), comparing solutions with one to nine latent classes specified. The plot illustrates a a distinct improvement improvement in model fit moving from a 1 to 3 class solution, with diminishing improvement from additional classes

Table 13.3 Mean probability of latent class membership for individuals assigned to their most likely latent class (highest posterior probability). For example, among individuals from whom membership in class 1 is most likely (row 1), the mean probability of being in that class is 81% (column 1), while their mean probability of being in class 2 is 5.3% (column 2), and so on

	Latent class					
Assigned latent class	1	2	3	4	5	6
1	**0.807**	0.053	0.057	0.002	0.022	0.058
2	0.026	**0.874**	0.000	0.000	0.026	0.074
3	0.063	0.020	**0.911**	0.000	0.002	0.003
4	0.000	0.000	0.000	**0.952**	0.048	0.000
5	0.010	0.026	0.004	0.012	**0.904**	0.044
6	0.050	0.055	0.002	0.001	0.044	**0.848**

13.4.3 Adding Covariates

We then added covariates, including distal health outcomes. It is important to note that the addition of covariates can result in changes to model fit, as well as how individuals are classified. Thus it is important to reevaluate the optimum number of latent classes once covariates are added. However, for brevity we will simply continue to expand on the 6-class solution.

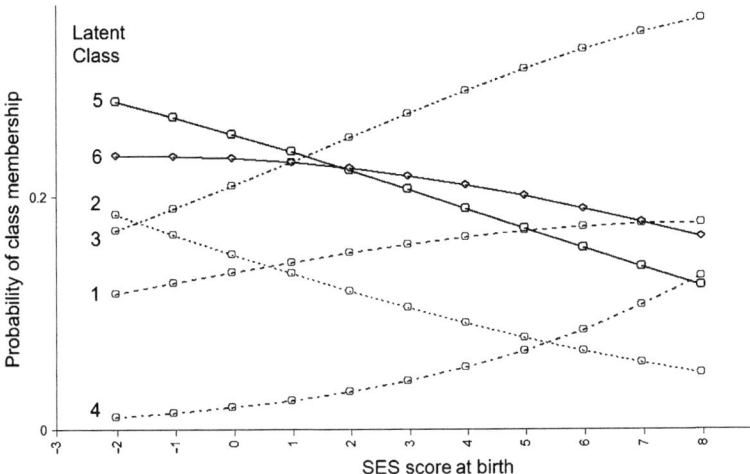

Fig. 13.5 Estimated probabilities of latent class membership as a function of SES at birth (13.4.3). With increasing SES, probability of membership in classes 2, 4, and 5 increases; while probability of membership in classes 1, 3, and 6 decreases

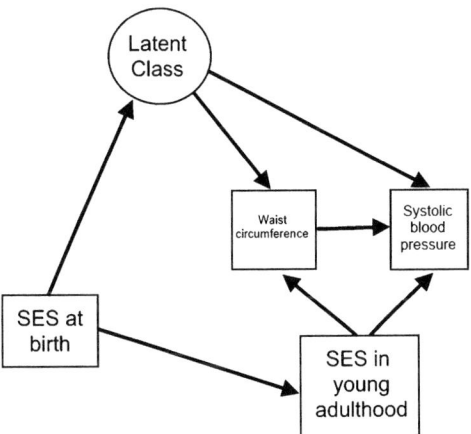

Fig. 13.6 Schematic for the final model in the latent class growth analysis (13.4.3)

SES at birth was modeled as a determinant of SES in adulthood and the probability of latent class membership. Both of these were modeled as determinants of waist circumference and systolic blood pressure in young adulthood. Lastly, waist circumference was modeled as an influence on systolic blood pressure. A schematic of the final model is given in Fig. 13.5.

This relationship between SES score at birth and class membership is estimated by a multinomial logistic regression. The results from this part of the model are best summarized by plotting the estimated probabilities of latent class membership as a function of SES at birth (Fig. 13.6). Individuals with higher SES at birth were more likely to be assigned into classes 2, 4 and 5, and less likely to be in classes 1, 3, and 6.

The following relationships are estimated with linear regressions: SES score at birth was positively associated with SES score in adulthood ($\beta = 0.68$ SES/SES; 95% CI: 0.59 to 0.77), which in turn was a positive predictor of waist circumference ($\beta = 0.70$ cm/SES; 95% CI: 0.52 to 0.89) but not systolic blood pressure (-0.05 mmHg/SES; 95% CI: -0.29 to 0.20); waist circumference was positively associated with systolic blood pressure (0.47 mmHg/cm; 95% CI: 0.37 to 0.56).

Lastly, we can look at the estimated intercepts of waist circumference and systolic blood pressure within each latent class, which are displayed in Fig. 13.7. These intercepts reflect the mean values of the outcomes within each class, independent of the linear influence of other predictor variables (SES for waist circumference; SES and waist circumference for systolic blood pressure). There are no apparent differences in the systolic blood pressure intercepts, although class 3, which was characterized by very poor growth in early life, had the lowest value (80.27 mmHg, 95% CI: 73.12 to 87.42). Classes 4 and 5 have the largest WC intercepts (79.98 cm, 95% CI: 71.49 to 88.46; and 74.63, 95% CI: 73.38 to 75.88, respectively). Both groups are characterized by relatively large BMI values at birth, rapid early BMI gains, and have the largest BMI values at 24 months.

13.5 Conclusion

Perhaps contrary to expectations, we did not identify an early life BMI trajectory that was clearly associated with systolic blood pressure in this sample of young adult Filipino males, independent of waist circumference and SES. While we did identify a subgroup characterized by larger waist circumferences, the small numbers of individuals falling in to this group prevented us from drawing any confident conclusions. Given that this was an abridged analysis, there are a number of important caveats needing exploration. Some of these, which we include as food for thought, are:

- What is the impact of non-normality in BMI measures on the model (see Bauer and Curran 2003)?
- Should raw scores be used, or are z-scores (internal or externally referenced) more appropriate?
- Should the model focus on growth velocity, or acceleration, versus growth distance?
- Would a model which includes both height and weight (adjusted for height) be more appropriate?
- What is the impact when measurements are not evenly spaced? For example, if we had many early measures and few later measures, would results be disproportionally driven by the former? Would it then make more sense to look for groups based on two or more latent categorical variables, each capturing parts of the total trajectory?

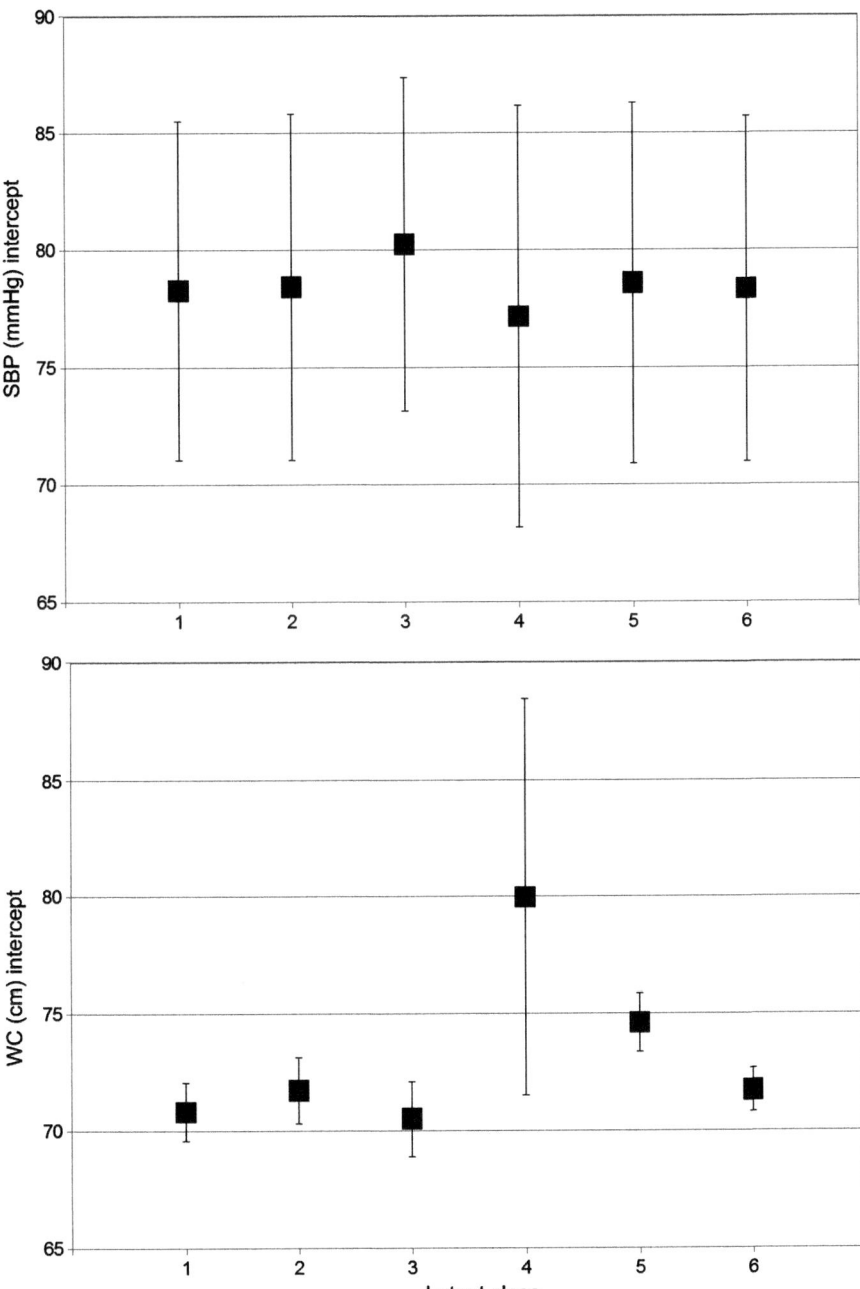

Fig. 13.7 Systolic blood pressure and waist circumference and intercepts (and 95% confidence intervals) by latent class (13.4.3)

- Should the models include autocorrelation structures or additional latent variables that account for additional sources of shared variation over specific periods of time (infancy, childhood, etc.)?
- What is the impact of constraining the intercept and error variances at zero? While freeing these parameters likely leads to improvement in model fit (which can of course be tested), what would be the impact on theoretical interpretation of the classes?
- How can the models be specified to account for important developmental "signposts," such as puberty, that occur at different ages?
- What is the best way to account for the fact that individuals are not actually measured at the exact same ages during each survey?

Individuals wanting to learn more about mixture modelling and growth mixture modelling should start with the citations from this chapter, many of which were included because they provide excellent overviews of these topics. Of particular interest are Jones et al. (2001); Li et al. (2001); McLachlan and Peel (2000); Muthén (2001); Muthén and Muthén (2000); Nagin (1999); and Pickles and Croudace (2010).

Appendix 1

13.4.1: Latent Growth Curve Model for Mplus

! Factor loadings defining the growth curve

i1 s1 | bmi0@0 bmi2@1 bmi4* bmi6* bmi8* bmi10* bmi12* bmi14* bmi16* bmi18* bmi20* bmi22* bmi24*;

! Freely estimated factor variances, means, and covariance

i1*;
s1*;
[i1*];
[s1*];
i1 WITH s1*;

! Freely estimated error variances

bmi0*;
bmi2*;
bmi4*;
bmi6*;
bmi8*;
bmi10*;
bmi12*;

bmi14*;
bmi16*;
bmi18*;
bmi20*;
bmi22*;
bmi24*;

Appendix 2

13.4.2: 2-Class Latent Class Growth Analysis for Mplus

Variable:
Classes = c (2); ! Increase this for more classes

Analysis:
Type = Mixture ;
STARTS = 100 20;
STITERATIONS = 20;

Model:
%OVERALL%
! Factor loadings defining the growth curve

i1 s1 | bmi0@0 bmi2@1 bmi4* bmi6* bmi8* bmi10* bmi12* bmi14* bmi16* bmi18* bmi20* bmi22* bmi24*;

! Freely estimated factor means; variances constrained as zero

i1@0;
s1@0;
[i1*];
[s1*];

! Freely estimated error variances

bmi0*;
bmi2*;
bmi4*;
bmi6*;
bmi8*;
bmi10*;
bmi12*;
bmi14*;
bmi16*;
bmi18*;
bmi20*;

bmi22*;
bmi24*;
%c#1%

[Repeat code from OVERALL model]
%c#2%

[Repeat code from OVERALL model]
! Add more class models as needed

Appendix 3

13.4.3: 6-Class Latent Class Growth Analysis with Covariates for Mplus

Variable:
Classes = c (2);

Analysis:
Type = Mixture ;
STARTS = 100 20;
STITERATIONS = 20;

Model:
! Factor loadings defining the growth curve

i1 s1 | bmi0@0 bmi2@1 bmi4* bmi6* bmi8* bmi10* bmi12* bmi14* bmi16* bmi18* bmi20* bmi22* bmi24*;

! Freely estimated factor means; variances constrained as zero

i1@0;
s1@0;
[i1*];
[s1*];

! Freely estimated error variances

bmi0*;
bmi2*;
bmi4*;
bmi6*;
bmi8*;
bmi10*;
bmi12*;
bmi14*;

```
bmi16*;
bmi18*;
bmi20*;
bmi22*;
bmi24*;
```

! Covariates

! Multinomial logit of C on SES
c ON ses0;

! Linear regression of SES in young adulthood on SES at birth
ses258 ON ses0;

! Linear regression of systolic blood pressure on SES and waist circumference
sys258 ON waist258 ses258;

! Linear regression of waist circumference on SES
waist258 ON ses258;

References

Adair, L. S., Martorell, R., Stein, A. D., Hallal, P. C., Sachdev, H. S., Prabhakaran, D., Wills, A. K., Norris, S. A., Dahly, D. L., & Lee, N. R. (2009). Size at birth, weight gain in infancy and childhood, and adult blood pressure in 5 low-and middle-income-country cohorts: When does weight gain matter? *American Journal of Clinical Nutrition, 89*, 1383.

Adair, L. S., Popkin, B. M., Akin, J. S., Guilkey, D. K., Gultiano, S., Borja, J., Perez, L., Kuzawa, C. W., McDade, T., & Hindin, M. J. (2010). Cohort profile: The Cebu longitudinal health and nutrition survey. *International Journal of Epidemiology*. doi:10.1093/ije/ dyq085.

Baird, J., Fisher, D., Lucas, P., Kleijnen, J., Roberts, H., & Law, C. (2005). Being big or growing fast: Systematic review of size and growth in infancy and later obesity. *British Medical Journal, 331*, 929.

Barker, D. J. P. (2001). *Fetal origins of cardiovascular and lung disease*. New York: M. Dekker.

Barker, D. J. P. (2004). The developmental origins of adult disease. *Journal of the American College of Nutrition, 23*, 588–595.

Bauer, D. J., & Curran, P. J. (2003). Distributional assumptions of growth mixture models: Implications for overextraction of latent trajectory classes. *Psychological Methods, 8*, 338.

Ben-Shlomo, Y., & Kuh, D. (2002). *A life course approach to chronic disease epidemiology: Conceptual models, empirical challenges and interdisciplinary perspectives*. London: IEA. Int. J. Epidemiol. (2002) 31 (2): 285–293. doi: 10.1093/ije/31.2.285.

Ben-Shlomo, Y., McCarthy, A., Hughes, R., Tilling, K., Davies, D., & Davey Smith, G. (2008). Immediate postnatal growth is associated with blood pressure in young adulthood: The Barry Caerphilly Growth Study. *Hypertension, 52*, 638.

Bollen, K. A., & Curran, P. J. (2006). *Latent curve models: A structural equation perspective*. Hoboken: Wiley-Interscience. http://onlinelibrary.wiley.com/doi/10.1002/0471746096.fmatter/pdf.

Celeux, G., & Soromenho, G. (1996). An entropy criterion for assessing the number of clusters in a mixture model. *Journal of Classification, 13*, 195–212.

Cole, T. J., Bellizzi, M. C., Flegal, K. M., & Dietz, W. H. (2000). Establishing a standard definition for child overweight and obesity worldwide: International survey. *British Medical Journal, 320*, 1240.

De Stavola, BL and Nitsch, D and Silva, ID and McCormack, V and Hardy, R and Mann, V and Cole, TJ and Morton, S and Leon, DA (2006) Statistical issues in life course epidemiology. AM J EPIDEMIOL, 163(1) 84–96. 10.1093/aje/kwj003.

Dolan, C. V., Schmittmann, V. D., Lubke, G. H., & Neale, M. C. (2005). Regime switching in the latent growth curve mixture model. *Structural Equation Modeling, 12*, 94–119.

Eriksson, J. G., Forsén, T., Tuomilehto, J., Osmond, C., & Barker, D. J. P. (2001). Early growth and coronary heart disease in later life: Longitudinal study. *British Medical Journal, 322*, 949.

Eriksson, J. G., Forsen, T. J., Osmond, C., & Barker, D. J. P. (2003). Pathways of infant and childhood growth that lead to type 2 diabetes. *Diabetes Care, 26*, 3006.

Gale, C. R., O'Callaghan, F. J., Bredow, M., & Martyn, C. N. (2006). The influence of head growth in fetal life, infancy, and childhood on intelligence at the ages of 4 and 8 years. *Pediatrics, 118*, 1486.

Garrett, E. S., & Zeger, S. L. (2000). Latent class model diagnosis. *Biometrics, 56*, 1055–1067.

Gillman, M. W. (2005). Developmental origins of health and disease. *The New England Journal of Medicine, 353*, 1848–1850.

Gluckman, P. D., & Hanson, M. A. (2004). Developmental origins of disease paradigm: A mechanistic and evolutionary perspective. *Pediatric Research, 56*, 311–317.

Hall, D. M. B., & Cole, T. J. (2006). What use is the BMI? *Archives of Disease in Childhood, 91*, 283–286.

Healy, M. J. R. (1974). Notes on the statistics of growth standards. *Annals of Human Biology, 1*, 41–46.

Hermanussen, M., & Meigen, C. (2007). Phase variation in child and adolescent growth. *International Journal of Biostatistics, 3*, 9.

Jackson, D. A. (1993). Stopping rules in principal components analysis: A comparison of heuristical and statistical approaches. *Ecology, 74*, 2204–2214.

Jones, B. L., Nagin, D. S., & Roeder, K. (2001). A SAS procedure based on mixture models for estimating developmental trajectories. *Sociological Methods & Research, 29*, 374.

Jung, T., & Wickrama, K. A. S. (2008). An introduction to latent class growth analysis and growth mixture modeling. *Social and Personality Psychology Compass, 2*, 302–317.

Keijzer-Veen, M. G., Euser, A. M., van Montfoort, N., Dekker, F. W., Vandenbroucke, J. P., & van Houwelingen, H. C. (2005). A regression model with unexplained residuals was preferred in the analysis of the fetal origins of adult diseases hypothesis. *Journal of Clinical Epidemiology, 58*, 1320–1324.

Kreuter, F., & Muthén, B. (2008). Analyzing criminal trajectory profiles: Bridging multilevel and group-based approaches using growth mixture modeling. *Journal of Quantitative Criminology, 24*, 1–31.

Kuh, D., & Ben-Shlomo, Y. (2004). *A life course approach to chronic disease epidemiology*. Oxford: Oxford University Press. http://books.google.co.uk/books?id=o_CFOTYglHsC&printsec=frontcover&source=gbs_ge_summary_r&cad=0#v=onepage&q&f=false.

Kuh, D., Ben-Shlomo, Y., Lynch, J., Hallqvist, J., & Power, C. (2003). Life course epidemiology. *Journal of Epidemiology and Community Health, 57*, 778–783.

Li, F., Duncan, T. E., Duncan, S. C., & Acock, A. (2001). Latent growth modeling of longitudinal data: A finite growth mixture modeling approach. *Structural Equation Modeling: A Multidisciplinary Journal, 8*, 493–530.

Li, C., Goran, M. I., Kaur, H., Nollen, N., & Ahluwalia, J. S. (2007). Developmental trajectories of overweight during childhood: Role of early life factors. *Obesity, 15*, 760–771.

Lo, Y., Mendell, N. R., & Rubin, D. B. (2001). Testing the number of components in a normal mixture. *Biometrika, 88*, 767.

Lohman, T., Roche, A., & Martorell, R. (1988). *Anthropometric standardization reference manual*. Champaign: Human Kinetics Books.

McLachlan, G. J., & Peel, D. (2000). *Finite mixture models*. New York: Wiley-Interscience. http://espace.library.uq.edu.au/view/UQ:145685.

Meredith, W., & Tisak, J. (1990). Latent curve analysis. *Psychometrika, 55*, 107–122.

Monteiro, P. O. A., & Victora, C. G. (2005). Rapid growth in infancy and childhood and obesity in later life-a systematic review. *Obesity Reviews, 6*, 143–154.

Muthén, B. (2001). Second-generation structural equation modeling with a combination of categorical and continuous latent variables: New opportunities for latent class/latent growth modeling. *New methods for the analysis of change* (pp. 291–322).

Muthén, B., & Muthén, L. K. (2000). Integrating person-centered and variable-centered analyses: Growth mixture modeling with latent trajectory classes. *Alcoholism, Clinical and Experimental Research, 24*, 882.

Nagin, D. S. (1999). Analyzing developmental trajectories: A semiparametric, group-based approach. *Psychological Methods, 4*, 139.

Nylund, K. L., Asparouhov, T., & Muthen, B. O. (2007). Deciding on the number of classes in latent class analysis and growth mixture modeling: A Monte Carlo simulation study. *Structural Equation Modeling, 14*, 535–569.

Ong, K. K., & Loos, R. J. F. (2006). Rapid infancy weight gain and subsequent obesity: Systematic reviews and hopeful suggestions. *Acta Paediatrica, 95*, 904–908.

Østbye, T., Malhotra, R., & Landerman, L. R. (2011). Body mass trajectories through adulthood: Results from the National Longitudinal Survey of Youth 1979 Cohort (1981–2006). *International Journal of Epidemiology, 40*, 240.

Pickles, A., & Croudace, T. (2010). Latent mixture models for multivariate and longitudinal outcomes. *Statistical Methods in Medical Research, 19*, 271.

Pickles, A., Maughan, B., & Wadsworth, M. (2007). *Epidemiological methods in life course research*. Oxford: Oxford University Press. http://books.google.co.uk/books?id=GfUeCFLDMdYC&printsec=frontcover&source=gbs_ge_summary_r&cad=0#v=onepage&q&f=false.

Stein, A. D., Thompson, A. M., & Waters, A. (2005). Childhood growth and chronic disease: Evidence from countries undergoing the nutrition transition. *Journal compilation, 1*, 177–184.

Stettler, N. (2007). Nature and strength of epidemiological evidence for origins of childhood and adulthood obesity in the first year of life. *International Journal of Obesity, 31*, 1035–1043.

Tu, Y. K., Woolston, A., Baxter, P. D., & Gilthorpe, M. S. (2010). Assessing the impact of body size in childhood and adolescence on blood pressure: An application of partial least squares regression. *Epidemiology, 21*, 440.

Victora, C. G., & Barros, F. C. (2001). *Commentary: The catch-up dilemma-relevance of Leitch's 'low-high' pig to child growth in developing countries*. London: IEA. Int. J. Epidemiol. (2001) 30(2): 217–220. doi: 10.1093/ije/30.2.217.

Victora, C. G., Adair, L., Fall, C., Hallal, P. C., Martorell, R., Richter, L., & Sachdev, H. S. (2008). Maternal and child undernutrition: Consequences for adult health and human capital. *The Lancet, 371*, 340–357.

Vyas, S., & Kumaranayake, L. (2006). Constructing socio-economic status indices: How to use principal components analysis. *Health Policy and Planning, 21*, 459.

Chapter 14
G-estimation for Accelerated Failure Time Models

Kate Tilling, Jonathan A.C. Sterne, and Vanessa Didelez

14.1 Time-Varying Confounding

There is an increasing interest in life-course epidemiology (Ben-Shlomo 2007; Ben-Shlomo and Kuh 2002), with the quantification of the effects of exposures over long periods of time. For example, several papers recently have examined the effects of socioeconomic position at different stages of life, and changes in that exposure between these stages, on outcomes including risk of stroke and respiratory function, and health behaviours including midlife drinking and smoking patterns (Amuzu et al. 2009; Glymour et al. 2008; Tehranifar et al. 2009; Tennant et al. 2008).

In longitudinal studies, the effects of risk factors on outcome may be estimated in different ways, with different interpretations. The usual approach is to examine the relationship between baseline exposure and rates of disease or death. For reasonably constant exposures, this estimates the cumulative effects of exposure. For example, in a longitudinal study the association between baseline diabetes and subsequent mortality represents the association of lifetime diabetes with mortality. Alternatively we may estimate time-varying effects of exposure. For example, subjects may take up smoking or quit smoking at various stages during the longitudinal study (usually we assume that the exposure level remains constant from one measurement occasion to the next). Here, the time-varying association between smoking and mortality represents the relationship between smoking at a given visit and mortality after that visit. If follow-up is fairly short this represents the instantaneous association between smoking and mortality and can be investigated using standard regression methods (e.g. survival models, structural

---

K. Tilling (✉) • J.A.C. Sterne
School of Social and Community Medicine, University of Bristol, Bristol, UK
e-mail: kate.tilling@bristol.ac.uk

V. Didelez
School of Mathematics, University of Bristol, Bristol, UK

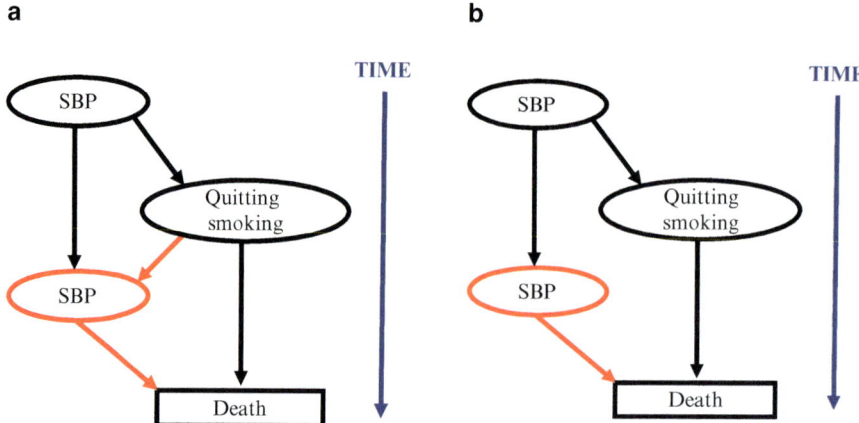

Fig. 14.1 (a) Time-varying confounding by SBP of the effect of quitting smoking on mortality. (b) Non time-varying confounding by SBP of the effect of quitting smoking on mortality

equation models, etc.). However, increased interest in exposures, confounders and outcomes which vary over time highlights a potential problem, referred to as *time-varying confounding*.

A covariate is a *time-varying confounder* (Mark and Robins 1993; Robins 1986; Young et al. 2010) for the effect of exposure on outcome if it is

1. a time-dependent confounder, i.e. past covariate values predict current exposure and current covariate value independently predicts outcome and also
2. past exposure predicts current covariate value.

As an example, suppose smokers (*exposed*) with high blood pressure are advised to quit smoking, so are less likely to smoke in future (condition 1 above). Suppose also that smoking raises blood pressure (condition 2), and that high blood pressure is a risk factor for death by another pathway other than through smoking (condition 1). In this situation, high blood pressure is a time-varying confounder for the effect of smoking on mortality. Figure 14.1a shows a directed acyclic graph (DAG, see Chaps. 1 and 11) for this example of time-varying confounding. The possible interplay between past and future exposure and confounders makes this very different from the usual definition of a confounder (Chap. 10) where a confounder is always assumed to precede exposure (with DAG for non time-varying confounding shown in Fig. 14.1b). The added complications due to time-varying confounding are twofold. Firstly, if a future covariate is affected by past exposure and independently predicts outcome, then it has the role of a mediator for the effect of past exposure and we do not want to adjust for mediators when estimating the total effect, but at the same time we have to adjust for it because it may confound future exposure and outcome. Secondly, if a covariate is affected by past exposure and other unobserved variables that also predict outcome (e.g. blood pressure may be affected by diet which also predicts survival), then adjusting for this covariate may introduce selection bias (Hernan et al. 2004), but again, we have to adjust for it if it confounds future exposure and outcome. Hence the question is how to adjust for time-varying confounding without interrupting mediated effects nor introducing selection bias. Standard statistical methods for the analysis of cohort studies (for example Cox or Poisson regression) often get this wrong and yield biased estimates (Robins et al. 1992a), while G-estimation provides a valid method.

We illustrate the problem with an example. When analysing the effect of smoking on mortality we could employ several possible strategies, including: examining the effect of baseline smoking; examining the effect of time-updated smoking; controlling for baseline covariates; and controlling for time-updated covariates.

The unadjusted estimate of the effect of baseline smoking will be biased (favouring smoking, in this case), because those who are both smokers and have high blood pressure (and therefore have the highest mortality risk) will tend to quit subsequently, and thus will reduce their mortality risk. Controlling for baseline covariates such as blood pressure which are measured at the start of the study will still give biased estimates of the effect of smoking, because it ignores the fact that individuals who quit after the start of the study will tend to be those whose blood pressure increased over time.

Controlling for time-updated measurements of covariates such as blood pressure will still give biased estimates of the effect of smoking, because smoking acts on mortality at least partly by raising blood pressure. Controlling for a variable (e.g. blood pressure) which is intermediate on the pathway between the exposure (e.g. smoking) and the outcome (e.g. mortality) will estimate only the direct effect of the exposure (ignoring the effect mediated through the covariate) and may additionally introduce selection bias (Hernan et al. 2004).

Example 1 To illustrate the bias of the usual survival analysis in the situation described above, we simulated data for 2,000 people with four assessment occasions (visits) 3 years apart. Each person had a randomly-generated (log-normally distributed) survival time representing how long they would survive if never exposed, which was then decreased by high blood pressure or smoking. Survival time for a smoker was 0.67 of survival time for a non-smoker with the same covariate history, and survival time decreased by 4% per 1 mmHg increase in current blood pressure. Blood pressure increased by 2 mmHg for current smokers, and by 1 mmHg for ex-smokers (i.e. if an individual smoked at the previous visit but not the current visit, blood pressure was 1 mmHg higher than if they had been a non-smoker at both visits). The odds of smoking were decreased by 0.3 if the participant had high blood pressure at the previous visit. All 2,000 participants were "followed up" until either they died (n = 1,672) or until 3 years after the fourth visit. We took visit 1 to be a baseline visit, and measured time to event/censoring from visit 2. Table 14.1 shows the simulated number at each visit, together with number smoking at that visit and average blood pressure at that visit.

The data were analysed using a Weibull model with the accelerated failure time parameterisation, because this is the parameterisation which corresponds to g-estimation (i.e., calculating the survival ratio rather than the hazard ratio).

Table 14.1 Simulated data for Example 1

Visit	N	N smokers (%)	Mean blood pressure (sd)
1	2,000	140 (7)	142 (4.70)
2	2,000	139 (7)	143 (4.87)
3	1,880	108 (6)	143 (3.80)
4	1,153	67 (6)	141 (4.27)

The accelerated failure time model assumes for the individual failure times T_i with covariates x_i that:

$$T_i = \exp(\theta^T x_i + \varepsilon_i)$$

where ε_i has a standard extreme value distribution with scale parameter $1/\gamma$, where γ is the shape parameter.

Survival models including current smoking, current smoking and blood pressure, current smoking plus baseline smoking and blood pressure, and smoking and blood pressure at current and previous visits, were all fitted. The model including current smoking only estimated the survival time ratio for smokers compared to non-smokers as 1.14 (95% CI 1.06–1.23), concluding that smoking had little (possibly even a positive) effect on survival. The model including current smoking and current blood pressure estimated the ratio as 0.87 (95% CI 0.84–0.89), that including current smoking and baseline smoking and blood pressure as 0.93 (95% CI 0.90–0.96) and that including all time-updated variables as 0.93 (95% CI 0.91–0.94). Thus all these standard analyses under-estimated the true adverse effect of smoking on mortality (a mortality ratio of 0.67).

14.2 Investigating Time-Varying Confounding

Relationships between time-varying exposures and covariates can be examined using a logistic regression of exposure on concurrent values of the other covariates, values of all exposures and covariates at the previous visit and at baseline (visit 1), and non time-varying covariates. All data from all n visits should be used, so each individual can contribute multiple observations to the model for an exposure. This model will examine condition (1) above. The other part of Condition 1 (whether the covariate affects outcome) can be examined using a model relating outcome to exposure and covariates (e.g. a survival model in the above example, where mortality is the outcome). Condition (2), whether past exposure predicts current covariate values, can be examined using similar logistic regression models of each time-varying covariate on concurrent values of the other covariates and exposure, values of all exposures and covariates at the previous visit and at baseline (visit 1), and non time-varying covariates.

14.2.1 G-estimation

G-estimation of causal effects was proposed by Robins (see e.g. Robins et al. 1992a; Witteman et al. 1998) as one method to allow for confounders which are also on the causal pathway, i.e. time varying confounding. G-estimation has been used in various applications, to estimate the causal association between: quitting smoking and time to death or first CHD (Mark and Robins 1993); isolated systolic hypertension and cardiovascular mortality (Witteman et al. 1998); therapy and survival for HIV-positive men (Joffe et al. 1997, 1998); graft versus host disease and relapse after bone marrow transplants in leukaemia (Keiding et al. 1999); various cardiovascular risk factors and mortality (Tilling et al. 2002); to estimate the total causal effect of highly active antiretroviral therapy (HAART) on the time to AIDS or death among those infected with immunodeficiency virus (HIV) (Hernan et al. 2005); and to correct for non-compliance in clinical trials (Korhonen et al. 1999). G-estimation has also been implemented as a Stata programme (Sterne and Tilling 2002).

14.2.2 Counterfactual Failure Time

The unbiased estimation of causal effects usually requires the assumption of *no unmeasured confounding* (Lok et al. 2004; Robins 1992). Roughly speaking this means that we have measured and included in the model all variables that determine whether a subject is exposed at each measurement occasion and which are also (directly or indirectly) associated with the outcome. G-estimation exploits the assumption of no unmeasured confounding in the following way.

For each subject i, U_i is defined as the time to failure if the subject was not exposed throughout follow-up. This time (the *counterfactual* failure time (Mark and Robins 1993; Robins et al. 1992a; Witteman et al. 1998)) is unobservable for subjects with any exposure. The assumption of no unmeasured confounding (which cannot be tested using the observable data) implies that the exposure for an individual i at a given time will be independent of their counterfactual failure time, U_i, conditional on covariate and exposure history so far. G-estimation proceeds by reconstructing U_i from the observed data and then determining the value of the causal parameter as the one for which this conditional independence is true. An example of this assumption is that, conditional on past weight, smoking status, blood pressure and cholesterol measurements, the decision of an individual to quit or start smoking is independent of what his/her survival time would have been had he/she never smoked. A violation of this assumption would typically occur if the decision depends on unobserved factors, e.g. alcohol consumption, that are informative for the counterfactual survival time U_i. Exposure does not have to be independent of subjects' *current* life expectancy (smokers may choose to quit precisely because they recognise that smoking reduces their life expectancy).

Table 14.2 Simulated data for three individuals in Example 2

Individual	Smoking status				Observed survival time (years)
	Visit 1	Visit 2	Visit 3	Visit 4	
A	1	1			4.88
B	1	1	1	0	11
C	1	1	0	0	14

In its simplest version, G-estimation proceeds by assuming that exposure accelerates failure time by $\exp(-\Psi)$, i.e. $U_i \exp(-\Psi) = T_i^a$ where T_i^a is the survival time for subject i if they are exposed throughout. The actually observed failure time T_i will typically be in between U_i and T_i^a for subjects who have been exposed for some but not all the time. For a given Ψ, the counterfactual survival time $U_{i,\Psi}$ can be calculated backwards from the observed data for subjects who experience an event at time T_i by:

$$U_{i,\Psi} = \int^{T_i} \exp(\Psi \times e_{i,t}) \, dt \quad (14.1)$$

where $e_{i,t}$ is 1 if subject i is actually exposed at time t and 0 if subject i is unexposed. Note that the above model that links the counterfactual survival time $U_{i,\Psi}$ with the observed survival time T_i can be generalised by choosing a more flexible function inside the integral.

For the case where we follow individuals for n follow-up visits (where the first is the baseline visit), we could calculate the counterfactual survival time for subjects who experience an event by:

$$U_{i,\Psi} = \sum_{v=1}^{n} \left[(t_v) \times \exp(\Psi \times e_{i,v}) \right]$$

where t_v is the time from visit v to either the event or the next visit.

Example 2 The simulated data on smoking and blood pressure used in example 1 were analysed using g-estimation. We had four visits, of which the first was the baseline. Thus, for a given value of Ψ, the estimated counterfactual survival time for an individual is given by $U_{i,\Psi}$ where

$$U_{i,\Psi} = \sum_{v=1}^{4} \left[(t_v) \times \exp(\Psi \times e_{i,v}) \right]$$

where t_v is the time from visit v to either the event or the next visit and $e_{i,v}$ = whether individual i smoked at visit v. Data from three simulated individuals are shown in Table 14.2:

The first individual in this simulated dataset (individual A) was a smoker at visits 1 and 2, and survived for a total of 4.88 years (i.e. 1.88 years from visit 2).

Suppose we assume that smoking halves life expectancy, i.e. $\exp(-\Psi)=0.5$, so $\Psi=0.69$. Then the counterfactual survival time for this individual at visit 1 (i.e. the length of time they would have survived from visit 1 had they not been a smoker at visit 1 and visit 2) is: $(3 \times \exp(\Psi \times 1)) + (1.88 \times \exp(\Psi \times 1)) = 9.76$ years.

The second individual in this simulated dataset (individual B) was a smoker at visits 1, 2 and 3, then gave up and survived for a further 2 years. Again assuming that smoking halves life expectancy then the counterfactual survival time for this individual at visit 1 (i.e. the length of time they would have survived from visit 1 had they not been a smoker at visits 1, 2 and 3) is: $(3 \times \exp(\Psi \times 1)) + (3 \times \exp(\Psi \times 1)) + (3 \times \exp(\Psi \times 1)) + (2 \times \exp(\Psi \times 0)) = 20$ years.

Thus, for all individuals who are followed up until death, the counterfactual survival time can be calculated in a similar way.

14.2.3 Definition of G-estimation

G-estimation uses the assumption of no unmeasured confounders to estimate the effect of exposure on survival by examining a range of values for Ψ, and choosing the value Ψ_0 for which current exposure is independent of counterfactual survival time U_i (Mark and Robins 1993; Robins 1992; Robins et al. 1992a; Witteman et al. 1998). This can be done by fitting a series of logistic regression models relating current exposure $e_{i,v}$ to $U_{i,\Psi}$, controlling for all confounders (this still assumes that there was no censoring):

$$\text{logit}(e_{i,v}) = \mu U_{i,\Psi} + \sum_{k=0} \alpha_k x_{ik} + \sum_j \beta_j c_{ij,v} + \sum_{j=1} \delta_j c_{ij,v-1} + \sum_{j=1} \lambda_j c_{ij,1} \quad v = 2,...,n$$

for different values of Ψ, where $c_{ij,v}$ are the time-varying confounders and x_{ik} the time-invariant confounders. Alternatively, one logistic model could be fitted including data from all visits, with allowance made for clustering within individuals (e.g. by using a GEE). The time-varying confounders may include the values of exposure at previous time-points and at baseline. In fact, the above model for exposure can be generalised and should be chosen according to what is judged appropriate based on subject matter knowledge about the exposure process. For example when exposure is treatment, we may have specific information on the rules according to which treatment was administered. Subjects contribute an observation for each occasion at which their exposure was assessed. The g-estimate Ψ_0 is the value of Ψ for which the Wald statistic of μ in this logistic regression is zero (P value 1, i.e. no association between current exposure and U_{ij,Ψ_0}). The upper and lower limits of the 95% confidence interval for Ψ_0 are the values of Ψ for which the two-sided P-value for the Wald statistic of μ in this logistic regression is 0.05.

This g-estimate Ψ_0 is minus the log of the "causal survival time ratio". Thus $\exp(-\Psi_0)$ estimates the ratio of the survival time of a continuously exposed person to that of an otherwise identical person who was never exposed. If $\exp(-\Psi_0)>1$ then exposure is beneficial (i.e. exposure increases time to the outcome event).

14.3 Censoring – Type I – End of Study

The counterfactual survival time $U_{i,\psi}$ can only be derived from the observed data for a subject who experiences the event. If the study has a planned end of follow-up (at time C_i for individual i) that occurs before all subjects have experienced the outcome event, not all subjects' counterfactual failure times will be estimable. If C_i is independent of the counterfactual survival time, then this problem can be overcome by replacing $U_{i,\psi}$ with an indicator variable ($\Delta_{i,\psi}$) for whether the event would have been observed both if the person had been exposed throughout follow-up and if they had been unexposed throughout follow-up, as described by Witteman et al. (1998).

$$\Delta_{i,\psi} = \mathrm{ind}(U_{i,\psi} < C_{i,\psi})$$

where $C_{i,\psi} = C_i$ if $\Psi \geq 0$ and $C_{i,\psi} = C_i \times \exp(\Psi)$ if $\Psi < 0$. Thus $\Delta_{i,\psi}$ is zero for all subjects who do not experience an event during follow-up, and may also be zero for some of those who did experience an event.

Example 3 Continuing with the data from example 1, this study had a planned end of follow-up 12 years after visit 1. Suppose we assume that smoking halves life expectancy, i.e. $\exp(-\Psi)=0.5$, so $\Psi=0.69$. Then for each individual, the indicator variable $\Delta_{i,0.69}$ is equal to 1 if the counterfactual failure time (given $\Psi=0.69$) is less than 12 years and 0 otherwise. The first individual in this simulated dataset (A, above) was a smoker at visits 1 and 2, and survived for 4.88 years from visit 1. The counterfactual survival time for this individual (see example 2) is 9.76 years, and thus the indicator variable $\Delta_{i,0.69}$ takes the value 1 for this individual. The counterfactual failure time for individual B, who smoked at visits 1, 2 and 3 then gave up and survived for another 5 years, was 20 years. Thus the indicator variable $\Delta_{i,0.69}$ takes the value 0 for this individual. Another individual (C) smoked at visits 1 and 2, then gave up and survived until the end of follow-up (dying 14 years after visit 1). As this individual did not experience an event during follow-up, their value for the indicator variable $\Delta_{i,0.69}$ is 0. The value of the indicator variable $\Delta_{i,\psi}$ can be calculated for all individuals, whether or not they experienced an event during follow-up.

Once the value of the indicator variable has been calculated for each individual, for a given value of Ψ, then the g-estimation can proceed by performing a logistic regression of the exposure of each individual at each timepoint on their

Table 14.3 Simulated data for three individuals in Example 3

Individual	Smoking status				Observed survival time (years)	$\Delta_{i,0.69}$
	Visit 1	Visit 2	Visit 3	Visit 4		
A	1	1			4.88	1
B	1	1	1	0	11	0
C	1	1	0	0	14	0

counterfactual failure time. The data for individuals A, B and C are shown in Table 14.3, assuming that smoking halves life expectancy):

Each individual i then contributes n_i observations to a logistic regression model with exposure as the outcome, where n_i is the number of visits at which that individual has observations. Thus in the example above, individuals A, B and C contribute 1, 3 and 3 observations respectively. In each case, the logistic regression relates their exposure to all their baseline covariates, and previous covariates and exposures, and to the indicator variable for their counterfactual failure time ($\Delta_{i,\psi}$).

We used g-estimation to estimate the effect of smoking on mortality using the entire simulated dataset. The g-estimate of Ψ was 0.41 (95% CI 0.37–0.44), and the g-estimated survival ratio was 0.66 (95% CI 0.64–0.69) compared to the true value of 0.67. This is closer to the true value than all the other (biased) models (see Example 1), and also has a slightly narrower confidence interval. In this one hypothetical example, g-estimation performs better than the usual survival analysis.

14.4 Censoring – Type II – Competing Risks

Censoring by competing risks can occur when subjects leave the study early or, in the case of cause-specific mortality models, die from other causes. For example, in models where systolic or diastolic blood pressure are the exposures, individuals might be censored when they first reported use of anti-hypertensive medication (Tilling et al. 2002). Subjects could also withdraw from the study because they felt too ill to participate in further follow-ups. In each of these cases, censoring is not independent of the underlying counterfactual survival time. Thus the above method for dealing with censoring by the planned end of a study cannot be used to deal with censoring by competing risks.

As outlined by Witteman et al. (1998), censoring by competing risks is dealt with by modelling the censoring mechanism, and using each individual's estimated probability of being censored to adjust the analysis. This is a similar idea to using weighting for non-response to adjust for missing data (Little and Rubin 2002). Multinomial (if there are several censoring mechanisms) or logistic regression (if there is only one censoring mechanism), based on all available data, is used to relate the probability of being censored at each measurement occasion to the exposure and covariate history. The probability of being uncensored to the end of the study for each individual is then estimated. The inverse of this probability is used to weight the contributions of individuals to the logistic regression models used in the g-estimation process, to which now only uncensored individuals contribute. This can be done by using probability weights, or by replacing $\Delta_{i,\psi}$ by $\frac{\Delta_{i,\psi}}{p(\text{not censored})}$. This approach means that observations within the same individual are no longer independent, so the logistic regression models for the g-estimation process use robust standard errors allowing for clustering within individuals (using the Huber-White sandwich estimator (Stata Corporation 2007)). This is equivalent to the procedure suggested by Witteman et al., to use a robust Wald test from a generalized estimating equation with an independence working correlation matrix (Witteman et al. 1998). The confidence intervals obtained using this procedure are conservative.

For example, suppose we are examining the effect of systolic and diastolic blood pressure (as exposures) on mortality, and that individuals were censored when they first reported use of anti-hypertensive medication. The probability of being censored at each visit will depend on blood pressure at previous visits, and is likely to be related to other factors also (e.g. smokers may be more likely to have other health problems and therefore to visit the GP). The censoring process is modelled, using logistic regression, with whether the individual was censored (i.e. prescribed anti-hypertensive medication) at each occasion as the outcome. This logistic regression model is then used to derive, for each individual, the probability that they remained uncensored to the end of the study. The inverse of this probability is used to weight all of that individual's contributions to the g-estimation model (using probability weights as before). For example, suppose a person with high initial blood pressure has a chance of 0.25 of being uncensored at the end of the study. In g-estimation the contribution of such a person to the model is multiplied by 4, representing the 'total' of 4 people with high blood pressure, 3 of whom were censored before the end of the study.

14.5 Converting to Survival Analysis

The parameter estimated by the g-estimation procedure, the causal survival time ratio, describes the association between exposure and survival using the accelerated failure time parameterisation. In epidemiology, the more usual parameterisation for survival analysis is that of proportional hazards. It would thus be useful to be able to express the causal survival time ratio in the proportional hazards parameterisation. One obvious way to do this is via the Weibull distribution, as this can be expressed in either parameterisation.

The Weibull hazard function at time t is $h(t) = \phi\gamma t^{\gamma-1}$, where ϕ is referred to as the scale parameter and γ as the shape parameter. If the vector of covariates x_i does not affect γ, the Weibull regression model can be written as either the usual epidemiological proportional hazards:

$$h(t, x_i) = h_0(t) \exp(\beta^T x_i)$$

or accelerated failure time, using the expected failure time:

$$T_i = \exp(\theta^T x_i + \varepsilon_i)$$

where ε_i has a standard extreme value distribution with scale parameter $1/\gamma$. The Weibull shape parameter γ can thus be used to express results from the accelerated failure time parameterisation as proportional hazards: $\theta = -\beta/\gamma$. If the underlying survival times follow a Weibull distribution, the Weibull shape parameter can be estimated from the survival data and used to express the g-estimated survival ratio as a hazard ratio for the exposure (Witteman et al. 1998).

The 95% confidence intervals for g-estimated effects are generally wider than those for corresponding Weibull estimates, particularly with rare outcomes and for estimates close to 1. This is because G-estimation discards information when censoring, by dichotomising the outcome variable.

Example 4 G-estimation has been used to examine the effects of changes in cardiovascular risk factors in mid-life on all-cause mortality and incidence of coronary heart disease (CHD) (Tilling et al. 2002). Cardiovascular risk factors (systolic and diastolic blood pressure, smoking, diabetes, HDL and LDL cholesterol) were measured four times, with the first measure being used as the baseline in the g-estimation model.

To identify the extent of time-varying confounding, the relationships between each exposure and past and current values of all covariates were examined. This was done using one regression model for each exposure, to which each individual could contribute up to three observations. These models showed that there was substantial time-varying confounding, with inter-relationships among most of the time-varying exposures. Weibull survival analysis (with the accelerated failure time parameterisation) was used to relate all the covariates to survival, and the shape parameter from this model (1.26, 95% CI 1.17–1.36) was later used to express the g-estimated survival ratios as hazard ratios for each exposure.

Separate g-estimation models were fitted for each exposure. In each g-estimation model all risk factors (other than the exposure of interest) were included as time-varying covariates. Baseline variables (e.g. age and sex) were included as non time-varying covariates. In the models for systolic and diastolic blood pressure, individuals were censored when they first reported use of anti-hypertensive medication. The probability of being on anti-hypertensive medication at each visit was dependent on blood pressure at baseline and previous visits, and was also related to baseline and time-varying values of BMI, smoking and diabetes, and to age and sex. This censoring process was modelled, using logistic regression, and the probability of each individual being censored was taken into account in the g-estimation method.

Table 14.4 (modified from (Tilling et al. 2002) with permission of Oxford University Press and the Society for Epidemiologic Research) shows the baseline,

Table 14.4 Baseline and time-varying Weibull survival analysis and G-estimated relations between time-varying cardiovascular risk factors and survival for Atherosclerosis Risk in Communities participants with data from at least the first two visits (1987–1989 and 1990–1993) (Modified with permission of the Oxford University Press and the Society for Epidemiologic Research from Tilling et al. (2002))

Variable	Reference group	Baseline HR	95% CI	Time-varying HR	95% CI	G-estimated HR	95% CI
SBP $\geq$ 140 mmHg	SBP < 140 mmHg	2.08	1.43, 3.03	1.72	1.23, 2.40	1.79	1.38, 2.24
DBP $\geq$ 90 mmHg	DBP < 90 mmHg	1.58	0.79, 3.17	1.91	1.02, 3.56	1.98	0.97, 28.56
Diabetes	No diabetes	2.04	1.67, 2.49	1.26	0.98, 1.62	1.62	1.06, 1.98
BMI (kg/m^2)	BMI 20–30 kg/m^2						
$\leq$20		2.58	1.89, 3.53	3.09	2.03, 4.71	2.07	1.39, 3.64
$\geq$30		1.01	0.85, 1.20	0.83	0.64, 1.07	0.71	0.51, 1.12

HR hazard ratio, *CI* confidence interval, *SBP* systolic blood pressure, *DBP* diastolic blood pressure, *BMI* body mass index, *HDL* high density lipoprotein, *LDL* low density lipoprotein time-varying and g-estimated hazard ratios for mortality for selected cardiovascular risk factors. The comparisons of the results for the usual survival analysis (relating exposure at baseline to mortality) and g-estimation shed some light on the likely mechanisms for each exposure. Diabetes at baseline was associated with a hazard ratio of 2.04 (Tilling et al. 2002). The g-estimated hazard rate ratio for time-varying diabetes (1.62) was weaker than that for baseline diabetes, indicating that the cumulative effect of diabetes is stronger than the instantaneous effect. The time-varying effect of diabetes was underestimated by the standard analysis (hazard ratio = 1.26). The g-estimated hazard ratio for systolic blood pressure was again weaker than the baseline effect, showing that the effect of blood pressure on mortality was long-term rather than instantaneous. G-estimation and Weibull analysis showed a higher risk of death for those with low BMI and no evidence of increased mortality among subjects with high BMI. The validity of G-estimation depends on there being no unmeasured confounders. Confounders not included here, such as comorbid conditions, may influence the relation between BMI and mortality. Alternatively, BMI may have a cumulative effect, and so short-term changes in weight (assessed by these time-varying models) have a different relation to mortality than long-term weight.

For blood pressure and diabetes, the time-varying effects of exposure were underestimated by the usual survival analysis, whereas the adverse effect of low BMI appeared to be over-estimated by the usual survival analysis. Thus the time-varying confounding present in this example led to biases in the estimation of the effects of time-varying exposures. The confidence intervals for the g-estimated hazard ratios were wider than those for the Weibull estimates, because g-estimation discards information when dichotomising the outcome variable to deal with censoring.

14.6 Extensions to G-estimation

G-estimation (as described above) assumes a binary exposure. The effect of trichotomous exposures on outcome has been estimated using g-estimation and an iterative procedure (Tilling et al. 2002). For each exposure, the middle category was chosen as the reference. One of the other two categories was selected, and the effect of the dichotomous exposure defined by that category and the middle category estimated using g-estimation. This estimate was then included as a fixed value in the g-estimation of the effect of the dichotomous exposure defined by the third category and the middle category. This procedure was iterated to convergence. The standard errors for the effects of variables with three categories estimated in this way may be under-estimated, because each iteration assumes that the effect of the other category on survival is known (rather than estimated). Ideally, both parameters should be estimated simultaneously and a 95% confidence region for their joint distribution calculated. However, this has not yet been carried out in practice. Similarly, there has to date been no extension of g-estimation to continuous exposures.

The parameterisation used in the g-estimation procedure described above assumes that the effect of exposure is both immediate and unlimited. Thus we assume that quitting smoking affects survival from the moment of quitting, and that this effect remains throughout the rest of the non-smoking lifecourse. Alternative models are possible (Lok et al. 2004), for example by generalisations of the integral in Eq. 14.1. They include examining a lagged effect of exposure, or allowing exposure to be related to outcome immediately after exposure, with a lesser effect after a period of time (Joffe et al. 1998). For example, one could hypothesise that the effect of quitting smoking on lung cancer mortality might be lagged, so might not start until 5 years after quitting smoking. The effects of a treatment could also be limited in time – the effect of a particular treatment on outcome may be different in the short and long term (say, before and after 30 months) for example (Joffe et al. 1998). The way in which the counter-factual survival time depends on the exposure can be easily amended to take these alternative hypotheses into account (Joffe et al. 1998).

The use of g-estimation is not restricted to survival outcomes – for example, g-estimation has been used to examine the effects of treatment regimes on non-survival outcomes in randomised clinical trials, allowing for non-compliance (Toh and Hernan 2008). The principle of g-estimation, exploiting the conditional independence between a baseline counterfactual and exposure, has also been used for estimating direct/indirect effects (Goetgeluk et al. 2008), genomic control (Vansteelandt et al. 2009), and for finding optimal treatment strategies (Robins 2004).

14.7 Unmeasured Confounding

G-estimation depends crucially on the assumption of no unmeasured confounding. In particular, it relies on having all variables determining exposure both observed and included in the model. However, in many cohort studies, the factors related to exposure are not measured. For example, when looking at smoking as an exposure there may be many factors related to an individual's decision to quit and success in quitting smoking, which may also be related to the outcome. If these are not all recorded, then there may still be bias in the G-estimation of the effect of smoking. Thus, in order for G-estimation to be used successfully, the factors determining treatment decisions need to be well standardised and well measured. The assumption of no unmeasured confounding is, of course, necessary for the validity of all observational epidemiological analyses.

14.8 Alternatives to G-estimation

Marginal structural models (MSMs) are one type of alternative to g-estimation for analysing longitudinal data (Hernan et al. 2000, 2002; Young et al. 2010). In these models each observation is weighted by the probability of exposure based on past covariate and exposure history, and a model is then fitted to the weighted data and coefficients interpreted as in a standard analysis. For example, weighted Cox proportional hazards models were used to estimate the joint effect of zidovudine (AZT) and prophylaxis therapy for *Pneumocystis carinii* pneumonia on the survival of HIV-positive men, controlling for time-dependent confounding (Hernan et al. 2001), and the effect of zidovudine therapy on mean CD4 count among HIV-infected men (Hernan et al. 2002; Sterne et al. 2005). The weights were based on the inverse of each patient's probability of the treatment history they actually had, given their covariate history. These inverse probability weights were stabilised and modified to adjust for censoring (Hernan et al. 2001). MSMs were designed to estimate marginal causal parameters and are difficult to adapt to situations where exposure or treatment interacts with covariates. G-estimation in contrast can relatively simply be adapted to include such interactions by modifying the function in the integral and hence the way U_i is calculated back from T_i.

A second alternative to G-estimation is G-computation; also referred to as (parametric) G-formula (Robins et al. 1999; Taubman et al. 2009). The G-formula computes the causal effect of a given exposure or treatment sequence by assuming regression models for all covariates that we wish to adjust for at all measurement time points given the past as well as an outcome regression model, and then integrating out the covariates. In practice this integral needs to be approximated by Monte Carlo simulation. The G-formula is somewhat cumbersome to implement, but has been successfully implemented (Robins et al. 1999; Taubman et al. 2009) and interest in its use is growing (Snowden et al. 2011). The G-formula can also be derived from a decision-theoretic point of view avoiding counterfactuals (Dawid and Didelez 2010).

All three approaches, G-estimation, MSMs, and G-formula, correctly adjust for time-varying confounding but require the same no unmeasured confounding assumption; they differ in that the former two require a valid exposure model in addition to the outcome model, while the latter requires valid models for the time-varying covariates in addition to the outcome model.

14.9 Conclusions and Further Reading

Time-varying confounding may occur in longitudinal studies where exposure and covariates change over time. Where time-varying confounding occurs, it may cause bias in the results of usual survival analyses. G-estimation is one possible method used to overcome this problem, and has been shown to reduce bias in some cases. For those interested in exploring g-estimation further, the following references may be helpful: (Hernan et al. 2005, 2006; Robins 1992, 2008; Robins et al. 1992b, 2007; Tanaka et al. 2008; Yamaguchi and Ohashi 2004; Young et al. 2010). An overview and comparison of three methods of analysing data with time-dependent confounding (marginal structural models and two forms of g-estimation) is provided by Young et al. (2010). A summary of confounding, in particular time-dependent confounding (in the context of marginal structural models) demonstrated using causal diagrams may be found in Robins et al. (2000).

References

Amuzu, A., Carson, C., Watt, H. C., Lawlor, D. A., & Ebrahim, S. (2009). Influence of area and individual lifecourse deprivation on health behaviours: Findings from the British Women's Heart and Health Study. *European Journal of Cardiovascular Prevention and Rehabilitation, 16*(2), 169–173.

Ben-Shlomo, Y. (2007). Rising to the challenges and opportunities of life course epidemiology. *International Journal of Epidemiology, 36*(3), 481–483.

Ben-Shlomo, Y., & Kuh, D. (2002). A life course approach to chronic disease epidemiology: Conceptual models, empirical challenges and interdisciplinary perspectives. *International Journal of Epidemiology, 31*(2), 285–293.

Dawid, A. P., & Didelez, V. (2010). Identifying the consequences of dynamic treatment strategies: A decision theoretic overview. *Statistics Surveys, 4*, 184–231.

Glymour, M. M., Avendano, M., Haas, S., & Berkman, L. F. (2008). Lifecourse social conditions and racial disparities in incidence of first stroke. *Annals of Epidemiology, 18*(12), 904–912.

Goetgeluk, S., Vansteelandt, S., & Goetghebeur, E. (2008). Estimation of controlled direct effects. *Journal of the Royal Statistical Society Series B-Statistical Methodology, 70*, 1049–1066.

Hernan, M. A., Brumback, B., & Robins, J. M. (2000). Marginal structural models to estimate the causal effect of zidovudine on the survival of HIV-positive men. *Epidemiology, 11*(5), 561–570.

Hernan, M. A., Brumback, B., & Robins, J. M. (2001). Marginal structural models to estimate the joint causal effect of nonrandomized treatments. *Journal of the American Statistical Association, 96*(454), 440–448.

Hernan, M. A., Brumback, B. A., & Robins, J. M. (2002). Estimating the causal effect of zidovudine on CD4 count with a marginal structural model for repeated measures. *Statistics in Medicine, 21*(12), 1689–1709.

Hernan, M. A., Hernandez-Diaz, S., & Robins, J. M. (2004). A structural approach to selection bias. *Epidemiology, 15*(5), 615–625.

Hernan, M. A., Cole, S. R., Margolick, J., Cohen, M., & Robins, J. M. (2005). Structural accelerated failure time models for survival analysis in studies with time-varying treatments. *Pharmacoepidemiology and Drug Safety, 14*(7), 477–491.

Hernan, M. A., Lanoy, E., Costagliola, D., & Robins, J. M. (2006). Comparison of dynamic treatment regimes via inverse probability weighting. *Basic & Clinical Pharmacology & Toxicology, 98*(3), 237–242.

Joffe, M. M., Hoover, D. R., Jacobson, L. P., Kingsley, L., Chmiel, J. S., & Visscher, B. R. (1997). Effect of treatment with zidovudine on subsequent incidence of Kaposi's sarcoma. *Clinical Infectious Diseases, 25*(5), 1125–1133.

Joffe, M. K., Hoover, D. R., Jacobson, L. P., Kingsley, L., Chmiel, J. S., Visscher, B. R., & Robins, J. M. (1998). Estimating the effect of zidovudine on Kaposi's sarcoma from observational data using a rank preserving structural failure-time model. *Statistics in Medicine, 17*, 1073–1102.

Keiding, N., Filiberti, M., Esbjerg, S., Robins, J. M., & Jacobsen, N. (1999). The graft versus leukemia effect after bone marrow transplantation: A case study using structural nested failure time models. *Biometrics, 55*(1), 23–28.

Korhonen, P. A., Laird, N. M., & Palmgren, J. (1999). Correcting for non-compliance in randomized trials: An application to the ATBC Study. *Statistics in Medicine, 18*(21), 2879–2897.

Little, R. J. A., & Rubin, D. B. (2002). *Statistical analysis with missing data* (2nd ed.). Hoboken: Wiley.

Lok, J., Gill, R., van der Vaart, A., & Robins, J. (2004). Estimating the causal effect of a time-varying treatment on time-to-event using structural nested failure time models. *Statistica Neerlandica, 58*(3), 271–295.

Mark, S. D., & Robins, J. M. (1993). Estimating the causal effect of smoking cessation in the presence of confounding factors using a rank preserving structural failure time model. *Statistics in Medicine, 12*(17), 1605–1628.

Robins, J. (1986). A new approach to causal inference in mortality studies with a sustained exposure period – application to control of the healthy worker survivor effect. *Mathematical Modelling, 7*(9–12), 1393–1512.

Robins, J. M. (1992). Estimation of the time-dependent accelerated failure time model in the presence of confounding factors. *Biometrika, 79*(2), 321–334.

Robins, J. M. (2004). Optimal structural nested models for optimal sequential decisions. In D. Y. Lin & P. Heagerty (Eds.), *Proceedings of the Second Seattle Symposium on Biostatistics* (pp. 189–326). New York: Springer.

Robins, J. M. (2008). Causal models for estimating the effects of weight gain on mortality. *International Journal of Obesity, 32*(Suppl 3), S15–S41.

Robins, J. M., Blevins, D., Ritter, G., & Wulfsohn, M. (1992a). G-estimation of the effect of prophylaxis therapy for Pneumocystis carinii pneumonia on the survival of AIDS patients. *Epidemiology, 3*(4), 319–336.

Robins, J. M., Mark, S. D., & Newey, W. K. (1992b). Estimating exposure effects by modelling the expectation of exposure conditional on confounders. *Biometrics, 48*(2), 479–495.

Robins, J. M., Greenland, S., & Hu, F. C. (1999). Estimation of the causal effect of a time-varying exposure on the marginal mean of a repeated binary outcome. *Journal of the American Statistical Association, 94*(447), 687–700.

Robins, J. M., Hernan, M. A., & Brumback, B. (2000). Marginal structural models and causal inference in epidemiology. *Epidemiology, 11*(5), 550–560.

Robins, J. M., Hernan, M. A., & Rotnitzky, A. (2007). Effect modification by time-varying covariates. *American Journal of Epidemiology, 166*(9), 994–1002.

Snowden, J. M., Rose, S., & Mortimer, K. M. (2011). Implementation of G-computation on a simulated data set: Demonstration of a causal inference technique. *American Journal of Epidemiology, 173*(7), 731–738.

Stata Corporation. (2007). College Station, Texas.

Sterne, J., & Tilling, K. (2002). G-estimation of causal effects, allowing for time-varying confounding. *The Stata Journal, 2*(2), 164–182.

Sterne, J. A., Hernan, M. A., Ledergerber, B., Tilling, K., Weber, R., Sendi, P., Rickenbach, M., Robins, J. M., & Egger, M. (2005). Long-term effectiveness of potent antiretroviral therapy in preventing AIDS and death: A prospective cohort study. *The Lancet, 366*(9483), 378–384.

Tanaka, Y., Matsuyama, Y., & Ohashi, Y. (2008). Estimation of treatment effect adjusting for treatment changes using the intensity score method: Application to a large primary prevention study for coronary events (MEGA study). *Statistics in Medicine, 27*(10), 1718–1733.

Taubman, S. L., Robins, J. M., Mittleman, M. A., & Hernan, M. A. (2009). Intervening on risk factors for coronary heart disease: An application of the parametric g-formula. *International Journal of Epidemiology, 38*(6), 1599–1611.

Tehranifar, P., Liao, Y., Ferris, J. S., & Terry, M. B. (2009). Life course socioeconomic conditions, passive tobacco exposures and cigarette smoking in a multiethnic birth cohort of U.S. women. *Cancer Causes & Control, 20*(6), 867–876.

Tennant, P. W., Gibson, G. J., & Pearce, M. S. (2008). Lifecourse predictors of adult respiratory function: Results from the Newcastle Thousand Families Study. *Thorax, 63*(9), 823–830.

Tilling, K., Sterne, J. A., & Szklo, M. (2002). Estimating the effect of cardiovascular risk factors on all-cause mortality and incidence of coronary heart disease using G-estimation: The atherosclerosis risk in communities study. *American Journal of Epidemiology, 155*(8), 710–718.

Toh, S., & Hernan, M. A. (2008). Causal inference from longitudinal studies with baseline randomization. *The International Journal of Biostatistics, 4*(1), Article 22.

Vansteelandt, S., Goetgeluk, S., Lutz, S., Waldman, I., Lyon, H., Schadt, E. E., Weiss, S. T., & Lange, C. (2009). On the adjustment for covariates in genetic association analysis: A novel, simple principle to infer direct causal effects. *Genetic Epidemiology, 33*(5), 394–405.

Witteman, J. C., D'Agostino, R. B., Stijnen, T., Kannel, W. B., Cobb, J. C., de Ridder, M. A., Hofman, A., & Robins, J. M. (1998). G-estimation of causal effects: Isolated systolic hypertension and cardiovascular death in the Framingham Heart Study. *American Journal of Epidemiology, 148*(4), 390–401.

Yamaguchi, T., & Ohashi, Y. (2004). Adjusting for differential proportions of second-line treatment in cancer clinical trials. Part I: Structural nested models and marginal structural models to test and estimate treatment arm effects. *Statistics in Medicine, 23*(13), 1991–2003.

Young, J. G., Hernan, M. A., Picciotto, S., & Robins, J. M. (2010). Relation between three classes of structural models for the effect of a time-varying exposure on survival. *Lifetime Data Analysis, 16*(1), 71–84.

Chapter 15
Generalised Additive Models

Robert M. West

15.1 Introduction

The inclusion of continuous covariates in generalised linear models is common in epidemiological applications. For example, age and deprivation are very common confounders and so are often 'adjusted for'. Sometimes, although covariates are continuous, they are entered in discretised form. This is one method employed to account for nonlinearity and is discussed in more detail below. The issue concerning this chapter is that covariates need not enter a generalised linear model merely as linear terms.

Specifically consider the outcome variable to be mortality and that a logistic regression is used to model the effects of covariates. The model will be used to explain mortality rather than simply to predict mortality. Epidemiological study focuses on an exposure, which enters as a covariate. Age often has a clinically and statistically large impact on mortality and, although often just a nuisance variable, needs to be included as a covariate. It is sometimes, but not often, plausible that the log odds of mortality increases linearly with age. More commonly the relationship has greater complexity. If age is poorly modelled then the estimate of the exposure of interest will be less accurate and biased. The log odds of mortality and age is most likely to increase with age and is plausibly smooth: the question becomes how the best model fit is obtained. The answer might be to use a transformation of the covariate, consider higher-order terms, to fit splines, or to make use of the techniques employed in Generalised Additive Models (GAMs).

Nonlinearity is not the only consideration that motivates the use of GAMs. The difficulty of interactions, see Chap. 16, for continuous covariates has been noted. In particular determining the functional form of second- and higher-order

R.M. West (✉)
Division of Biostatistics, Centre for Epidemiology and Biostatistics, Leeds Institute
of Genetics, Health & Therapeutics, University of Leeds, Leeds, UK
e-mail: r.m.west@leeds.ac.uk

interactions is even more challenging than for a single main effect. The techniques available with GAMs provide a suitable means to tackle this ferocious challenge.

The first step however is to focus on the challenges of nonlinearity for a single main effect. Throughout this chapter data from a study of sympathetic nerve activity has been selected to illustrate issues and procedures.

15.2 Sympathetic Nerve Activity: Basic Model

Sympathetic nerve activity (*sna*) is known to increase with *age* and so is a convenient example for the topic of this chapter. Further, there is a complex relationship with systolic blood pressure (*sbp*) as well, so that there are two continuous covariates to explore in models of *sna* (Burns et al. 2007). The setting for this example is a study where 172 volunteers were recruited in order to investigate certain aspects of the variation of *sna* between individuals. For simplicity here only the effects of *sex*, *age*, and *sbp* on *sna* will be considered, and although the causal relationship might be debated, in this and the next chapter, *sna* is taken to depend upon the other variables.

The outcome *sna* is a measurement on a continuous scale, *sex* is a dichotomous covariate (factor), and as mentioned above, *age* and *sbp* are continuous covariates. A basic model will fit just linear terms as covariates. All modelling will be undertaken in R since this statistical language is widely available (R Development Core Team 2010) and has good capabilities, once the relevant libraries have been downloaded. In R, models are specified by notation suggested by Wilkinson and Rogers (1973), and is straightforward to follow. The basic model is specified by sna ~ as.factor(sex) + age + sbp and the fitted model yields the results given in Table 15.1.

Note that for this model the adjusted sum of squares is 0.60: 60% of variation is explained by the model. The errors were also explored through plots, and it was seen that the residual plot against the fitted values, the normal QQ plot, the scale location plot and the leverage plots were all satisfactory. This is also true for all the subsequent residual plots in this chapter.

For this basic model, the effects of *age* and *sbp* are clear: they are simply linear terms. For completeness, and to permit comparison with later plots, graphical representations are provided in Figs. 15.1 and 15.2. These include rug plots along the abscissas to indicate for which ages and SBPs measurements of *sna* have been recorded. Note also the ranges of the ordinates.

Table 15.1 Table of coefficients for the basic model

Coefficient	Estimate	95% CI	p-value
Intercept	−16.6	(−26.5, −6.6)	0.00123
Male	7.3	(3.8, 10.8)	5.37e-05
Age	0.70	(3.8, 10.8)	6.24e-12
SBP	0.25	(0.16, 0.33)	4.54e-08

15 Generalised Additive Models

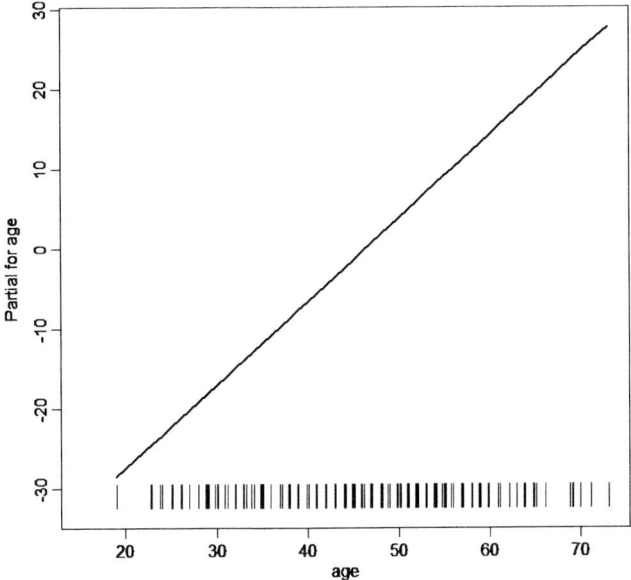

Fig. 15.1 Term plot for linear *age*

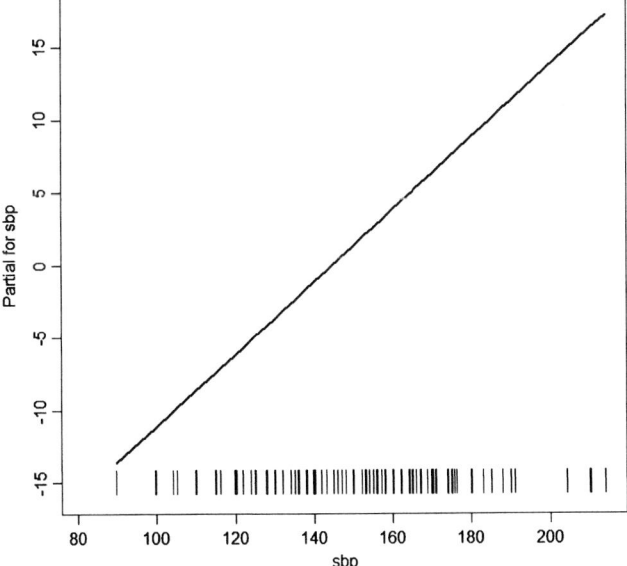

Fig. 15.2 Term plot for linear SBP

The use of discretisation of age into age groups has a long history. John Graunt (1662) is one of the earliest to publish material (life tables) and establish this methodology that has been exploited to great effect by modern insurance companies as just one example. As more data is available, the width of the age groups can be diminished, any errors due to discretisation will be minimal, and age can be considered to be modelled sufficiently well.

Such fine discretisation is not however undertaken throughout epidemiology, even when sample sizes are large: widths of age groups of 5 or 10 years can be found. There is an issue of parsimony in the model. If m age groups are to be used then $(m-1)$ variables are required to model age. Then a polynomial of degree $(m-1)$ is just as parsimonious and should be considered, see Sect. 15.4.

Discretisation might be favoured for reasons of interpretation, especially with logistic regression. For example age might be discretised as: Under 60, 60–69, 70–85, and Over 85 years. Then logistic regression delivers three odds ratios comparing the odds of mortality for persons in the three older groups with those in the youngest group. Interpretation is very simple in relation to the age effect. Effectively though, age has been modelled as a step function. An individual of age 69 steps up their risk on their seventieth birthday. There is certainly a discretisation error. The main concern though is that inaccuracy in modelling age will result in inaccuracy and bias for the role of other covariates including the exposure of interest.

Another concern about discretisation is that the number of groups and the group boundaries need to be chosen. There may be clinical or political reasons for specifying boundaries, such as achieving adult status at age 18, achieving retirement age at 65, etc. The results achieved for all covariate coefficients will differ when boundaries are changed. From a modelling perspective, the boundaries may be chosen for example by minimising the Akaike Information Criterion (AIC), although this may lead to what seem strange boundary values that once more lead to interpretation difficulties, albeit a fascinating challenge to obtain an interpretation.

Where there is a choice of the number of groups and their boundaries, there is 'temptation' to choose them to deliver the coefficient values of other covariates that are most favoured—especially if the main exposure has a coefficient close to statistical significance, but these issues are always present in complex modelling situations.

When a continuous variable is discretised, it is easy to define a further category of 'missing' when values are not recorded for some participants. This has great appeal if such an approach is appropriate for the modelling of missing values—for example where values are missing at random. In other circumstances however this could be disastrous. Consider the case where age is withheld by either the very young or very old for reasons of identifiability of those with a rare disease. Then such a category is misleading and it might be more appropriate to consider an imputation technique to handle missingness.

It is possible that some continuous covariates are discretised due to doubt about their true nature. An example might be a score from a psychometric test, which is not truly continuous, being the sum of (weighted) responses to a questionnaire.

Established thresholds might be used, for example defining a patient as depressed if he/she scores over a certain value on a depression scale. The underlying scale may not regarded by all as ordinal, let alone continuous. It is not clear if the use of the established thresholds improves matters. Information is lost regarding a variable whenever it is discretised and so error is introduced into the model, and the model cannot be improved by adding discretisation error. In such circumstances the variable might be considered as measured with error: refer to Chap. 3.

Deprivation scores are also composites and their full validity is sometimes in doubt: specifically the deprivation score of an area is associated with an individual. Often in epidemiological studies continuous measures of deprivation such as the Index of Multiple Deprivation or Townsend Score, are divided into fifths. This allows for nonlinearity but again there must be discretisation error as well as measurement error. The discretisation error might be avoided by using higher-order terms of deprivation scores: polynomial expressions of deprivation. Plots of the impact of deprivation on the modelled outcome will be required to facilitate interpretation as seen below in Sect. 15.4.

15.3 Sympathetic Nerve Activity: Discretisation

The basic model provided a fit for all three covariates with highly significant values for the three coefficients, but nonlinearity does potentially exist and an investigation is warranted. Here both *age* and *sbp* are discretised into five categories forming the new variables *agegp* and *sbpgp*. Cut points for *age* were taken as 30, 40, 50, and 60 years. Those for *sbp* were taken as 120, 140, 160, 180 mm Hg. For both variables the categories are all reasonably evenly populated whilst the cut points are easy to interpret. Values of *sbp* above 140 mm Hg suggest hypertension and so 140 mm Hg has some clinical meaning.

The model is specified by sna ~ as.factor(sex) + as.factor(agegp) + as.factor(sbpgp), and results given in Table 15.2.

The contributions of the covariates *age* and *sbp* are expressed graphically in Figs. 15.3 and 15.4. Note that one clear effect is that the ranges of the effects are much reduced from those in the basic model: compare the graphs. For this model with discretised covariates, the adjusted $R^2 = 0.63$, so that on the basis of the proportion of variation that is represented, the model with discretised *age* and *sbp* is preferred to the basic model.

From Table 15.2 it is strongly tempting to coalesce some categories, thus improving the adjusted R^2. In particular the exact match of the category boundary for *sbp* with the definition of hypertension $sbp = 140$ mm Hg, is extremely tempting. Such a data-driven approach however can be regarded as over-fitting to the dataset. If disctretisation is to be employed, it is advisable to fix the boundaries of all categories before fitting to the data.

Table 15.2 Table of coefficients for the model with discretised covariates

Coefficient	Estimate	95% CI	p-value
Intercept	25.0	(20.1,29.9)	< 2e-16
Male	7.3	(4.0,10.7)	2.93e-5
Age [30,40)	13.4	(6.8,20.0)	9.33e-5
Age [40,50)	20.3	(3.9,26.7)	2.99e-9
Age [50,60)	22.7	(15.9,29.4)	5.13e-10
Age $\geq$ 60	28.8	(20.5,37.1)	1.51e-10
SBP [120,140)	2.2	(−3.1,7.5)	0.413
SBP [140,160)	17.9	(12.1,23.7)	7.29e-9
SBP [160,180)	16.0	(10.3,21.7)	1.22e-7
SBP $\geq$ 180	15.0	(6.8,23.2)	0.000419

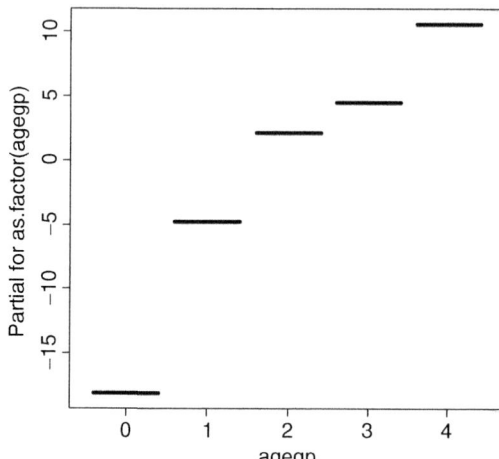

Fig. 15.3 Term plot for discretised *age*

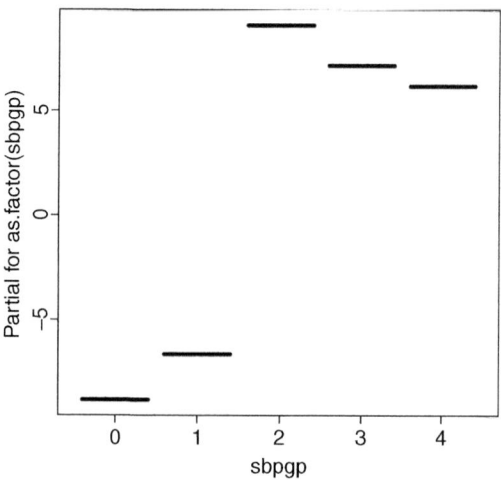

Fig. 15.4 Term plot for discretised *sbp*

15.4 Higher-Order Terms

A very straightforward way to check if a covariate should appear as a linear term only is to fit higher-order terms and test their significance. Thus if *age* has been entered as a linear term, then adding age^2 and age^3 will reveal if the relationship is more complex. Interpreting the contribution of that covariate is not so easy to from a table of coefficients. It will be necessary to construct the fitted polynomial and plot it in order to make the position clear.

A phrase attributed to George Box is commonly cited: 'all models are wrong'. By better fitting of covariates, the models will be improved and the effects of exposures better assessed. Hence the added complexity of polynomial terms can be justified. Measures of fit of models can be used to balance complexity against fit such as adjusted R^2, AIC, and others. There are often automated searches available within software packages to obtain the best fit against these criteria. For example, R has a function `R::leaps::regsubsets()`, Miller (2002), that can search for the best fit by adjusted R^2, and the functions `R::stats::step()` and `R::MASS::stepAIC()` Venables and Ripley (2002) to search for the best fit by AIC. So there can be few excuses for not exploring this approach.

Searching higher-order terms can be made more efficient and robust by using orthogonal polynomials, Kennedy and Gentle (1980), due to increased numerical stability and the ease with which the best degree can be determined: orthogonality helps. In R, the function `R::stats::poly()` provides this ability. The function `R::stats::termplot()` can be used to display the functional representation and its influence on the outcome variable.

15.5 Sympathetic Nerve Activity: Higher-Order Terms

For the illustrative example, orthogonal polynomials were chosen, the formula in the R code being `sna ~ as.factor(sex) + poly(age,3) + poly(sbp,3)`.

From Table 15.3, the impact of the covariates on the outcome *sna* is not immediately clear. This is where graphical representations become important. Figures 15.5 and 15.6 demonstrate the effect of *age* and *sbp* effectively. Comparing the graphical figures for each of the models that have been fitted, it appears that the effect of *age* gives the largest range of effect in the model with higher-order terms, the youngest age resulting in a sizable decrease in *sna*: see Sect. 15.6 below for further comment.

Inspecting Fig. 15.6, the final downturn in the effect of SBP can be seen from the rug plot to be based on just a few measurements where *sbp* is above 200 mm Hg. Considering also the marginal statistical significance ($p = 0.0744$) of the cubic term for *sbp*, many might consider refitting with only a quadratic polynomial for *sbp*. The cubic representation is chosen here to identify that there is an issue of how best to identify the degree of polynomial representations of covariates in general: this issue is dealt with in Sect. 15.8.

Table 15.3 Table of coefficients for model with higher-order terms of covariates

Coefficient	Estimate	95% CI	p-value
Intercept	52.6	(50.2,54.9)	< 2e-16
Male	6.3	(2.9,9.6,)	0.000265
Poly(age,3) 1	108.9	(81.4,136.4)	5.95e-13
Poly(age,3) 2	−27.3	(−49.9,−4.8)	0.0179
Poly(age,3) 3	42.2	(20.7,63.7)	0.000152
Poly(sbp,3) 1	85.7	(58.2,113.2)	5.60e-9
Poly(sbp,3) 2	−24.0	(−46.5,−1.5)	0.0364
Poly(sbp,3) 3	−19.4	(−40.7,1.9)	0.0744

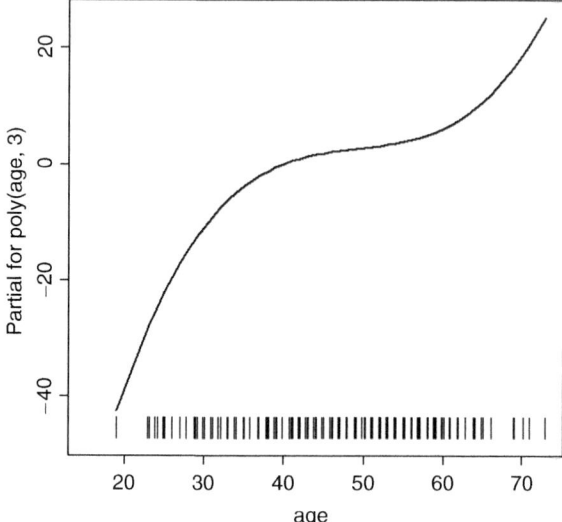

Fig. 15.5 Term plot for model with polynomial *age*

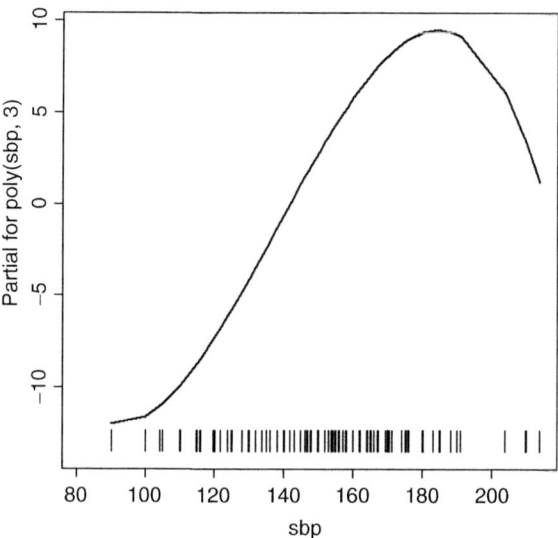

Fig. 15.6 Term plot for model with polynomial *sbp*

Note that for the model fitted with higher-order terms has two fewer parameters than the model for which the continuous covariates have been discretised. It is not only more parsimonious, but has an adjusted $R^2 = 0.65$, up from 0.63.

15.6 Splines

The complexity of the relationship between the continuous covariate and the modelled outcome may be efficiently represented using splines. These are low-order polynomials that are fitted locally but joined at knots smoothly, meaning that at the knots the function represented by the spline, and perhaps also some of its derivatives, are continuous. There are also advantages of numerical stability. The term spline derives from thin strips of flexible wood that have been used in construction to represent complex smooth curves. Fitting splines to covariates can be thought of as taking a nonparametric approach.

In the few situations where a small extrapolation might be considered, splines can often provide less extreme behaviour immediately beyond the range of the covariate. Note that this was a concern in the example above, where the model with higher-order terms predicted very low *sna* for the youngest subjects of the study. Similarly the sharp decline of *sna* with increasing *sbp* above 200 mm Hg provides a further reason to reconsider the model that was fitted. Runge's phenomenon, Runge (1901), which occurs with higher-order polynomials can become problematic. A very nice overview of splines together with a discussion is provided by Eilers and Marx (1996).

There are many ways to specify a basis for a spline fit, Wahba (1990), some examples are B-splines de Boor (1978), P-splines Eilers and Marx (1996), natural cubic splines, and O'Sullivan splines O'Sullivan et al. (1986). The order of the spline approximation must be chosen, as must the number and the location of knots. Penalised splines can be employed, see Sect. 15.8, and then further parameters are involved: the smoothness parameter and the derivative to be smoothed. Smoothing is not considered in this introductory section, but deferred until Sect. 15.8. Knots are often evenly spaced, or placed at certain percentiles of the covariate.

15.7 Sympathetic Nerve Activity: Splines

To illustrate the use of splines, natural cubic splines are selected. A single internal interpolation point is chosen as the median (50th percentile) for each of the two covariates. The end points of the range of a covariate are automatically used as knots, and without internal knots the spline degenerates to a polynomial fit. The formula for use with R is sna ~ as.factor(sex) + ns(age,knots = median(age)) + ns(sbp,knots = median(sbp)).

In tabulated form, the results of the fit are provided in Table 15.4. It is noted that the fit is not so satisfactory, with the adjusted $R^2 = 0.62$. The effects of the covariates are given graphically in Figs. 15.7 and 15.8.

Table 15.4 Table of coefficients for model with spline fits for covariates

Coefficient	Estimate	95% CI	p-value
Intercept	7.6	(−0.6,15.8)	0.0689
Male	6.2	(2.8,9.7)	0.000480
ns(age,knots = median(age)) 1	57.1	(41.5,72.6)	1.63e-11
ns(age,knots = median(age)) 2	20.7	(11.2,30.2)	2.80e-5
ns(age,knots = median(sbp)) 1	46.0	(29.0,63.1)	3.33e-7
ns(age,knots = median(sbp)) 2	20.7	(10.4,31.0)	0.000109

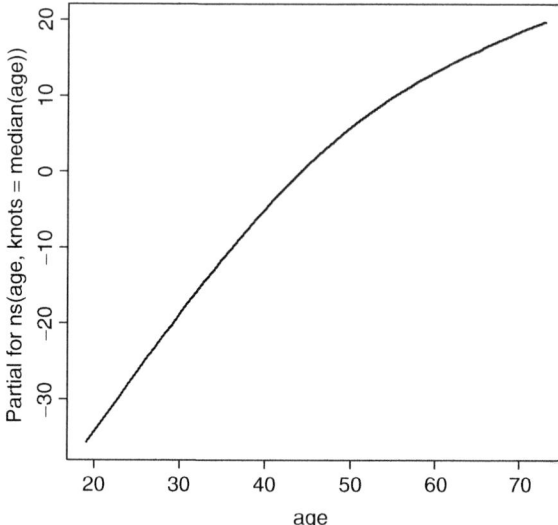

Fig. 15.7 Term plot for model with natural spline fit for *age*

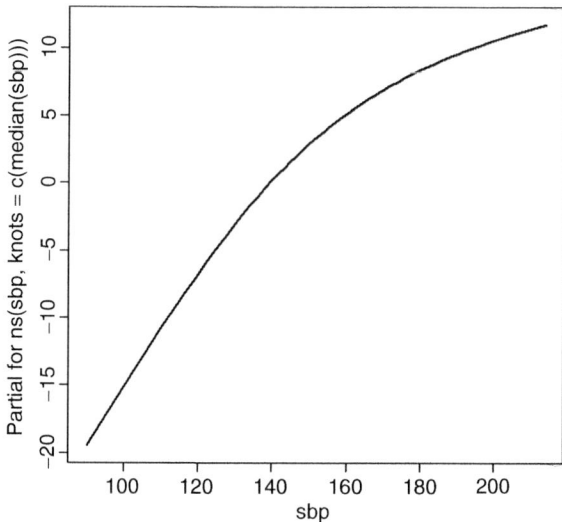

Fig. 15.8 Term plot for model with natural spline fit for *sbp*

By comparison of Figs. 15.7 and 15.8 with preceding ones, it can be seen that this particular spline fit gives rather different results for the effects of *age* and *sbp* than the other models considered. The fit is better than that of the basic model, but it is clear that there are challenges in finding the best spline representation. Those providing libraries for GAMs have also provided tools to make spline selection much easier and much more efficient: see Sect. 15.8.

15.8 Generalised Additive Models

Generalised additive models have continued to receive attention since their introduction by Hastie and Tibshirani, see Hastie and Tibshirani (1986, 1990). Additive models are ones where the effects of each covariate are added: there are no interaction terms and so the additivity of effects is assumed. This chapter focusses on nonlinearities whilst Chap. 16 enables the exploration of interactions. Hence here the initial attention has been to the representation of the effect of each covariate with a graphical representation of that effect to enable interpretation. GAMs continue this theme. The generalised term simply refers to the fact that the methodology of additive models (spline fits to covariates) can be just as easily applied to generalised models, such as logistic regression, as well as it can be applied to linear regression.

Given the large number of parameters that need to be selected for a spline fit, tools to provide automated choices save considerable effort and can provide some objectivity. The principle of parsimony where a model with fewer parameters is preferred to a more complex model is often to the forefront of automated procedures. A statistical epidemiologist will be concerned with estimating the effects of each covariate rather than intricate and subtle choices of parameters in spline fitting and will want to utilise developed software tools with automated choices rather than lavish time and resources on a general spline fit. There is software available to fit GAMs in several statistical packages but here attention is restricted to three libraries that are available in R and which provide more than enough material for discussion in a single book chapter.

15.9 Smoothed Low-Order Splines

The fitting of very low-order splines as an initial data-exploration technique is well established and often referred to as 'lowess' or 'loess'. This approach is available for covariates in generalised linear models and has been provided by Trevor Hastie in the function R::gam::gam. The default settings are for a spline with degree $= 1$ and span $= 0.5$ so that fitting is performed with a proportion of the data (span) equal to 0.5. Data points receive a tri-cubic weighting proportional to their distance from the estimation point. It is possible to change the degree to be in $\{0, 1, 2\}$ and the span to be in $(0,1]$. The best policy might be to accept the default settings unless there is evidence not to do so and focus attention on interpreting the effects of covariates.

With the same function in the R::gam library it is possible to fit penalised splines (smooths). The target number of degrees of freedom needs to be specified. Rather than expand this aspect here, smooths are considered with the R::mgcv package discussed in Sect. 15.11.

15.10 Sympathetic Nerve Activity: Loess Splines

The model was reformulated to include loess representation of the two continuous covariates through the formula sna ~ as.factor(sex) + lo(age) + lo(sbp). The fit is excellent with the adjusted $R^2 = 0.66$ and the significance of terms is given in Table 15.5 with the nonlinear nonparametric effects of the covariates shown in Figs. 15.9 and 15.10. Note that there is a facility to display the partial deviance residuals, which was exploited and that upper and lower pointwise twice-standard-error curves were included.

The fits obtained by R::gam::gam provide good material for an epidemiologist to consider. The main features of the fits should be explained. Smaller details that lead to a little jaggedness might be ignored in many cases. This approach to interpretation suggests that a smoother fit might be warranted.

Table 15.5 Table of coefficients for model with loess fits for covariates

Coefficient	Npar DF	Npar F	p-value
lo(age)	2.5	7.71	0.000232
lo(sbp)	3.1	6.88	0.000187

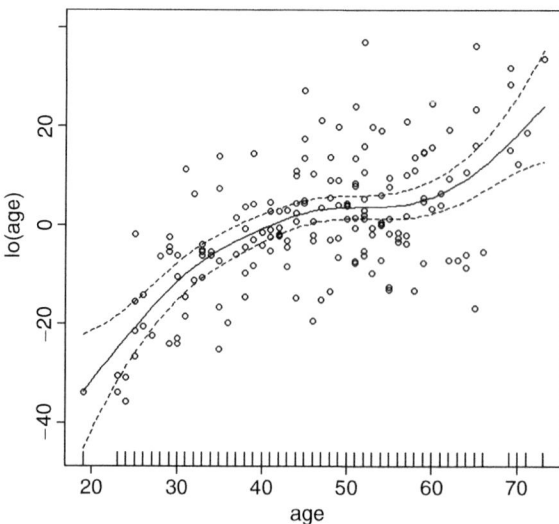

Fig. 15.9 Term plot for model with loess spline fit for *sbp*

15 Generalised Additive Models

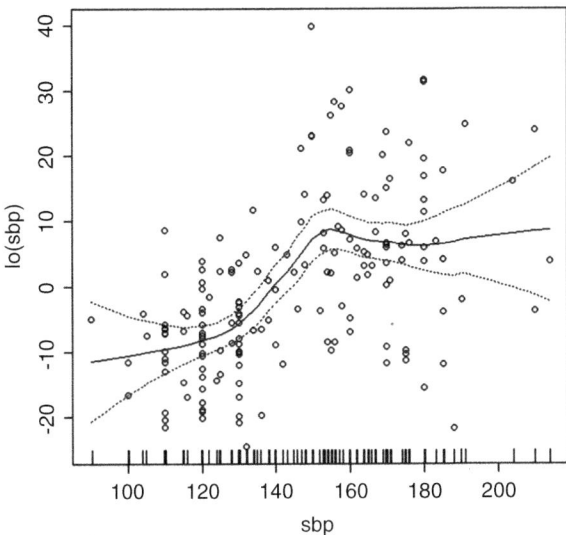

Fig. 15.10 Term plot for model with loess spline fit for *sbp*

15.11 Generalised Cross Validation

The advantages of automatic determination of parameters have been emphasised. Simon Wood (2006) has published a most useful library for automatically fitting GAMs with smooths for covariates, namely R::mgcv. Note that this library has a function R::mgcv::gam so that it is important to ensure that the correct library has been loaded into R.

A generalised linear model can be fitted by R::mgcv::gam identifying which covariates a smooth is to be used: see example below. By cross validation, the 'best' smoothing parameter is chosen, yielding a totally automated procedure. In fact the procedure used is generalised cross validation, which is numerically efficient and yields results close to those of cross validation. Hence a powerful tool is made available to explore smooth non-parametric nonlinearities in covariates for generalised linear models.

15.12 Sympathetic Nerve Activity: Cross Validation

The formula needed to indicate smooths for *age* and *sbp* that is used in R::mgcv::gam is sna ~ as.factor(sex) + s(age) + s(sbp) which reports significance of smooths as is Table 15.6. The effects are shown graphically in Figs. 15.11 and 15.12. Note the great similarity to the results with loess smoothing, although of course the representation of each covariate effect is much smoother, and perhaps therefore more credible in some circumstances. Partial residuals are shown, as are 'twice standard error' curves.

Table 15.6 Table of coefficients for model with smooths as covariates

Coefficient	edf	Ref. df	F	*p*-value
s(age)	4.289	4.789	16.41	1.05e-12
s(sbp)	4.812	5.312	10.39	5.40e-9

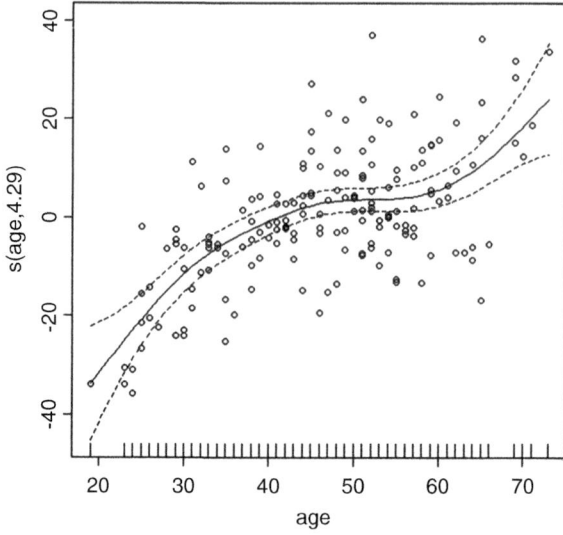

Fig. 15.11 Term plot for model with smooth for *age*

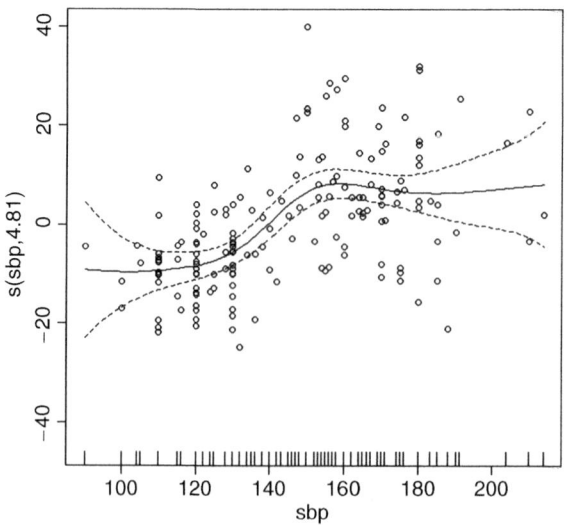

Fig. 15.12 Term plot for model with smooth for *sbp*

Although the main philosophy of GAMs is to assume additivity of covariate effects, modelling can be extended in dimension by fitting higher-dimensional splines to groups of covariates. This enables interactions to be visualised and compared to strictly additive models. For example two covariates might be suspected of interacting and it would then be appropriate to fit a two-dimension spline. The function R::mgcv::gam enables higher-dimensional splines.

15.13 Sympathetic Nerve Activity: Two-Dimensional GAM

The fit with a two-dimensional spline for *age* and *sbp* give the best fit to date with adjusted $R^2 = 0.69$ (Table 15.7). Thus there is evidence of an interaction between *age* and *sbp*, see Chap. 16 where this interaction effect is considered further.

Figure 15.13 shows that there are no younger participants with hypertension (high values of *sbp*) and no older participants with *sbp* in the normal range. This might have been a property of the recruiting strategy, or it may be that older people who volunteer for studies tend to have higher systolic blood pressure. The study is cross-sectional rather than longitudinal but there are longitudinal explanations that account for the relationship. Sympathetic nerve activity tends to increase with age and is higher for hypertensives. For younger participants with higher *sbp*, the increase of *sna* with age is more rapid (contours closer together).

Table 15.7 Table of coefficients for model with 2d smooth

Coefficient	edf	Ref. df	F	p-value
s(age,sbp)	12.82	13.32	26.15	<2e-16

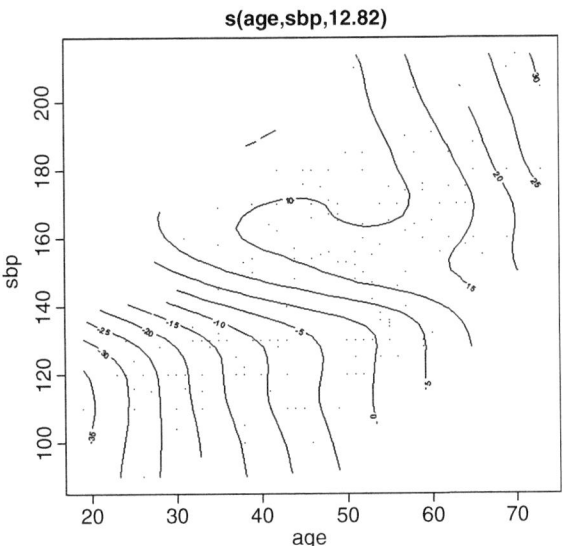

Fig. 15.13 Plot for model with 2d smooth of *age* and *sbp*

Note that standard error curves were omitted: the plot is already complex and needs full-colour treatment if further information is to be included. For the 2d plot, the standard se curves are ±1 standard error rather than ±2 standard errors as with the one-dimensional curves.

15.14 Further Aspects of GAMS

This chapter provides an introduction only to GAMs motivating their use through exploration of nonlinearities in covariate effects. Here is a brief mention of further aspects.

A third library is available in R, namely Vector Generalised and Additive Models, see Yee and Wild (1996). R::VGAM, that has been made available by Thomas Yee and makes use of B-splines and O'Sullivan splines that have certain advantages. The VGAM library is huge and there is a focus on multivariate outcomes for generalised linear models and generalised additive models.

Random effects can be included in GAMs through the function R::mgcv::gamm. Thus GAMs can be used in a multilevel context.

15.15 More on the Case Study

Further description of the case study of sympathetic nerve activity was delayed until this point as the primary interest was the methodology for exploring nonlinearities in covariates. Exploring different models however often helps to develop understanding of a situation, indeed that is one of the aims of modelling.

From each of the models it is clear that both *age* and *sbp* make significant contributions to *sna*, explaining well over 50% of the variation in results. Exploring residuals revealed nothing unusual so that for this application there was no indication that a linear model was unsuitable as regards the distribution of residuals. Discretisation of covariates provided little extra information other than indicating that the effect of *sbp* was far from linear. It is possible that a different discretisation would have produced different results: model fitting has challenges. Fitting higher-order terms was found to be no easier. By contrast the procedures for fitting GAMs made modelling far simpler.

Figures 15.10 and 15.12 show partial residuals. These again indicate that the distribution of residuals satisfy distributional assumptions of normality and homogeneity of variance. It is revealed also that there may be some digit preference for some of the participants: those with *sbp* values of 110, 120 and 130, possibly 100, whereas for other values there is no evidence of digit preference. Possibly a different sphygmomanometer was employed for these participants, at a time when younger normotensive volunteers were recruited to the study.

Fitting of statistical models cannot of course reveal biological mechanisms, but knowledge of biological mechanisms may aid in the interpretation of the statistical models. For example, a plausible biological mechanism is that a state of hypertension where *sbp* is constantly raised can result in thickening of the left ventricle and in central sympathetic nerve activity. This suggests that a step increase in *sna* is plausible for patients with *sbp* above the acknowledged threshold for hypertension of 140 mm Hg.

In Sect. 15.13 it was mentioned that the study was cross-sectional but the most plausible interpretation was longitudinal. This suggests that a longitudinal study on sympathetic nerve activity would be of interest. If *sna* is an indicator of progression of cardiovascular disease, then a longitudinal study recording *sna* and cardiovascular events is suggested with analysis using random-effect GAMs.

15.16 Chapter Summary

A range of methods to explore nonlinearity in covariates has been outlined and demonstrated with an example. There are considerable modelling challenges posed when there are so many modelling options, and automated procedures were advocated. Different approaches to modelling with GAMs were mentioned. In particular, loess fits can be exploited through R::gam::gam and smooths can be automatically selected through R::mgcv::gam. Both of these approaches with GAMs have been shown to be capable of producing good modelling results with the effects of covariates made clear through graphical plots.

References

Burns, J., Sivananthan, M. U., Ball, S. G., Mackintosh, A. F., Mary, D. A., & Greenwood, J. P. (2007). Relationship between central sympathetic drive and magnetic resonance imaging-determined left ventricular mass in essential hypertension. *Circulation, 115*, 1999–2005.

de Boor, C. (1978). *A practical guide to splines*. New York: Springer.

Eilers, P. H. C., & Marx, B. D. (1996). Flexible smoothing with B-splines and penalties. *Statistical Science, 11*, 89–121.

Graunt, J. (1662). *Natural and political observations on the bills of mortality*. London.

Hastie, T. J., & Tibshirani, R. J. (1986). Generalised additive models (with discussion). *Statistical Science, 1*, 295–318.

Hastie, T. J., & Tibshirani, R. J. (1990). *Generalised additive models*. Boca Raton: Chapman and Hall/CRC.

Kennedy, W. J., & Gentle, J. E. (1980). *Statistical computing*. New York.

Miller, A. J. (2002). *Subset selection in regression* (2nd ed.). Boca Raton: Chapman and Hall/CRC.

O'Sullivan, F., Yandell, B., & Raynor, W. (1986). Automatic smoothing of regression functions in generalised linear models. *Journal of the American Statistical Association, 18*, 96–103.

R Development Core Team. (2010). *R: A language and environment for statistical computing. R Foundation for Statistical Computing*, Vienna, Austria. ISBN 3-900051-07-0, URL http://www.R-project.org.

Runge, C. (1901). Uber empirische funktionen und die interpolation zwischen aquidistanten ordinaten. *Zeitschrift fur Mathematik und Physik, 46*, 224–243.

Venables, W. N., & Ripley, B. D. (2002). *Modern applied statistics with S* (4th ed.). NewYork: Springer Science and Business Media.

Wahba, G. (1990). *Spline models for observational data*. Philadelphia: SIAM.

Wilkinson, G., & Rogers, C. (1973). Symbolic description of factorial models for the analysis of variance. *Applied Statistics, 22*, 329–399.

Wood, S. N. (2006). *Generalised additive models: An introduction with R*. Boca Raton: Chapman and Hall/CRC.

Yee, T. W., & Wild, C. J. (1996). Vector generalised additive models. *Journal of the Royal Statistical Society, Series B, Methodological, 58*, 481–493.

Chapter 16
Regression and Classification Trees

Robert M. West

16.1 Introduction

Interactions in (generalised) linear models can be difficult, mainly due to the fact that there are so many potential interactions to consider when there are a number of covariates and factors in the model. For example, if a generalised linear model has four factors and each factor has four levels, then there are four main effects, six two-way terms, four three-way terms, and one four-way term to be considered: the four main effects and 11 interactions. Perhaps eight continuous covariates have been identified and it has been determined that they enter the model only in a linear manner, although if interactions have not yet been identified it is doubtful that there is any certainty about linearity of covariates, then there is 1 seven-way product, 7 six-way products, 21 five-way products and so on. Considering all interactions in a model with a large number of covariates and factors involves a huge number of terms and hence extensive modelling time.

One common approach to 'work around' this is to decide that such complexity is beyond reasonable modelling capabilities given the limited amount of data available. It is rare to encounter studies or trials that have been designed to investigate full details of all possible interactions. In that case an additive assumption may be made and additive models used: see Chap. 15 on generalised additive models.

The approach suggested in this chapter is to make use of regression trees and classification trees according to the nature of the outcome variable. In general specifying a model for datasets with multiple factors and covariates can be challenging. The idea here is to use trees to suggest viable models and in particular a shortlist of appropriate potential interaction terms.

R.M. West (✉)
Division of Biostatistics, Centre for Epidemiology and Biostatistics, Leeds Institute of Genetics, Health & Therapeutics, University of Leeds, Leeds, UK
e-mail: r.m.west@leeds.ac.uk

16.2 Trees

Regression trees, and classification trees, are simple models but are not familiar to all, hence this section is included to give some background to them. The popularity of classification trees and regression trees was greatly spurred by Breiman, Friedman, Stone, and Olshen; see Breiman et al. (1984), and this remains an excellent source for more detail. Trees will continue their popularity since there are numerous software tools available, which are easy to apply, and the resultant tree models are simple to implement and interpret, even for non-specialist users of statistics.

16.3 Regression Trees

First consider regression trees for continuous outcomes. Fitting is done by successively splitting the data two ways according to a single covariate or factor: branching. Start with the whole dataset and search through all the covariates and factors and all the possible cut points. For example a continuous covariate *age* might be split at any cut point that lies midway between two adjacent values for *age*. The split is chosen so that the difference between the two groups so defined gives maximal difference in the mean outcome variable. If the outcome is sympathetic nerve activity *sna* then the mean values of *sna* of the two groups is calculated. The residual sums of squares about those means are calculated and the two sums added to produce a residual sums of squares for that split (partition). The best split is the one that produces the smallest residual sum of squares: the means are maximally distinguished. The two groups defined by the first step are then each split again by the same procedure of searching through all variables and all cut points. The process continues and can continue until there are only single values at the end of each branch.

Note that linearity of covariates is not an issue for regression trees: there is no need to assume linearity, nor monotonicity. As will be seen, interactions can be revealed and need not pose any difficulties.

Regression trees (and classification trees) are restricted in the manner in which they are fitted. Splits can occur along only one axis (covariate or factor) at a time. A better fit might be obtained by considering multiple fits at each step: that is a multiple split may reduce the residual sums of squares significantly whereas a split on only one covariate or factor would achieve only a small RSS reduction.

16.4 R Libraries

Trees are relatively straightforward to programme and there is much software available to fit trees, including specialist code. Software aspects are discussed here through the statistical programming language R (R Development Core Team 2010), which is widely available and much used by statisticians and epidemiologists. There are two commonly used libraries in R that enable tree modelling, `R::tree` and `R::rpart`.

16.5 Sympathetic Nerve Activity

Often an example helps to demonstrate a methodology so here regression tree modelling is applied to the dataset considered in Chap. 15. The outcome, sympathetic nerve activity *sna*, was recorded with covariates *age* and systolic blood pressure *sbp*, as well as a factor, *sex* (male and female). Fitting a regression tree will indicate which covariates and factors (one in this case) are important for explaining variation in *sna*, if there may be nonlinearities, and if there might be interactions.

For this example the function R::rpart::rpart was used. With the default settings the two functions produce slightly different results and here the simpler one has been selected. The tree model produced is shown in Fig. 16.1. Note that:

- the length of the branch indicates the relative importance of the variable upon which the split has been made: the relative improvement of the fit
- the terminal nodes report the value of *sna* fitted by the model
- branch left if the rule is satisfied
- both *sbp* and *age* can be seen to offer important contributions
- there is a contribution from *sex* through some of the branches
- further pruning may be indicated by clinical judgement: older people with high *sna* are likely to be hypertensive, others may be distinguished just through overfitting.

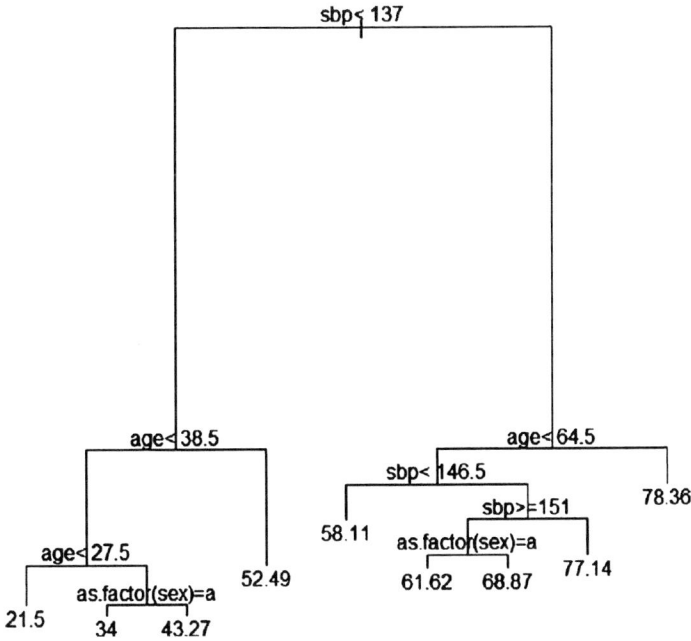

Fig. 16.1 Tree model for sympathetic nerve activity. Here the expression as factor(sex) = a is to be read as sex = female

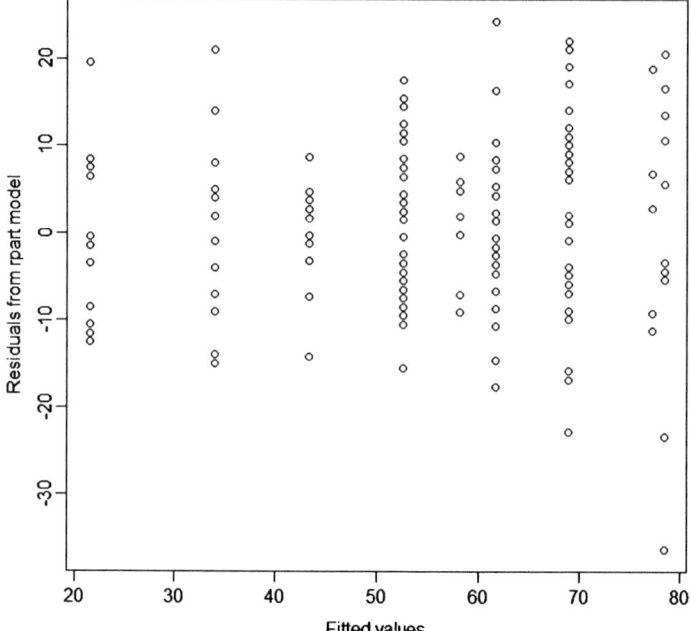

Fig. 16.2 Plot of residuals from the tree model fitted by R::rpart::rpart

As with linear modelling, attention should be given to the distribution of residuals. A plot of residuals against fitted values is shown in Fig. 16.2.

Since the branches in Fig. 16.1 show dependence upon both *sbp* and *age* before arriving at the terminal nodes, an interaction between *sbp* and *age* is suggested by the model: see Sect. 16.6.

Although a least squares fit does not require the residuals to be normally distributed to provide a pragmatic modelling tool, it is useful to also inspect residuals for normality. See Fig. 16.3. There is a suggestion, apart from one result, that the residuals do not depart from normality and therefore the residual sums of squares is an appropriate measure of fit for the model. The one 'outlier' might be inspected.

16.6 Interactions and Complexity

Discussion of interactions has been delayed until after the example on sympathetic nerve activity. In Fig. 16.1, the two most important covariates/factors are seen to be *sbp* and *age*. It is the early splits that involve these and the height/depth of

Fig. 16.3 QQ plot of residuals from the tree model fitted by R::rpart::rpart

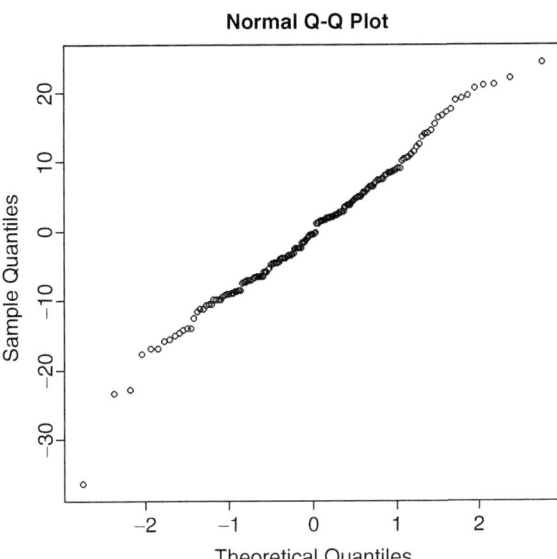

the branches for these splits is greater reflecting their greater contribution to the reduction of the residual sum of squares. Often when an interaction occurs between two variables, after the branch due to the first variable only one part of the tree branches according to the second. Thus the second variable is of greater importance for a certain range of the first: hence there is an interaction. In this example both sides of the tree split by *age* after the split by *sbp*, but the split by age is different on separate sides of the tree. Again an interaction is revealed, here between *age* and *sbp*.

Trees with a few branches are especially easy to interpret. As there are more branches, the complexity of the model is displayed. Thus trees are very useful for determining:

- which covariates and factors should be considered
- where interactions between covariates might occur
- how complex the model might be.

A way to quantify the complexity of a tree model is available with the R::rpart library through the function R::rpart::plotcp. Such a plot is provided in Fig. 16.4 for the sympathetic nerve activity example. It shows the relative gain in the reduction of the residual sums of squares (more broadly the objective function selected for the fit) for additional splits.

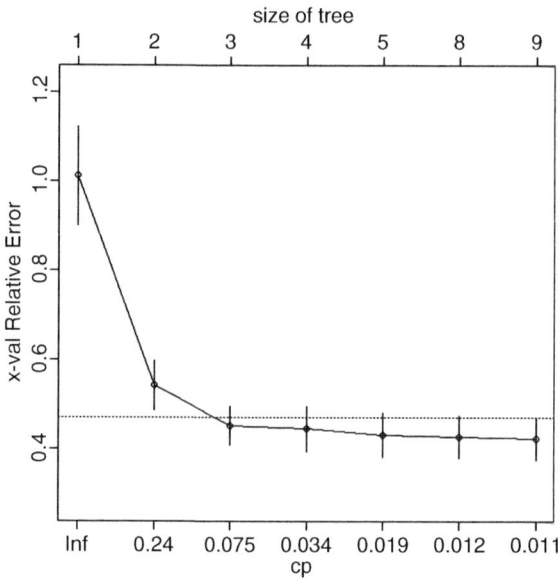

Fig. 16.4 Plot relative improvement of the fit of the tree model with increased complexity

16.7 Issues for Regression Trees

As with a linear model, if the outcome variable is transformed, then the model is changed: a different tree will be fitted since the residual sums of squares will be defined in a different way. Hence if the outcome is the concentration of a toxin in a urine sample, then the model will change if the logarithm of the concentration is taken as the outcome. The issues are the same as in least squares fitting of a linear model: are the residuals better represented on the original scale or the transformed one.

One of the largest issues is how to determine the best tree model. The tree with each terminal branch giving a unique value is in almost all circumstances overfitting the model.

The above fitting procedure can be regarded as the tree equivalent of linear modelling, being based on least squares. The procedure is generalised by defining deviance rather than a residual sum of squares for outcomes based on the binomial, Poisson, multinomial etc.

Missing values can be handled easily in some circumstances. For factors, missing values might be assigned another factor value/level. If missing values occur at random, then this approach is justified. If values are missing at random for a covariate, then a suitable weighting must be applied in order to compare splits between different covariates. The challenge as always with modelling is how to deal with missing values when missingness does not occur at random.

When there is a large dataset perhaps with many covariates and factors, then the number of splits to investigate rapidly becomes very large. So the are computational challenges for larger datasets. One option is to consider subsets of covariates and factors – see Sect. 16.9 on Random Forests.

16.8 Classification Trees

If the outcome variable is categorical, it has been mentioned that deviance can be used to consider partitions of the tree. Two alternatives are entropy and the Gini index. In the R::tree library, the default splitting method for R::tree::tree is deviance and an average deviance across the terminal modes is reported. The R::rpart::rpart function from the R::rpart library uses the Gini index as its default method.

For illustrative purposes, consider the new indicator variable defined from the sympathetic nerve activity dataset, namely the variable *ht* which takes the value 0 if $sbp < 140$ and 1 otherwise: that is *ht* indicates 'hypertension'. Taking *ht* as the outcome, a classification tree is required rather than a regression tree, but the modelling process is of course similar. With the default settings for R::tree::tree, the model resulting is shown in Fig. 16.5. Similar tree models are produced irrespective of the method of splitting, but the default settings provide different amounts of pruning. The deviance results, being the default for the R::tree::tree function are displayed in Fig. 16.5.

It is interesting to note that:

- the proportion of hypertensives is displayed at the terminal nodes
- sympathetic nerve activity *sna* and *age* are useful predictors of hypertension and interact
- The factor *sex* is not needed by the model and so has little impact on hypertensive status.

Close inspection of Fig. 16.5 with clinical expertise would suggest that further pruning would be merited, thus as seen with tree regression the default settings in this scenario provide a good starting point for the model but there is further work to be done.

16.9 Random Forests

As the number of covariates and factors increases, regression trees and classification tree become more difficult to handle. One way to facilitate data fitting would be to take subsets of the variables and fit with those. There are greater advantages obtained by taking this idea further and using random forests, see Breiman (2001).

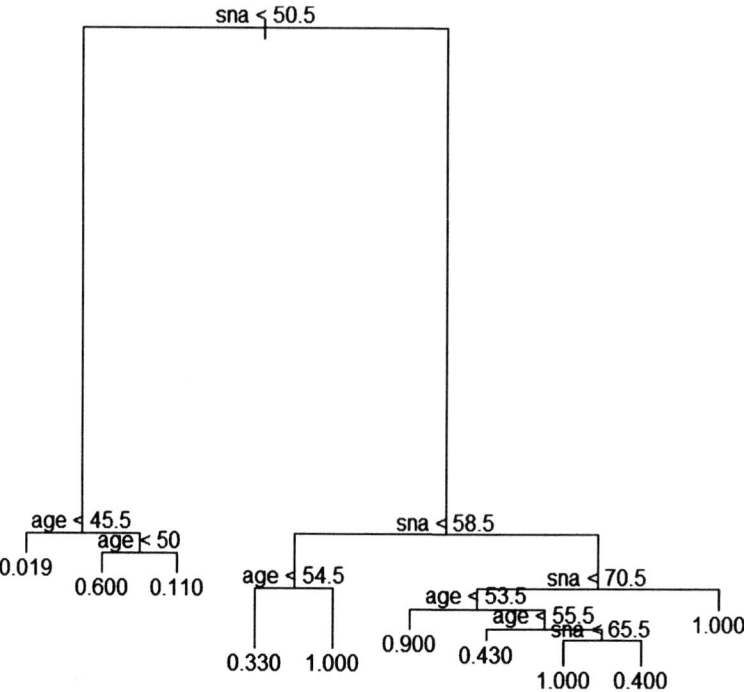

Fig. 16.5 Classification tree modelling hypertension

The algorithm for random forest fitting is as follows:

1. Draw bootstrap samples of size n_1 from the original samples of observations: sample with replacement and set n_1 be less than or equal to the original sample size. There will be n_2 such bootstrap samples.
2. For each of the n_2 samples grow a tree without any pruning and allow each split to be based on a subset of n_3 covariates and factors. It is suggested that n_3 is taken to be around one third of the total number of covariates and factors available.
3. Aggregate the tree produced by taking an average for a regression tree and taking the majority vote for a classification tree.

An interesting aspect of the random forest algorithm is that, for each bootstrap sample, there will (almost always) be observations that are not included, called out-of-bag samples. These can be used to cross validate the tree based on that sample. An average of the error rates over the n_1 bootstraps is often used. For regression the importance of covariates and factors can be quantified.

The downside of random forests is that interpretability is almost completely lost and this is a major drawback for statistical epidemiology. There is no tree output as there is for regression or for classification trees, prediction is from an average of many trees. The clearest outcomes from fitting a random forest are the importance of covariates and the proportion of variation that might be achieved. See the example below in Sect. 16.10.

16.10 Sympathetic Nerve Activity

The example of sympathetic nerve activity is not an ideal application for random forests since there is a very limited number of covariates and factors: just three. For completeness and to illustrate performance, a random forest was fitted using the function R::randomForest::randomForest. The sample size in each bootstrap n_2 was taken as 130 (the original sample size is 172), the default number of trees $n_2 = 500$ was used and the number of variables to consider at each node n_3 was restricted to 2. The resulting forest explains 62% of variation. Figure 16.6 shows how the error reduces as the number of trees in the forest increases: such a plot is a useful tool for indicating the number of trees to sample, in this case 200 trees appears sufficient. Figures 16.7 and 16.8 show how predictions vary from

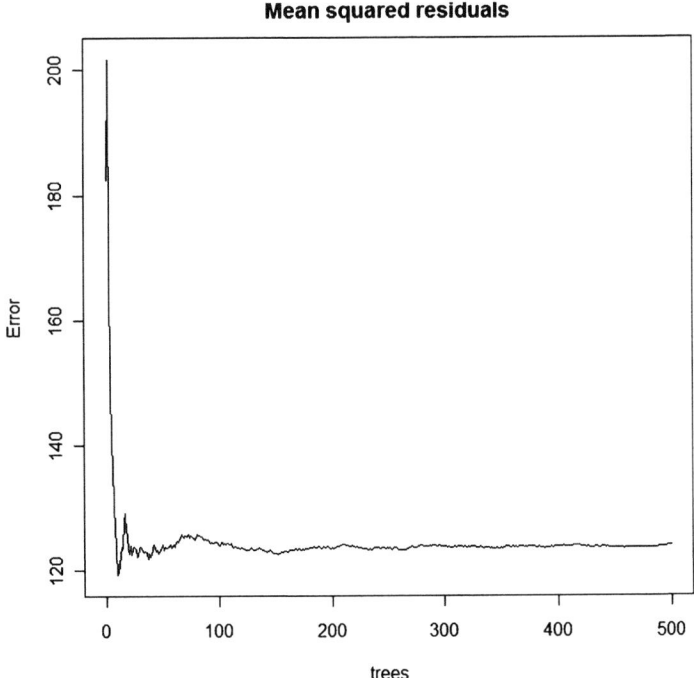

Fig. 16.6 Reduction in error with size of forest

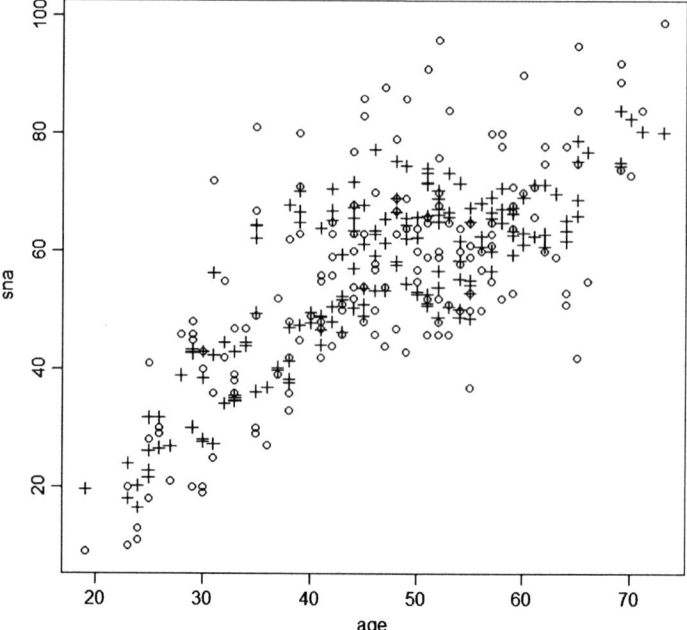

Fig. 16.7 Observed (o) and fitted (+) values

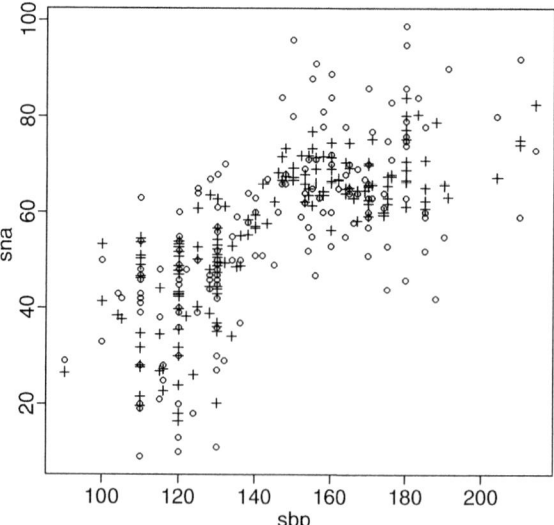

Fig. 16.8 Observed (o) and fitted (+) values plotted against *sbp*

Table 16.1 Importance of covariates and factors as indicated by fitting a random forest

Covariate or factor	% Increase in mean square error
sex	15.48
age	41.01
sbp	47.97

observed values. The importance of the covariates and factor are given in Table 16.1. It is clear that the two covariates *sbp* and *age* are the most important in agreement with the results from the regression tree and the generalised additive models fitted in Chap. 15.

16.11 Other Approaches

The subject of regression trees and, in particular, classification trees has interest to computer scientists as well as statisticians and associated with pattern recognition, classification, machine learning, and data mining. Consequently there are a large number of interested researchers developing the techniques and a wide variety of methods that can be exploited. Just couple of alternative approaches are considered here.

Boosting is a technique that can be used with a range of prediction methods including GAMs and trees, but is perhaps most commonly applied to trees. The idea of boosting for trees is to compute a sequence of simple trees with very few nodes, where each successive tree is built for the residuals of the preceding tree. Random forests can be thought to work in parallel and tree boosting thought to work in series. If a tree has difficulty with some cases then these will have larger residuals and have greater influence in the next tree, hence there is some focus on the more difficult cases.

Boosting for trees is implemented in R and one library is R::gbm based on the work of Friedman (2001) and others, see Hastie et al. (2001). Initial experimentation with the dataset for sympathetic nerve activity achieves a fit that is not very good in terms of least squares. Importance is reported with *sbp* being more important than *age* but *sex* not entering the model. There is little interpretable output.

Neural networks have been often used as black-box predictors and there is opportunity to use them in R through the library R::nnet. The black-box nature provides no understanding, but neither is any knowledge of the process necessary. One may to use R::scale() in order to standardise the scale of all variables before use. Neural nets can be effective for large datasets and are often good for prediction in those circumstances.

It is possible to plot marginal effects to obtain a little understanding of the effect of each covariate or factor. It can also be the case that a neural network model produces a very different model from a statistical model and this prompts effort to determine why this might be so.

16.12 Chapter Summary

Regression trees and classification trees were suggested as tools to be able to assess the appropriateness of covariates and factors, together with their interactions for linear models. The R libraries `R::tree` and `R::rpart` were briefly introduced and there is much software available for fitting tree models. Random forests, boosting and neural networks can also have benefits but their interpretability limits their use in statistical epidemiology.

References

Breiman, L. (2001). Random forests. *Machine Learning, 45*, 5–32.
Breiman, L., Friedman, J., Stone, C. J., & Olshen, R. A. (1984). *Classification and regression trees*. Boca Raton: Chapman and Hall/CRC, Monterey, CA.
Friedman, J. H. (2001). Greedy function approximation: A gradient boosting machine. *The Annals of Statistics, 29*, 1189–1232.
Hastie, T., Tibshirani, R., & Friedman, J. H. (2001). *The elements of statistical learning*. New York: Springer.
R Development Core Team. (2010). *R: A language and environment for statistical computing. R Foundation for Statistical Computing*, Vienna, Austria. ISBN 3-900051-07-0, URL http://www.R-project.org.
Ripley, B. D. (1996). *Pattern recognition and neural networks*. New York: Cambridge University Press.

Chapter 17
Statistical Interactions and Gene-Environment Joint Effects

Mark S. Gilthorpe and David G. Clayton

17.1 Overview

Statistical interactions are often employed within epidemiology, where one is exploring the joint association or action of putative causal agents in relation to a single outcome. Different language is occasionally used to describe such processes, e.g. effect modification. The concept of interaction is entirely separate from that of confounding, discussed in Chap. 4. An important example of a statistical interaction is the exploration of the joint effects of genes and environmental factors on disease risk. In this chapter, we explore the issue of gene-environment interactions specifically, with a view to highlight issues regarding the use and interpretation of statistical interaction in general.

We focus on gene-environment interactions because they are widely reported in the literature, but are not often used or interpreted correctly (Clayton 2009). Therefore, despite remaining quite basic in theoretical terms, this chapter addresses some important misunderstandings within modern epidemiological methods. Whilst dealing with these misconceptions, there is little complexity to what is discussed. Part of the discussion is more philosophical than theoretical, and controversy over statistical interaction will likely persist. However, no epidemiology book (modern or otherwise) is complete without discussing causality and, given the often implicit link, the interpretation of statistical interaction must then follow (Cox 1984).

M.S. Gilthorpe (✉)
Division of Biostatistics, Centre for Epidemiology and Biostatistics, Leeds Institute of Genetics, Health & Therapeutics, University of Leeds, Leeds, UK
e-mail: m.s.gilthorpe@leeds.ac.uk

D.G. Clayton
Juvenile Diabetes Research Foundation/Wellcome Trust Diabetes and Inflammation Laboratory, Cambridge University, Cambridge, UK

17.2 Biological vs. Statistical Interaction

Statistical interaction is a well-defined concept, but its interpretation in our everyday attempts to understand the world around us can prove troublesome. Seeking to combine biological insight and statistical models is not straightforward. This is particularly true for gene-environment interactions, in part because the different scientific communities use language differently to communicate biological and statistical ideas. It has been widely noted that statistical and biological interactions are different concepts that do not readily correspond to each other (Kupper and Hogan 1978; Rothman et al. 1980; Saracci 1980; Walter and Holford 1978). However, both concepts are often misunderstood, leading to incorrect conclusions being drawn from studies into the joint effects of genes and the environment. We therefore examine these concepts, building upon work in the context of multiple behavioural and environmental causes.

17.2.1 Gene-Environment Interaction

Although gene-environment interactions receive considerable attention in the literature, little reference is made to a lively debate amongst epidemiologists during the early 1980s, which focussed on the over-interpretation of statistical interaction, particularly in logistic regression models that are the main analytical tool in the epidemiology of multifactorial disease. Whilst many researchers acknowledged that a statistical interaction is only a product interaction term within a generalised linear model, how this maps onto biology remains ambiguous. Biologists use the word interaction rather loosely, in a mechanistic sense, and it is challenging, if not impossible, to project statistical model interpretations directly onto biological phenomenon.

In considering biological processes and wishing to describe the joint effects of genes and the environment, there are a plethora of biological processes that depict joint action. Separately, genetic and environmental effects can operate mechanistically in different ways, so their joint action is likely to be complicated. For instance, a genetic polymorphism may 'program' a condition to occur absolutely, e.g. cystic fibrosis occurs definitively as a consequence of the CFTR polymorphism on chromosome seven (Rowntree and Harris 2003). Alternatively, individuals might merely have a greater predisposition of developing a condition, e.g. deep vein thrombosis (DVT) is more likely, though not definitively, a consequence of Factor V Leiden genetic mutation on chromosome one (Vandenbroucke et al. 1994), and DVTs occur amongst normal individuals. The mechanism by which an outcome occurs therefore potentially involves multiple stages in biology, of which some steps may be necessary and sufficient whilst others attenuate the likelihood of occurrence.

To a statistician, where likelihood (probability between zero and one) is involved, this invokes the idea of an underlying *latent* (unobserved) process (e.g. *risk* of DVT) that is manifest in intermediate events (e.g. localised blood clot) or end point (e.g. DVT). We may consider these latent processes to be either categorical or continuous, though the underlying *risk* of an event occurring is more naturally thought of as a continuous concept. Although genetic and environmental factors may combine biologically in a cascade of processes, to describe these phenomena in some kind of statistical model requires the conceptual projection of a statistical model onto the underlying biology, or vice versa, and it may be a matter of convenience how the biological processes are represented. Even where a statistical model employs categorical variables, one cannot escape the inherent underlying latent complexity, which may be continuous. It is therefore a matter of subjectivity, driven by statistical convenience, as to which statistical analogue is used as a representation of the biological domain.

17.2.2 A Linear Regression Model

A model is *linear* because successive terms (covariates) are included additively. A model may be *linear* and yet represent *curvilinear* relationships between the outcome and covariates (such as where a quadratic term of the covariate is included in the model additively with the original form of the covariate). A *non-linear* model occurs if there is a *functional* relationship of a covariate, such as where the logarithm (or any other function) is applied to the covariate. A *functional* relationship that operates on the outcome is a *link function*. If the set of covariates remain *linear* (i.e. they are combined additively without transformation), one may have a *linear model* with a *non-identity link*. This is not a *non-linear model*, as is sometimes described (i.e. referring to the link function and not the covariates). The logistic regression model, a key analytical tool in the epidemiology of multifactorial disease, uses the *logit* link:

$$\text{logit}(\pi) = \ln\left(\frac{p}{1-p}\right) = \gamma_0 + \gamma_1 x_1 + \gamma_2 x_2 + \xi \qquad (17.1)$$

where p is the probability of disease (usually coded one), $1 - p$ is the probability of being disease-free, x_i and γ_i ($i = 1\ldots 2$) are covariates and associated regression coefficients, and the residual error (ξ) follows the binomial distribution with variance $\pi/\sqrt{3}$. The exponential of γ_1 is the odds ratio (OR) of disease, i.e. the odds of disease occurring if $x_1 = 1$ divided by odds of disease occurring if $x_1 = 0$. Most statistical regression methods evaluating genetic and environmental factors affecting disease outcomes are likely to be a linear logistic regression model using the *logit* link function.

17.2.3 Biological Interpretation of Interaction

Consider Factor V Leiden genetic mutation again, where individuals with the mutation have more coagulants in their blood and are thus at greater risk of DVT. Genetically normal individuals can develop DVT, but the risk is elevated amongst individuals with the genetic mutation. Amongst women, exposure to the combined oral contraceptive pill (COCP) brings about changes in hormone levels that can also raise levels of coagulant proteins and lower levels of anticoagulant proteins, thereby yielding an elevated risk of DVT (Vandenbroucke et al. 1996). Considering the joint action of the genetic mutation and the environmental impact of the combined pill, both exposures are binary (i.e. present or absent), as too is the outcome (DVT or no DVT), yet the putative causal process is best captured by the underlying *risk* of developing DVT, which is a continuum between zero and one. The genetic and environmental exposures operate jointly to affect the *risk* of DVT along this continuum, and the impact of either genetic or environmental exposure on the *risk* of DVT probably varies from woman to woman. To use a statistical model to describe this situation, one ought to acknowledge the continuous underlying latent risk *and* random variation amongst women. However, more often than not, a logistic model (with binary outcome of DVT present/absent) with two binary covariates (genetic and environmental exposures present/absent) is as an oversimplification of the underlying biology. The question becomes: what is the *biological* interpretation of the gene-environment statistical interaction in this scenario?

17.2.4 Statistical Interpretation of Interaction

Interpretation of statistical models in epidemiology is context-specific. Statistical interaction has only one mathematical form in a linear regression model, namely the *product interaction term*, and it describes deviation from additive effects on some context-driven predefined scale. For a statistician, the test for interaction between two factors is a test of the fit of a particular model of joint action and the extent of deviation from the additive model on the predefined scale. There is no *explicit* interpretation of biological mechanisms unless the statistical model has a biological analogue, in which case there may be *implicit* interpretation, though one needs to be careful in relating biological mechanistic processes to aspects of a statistical model. It is important within a regression model to recognise that the statistical interaction is both *linear* and *scale-dependent*. These two points are often overlooked, yet they are crucial in seeking to interpret statistical interactions meaningfully.

17.3 The Importance of Scale in Statistical Interaction

When modelling a continuous outcome using standard linear regression, the covariates in the model are included additively and these covariates operate on the outcome scale additively. Consider the following linear model (with *identity* link function):

$$y = \beta_0 + \beta_1 x_1 + \beta_2 x_2 + e \qquad (17.2)$$

where y is a continuous outcome, β_0 is the intercept (value of y when all covariates are zero), x_i and β_i ($i = 1\ldots 2$) are covariates and associated regression coefficients respectively, and e is residual error, which is assumed to be normally distributed with mean zero and variance σ^2.

If the values of x_1 and x_2 change by one unit, the outcome changes by $\beta_1 + \beta_2$, i.e. the effects of x_1 and x_2 are combined additively. Considering the logistic linear model in Eq. 17.1, however, whilst the effect on $logit(\pi)$ is additive (i.e. the effect of changing x_1 and x_2 by one unit each is to change $logit(\pi)$ by the amount $\gamma_1 + \gamma_2$), this transpires to a change in the original outcome via the inverse link function $logit^{-1}(\gamma_1 + \gamma_2)$. Denoting the odds ratio for x_1 as $c_1 = \exp(\gamma_1)$, the odds ratio for x_2 as $c_2 = \exp(\gamma_2)$, and denoting *change* in outcome probability as Δp, we have:

$$\ln\left(\frac{\Delta p}{1 - \Delta p}\right) = \gamma_1 + \gamma_2 \Rightarrow \Delta p = \frac{c_1 c_2}{(1 + c_1 c_2)} \qquad (17.3)$$

where change in outcome probability is constrained to ensure $0 \leq Pr(\pi = 1) \leq 1$. The property of the *logit* link is such that if x_1 changes by one unit, the *log odds* of the outcome changes *additively* by the factor γ_1, but the *odds* of the outcome changes *multiplicatively* by c_1; similarly for a unit change in x_2. Thus, if the values of x_1 and x_2 change by one unit, the *odds* of the outcome changes *multiplicatively* by the factor $c_1 \times c_2$. The choice of link function (*identity* vs. *logit*) therefore affects the scale upon which covariate changes are associated with outcome changes. Switching between the continuous model (*identity* link) and the binary model (*logit* link) changes the model scale from *additive* to *multiplicative*.

17.3.1 Example

We consider models with and without statistical interaction for these two link functions and illustrate the impact of model scale on perception of presence or absence of statistical interaction and its associated magnitude. This is a simple illustration of how we perceive and hence interpret the additive and multiplicative scales in linear models. For the example, initially we consider the continuous outcome *Blood Pressure* (*BP*) measured in millimetres mercury (mmHg). This is dichotomised across the threshold of 160 mmHg to create the binary outcome *Hypertension* (*Hyp*). We consider two covariates: a genetic binary variable (*G*) that depicts individuals to have a genetic mutation predisposing to hypertension (coded one if present or zero otherwise); and an environmental variable (*E*) that is recorded as a binary to depict high or low salt intake (coded one or zero respectively). We assume that both genetic mutation and high salt intake elevate blood pressure.

The *normal* linear model is:

$$BP = \beta_0 + \beta_1 G + \beta_2 E + \beta_3 GE + e \qquad (17.4)$$

The *binary* logistic model is:

$$\text{logit}(Hy) = \ln\left(\frac{p}{1-p}\right) = \gamma_0 + \gamma_1 G + \gamma_2 E + \gamma_3 GE + \xi. \qquad (17.5)$$

For no statistical interaction, $\beta_3 = 0$ in Eq. 17.4 and $\gamma_3 = 0$ in Eq. 17.5; for a synergistic interaction, $\beta_3 > 0$ in Eq. 17.4 and $\gamma_3 > 0$ in Eq. 17.5. We chart hypothetical data in two ways: (a) using a single chart for all model coefficients showing their relative effect sizes with reference to the genetic wild type and low salt intake group; (b) & (c) using two separate charts for high and low salt intake respectively, contrasting genetic mutation to the genetic wild type.

With no statistical interaction between genetic mutation and salt intake, the difference in blood pressure within the *normal* model between those with and without the genetic mutation is 10 mmHg and the difference between those with and without high salt intake is 15 mmHg, seen in both chart formats (Fig. 17.1a–c). With statistical interaction present, we note that greater elevated blood pressure occurs due to the genetic mutation amongst those with a high salt intake (20 mmHg) compared to those with a low salt intake (10 mmHg), again seen in both chart formats (Fig. 17.2a–c).

Considering the *logistic* model, something inconsistent happens in chart formats when plotting odds ratios (the exponential of the model coefficients). With no statistical interaction present, the absolute difference in the odds ratios for hypertension between low and high salt intake is 3.3 (Fig. 17.3a), not zero as anticipated. When the odds ratios for hypertension are plotted separately for low and high salt intake, however, their absolute difference is zero, as anticipated (Fig. 17.3b, c). With a *synergistic* statistical interaction present, the combined chart reveals a non-zero difference in the odds ratios for hypertension of 4.9 (Fig. 17.4a), and the separate charts for low and high salt intake indicate the absolute difference in the odds ratios for hypertension is only 2.0 (Fig. 17.4b, c). Therefore, how model coefficients are plotted can give rise to different indications

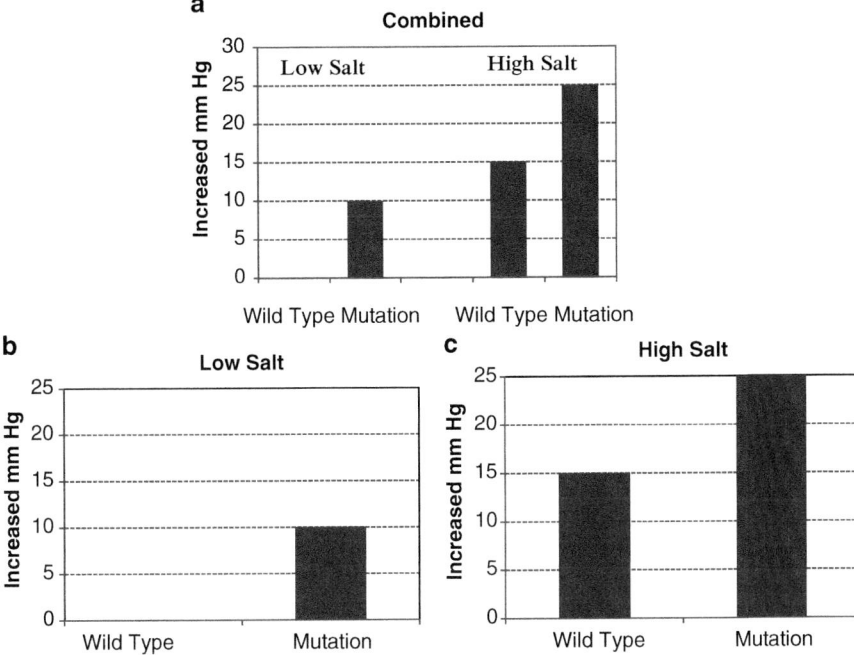

Fig. 17.1 Graphical display of a normal model for hypertension without statistical interaction showing model coefficients: (**a**) combined; and separately for low (**b**) and high (**c**) salt intake

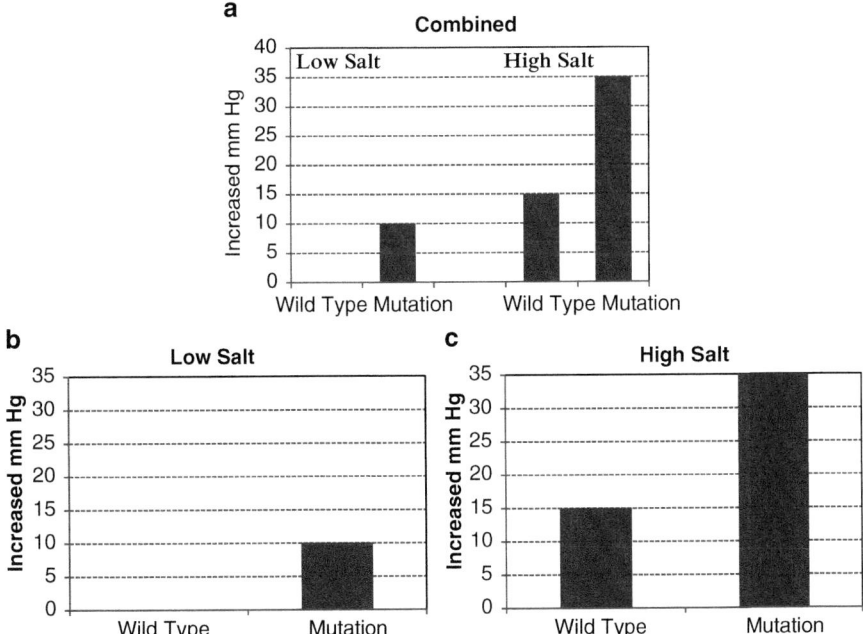

Fig. 17.2 Graphical display of a *normal* model for hypertension with synergistic statistical interaction showing model coefficients: (**a**) combined; and separately for low (**b**) and high (**c**) salt intake

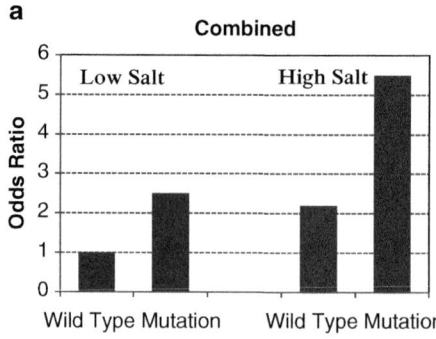
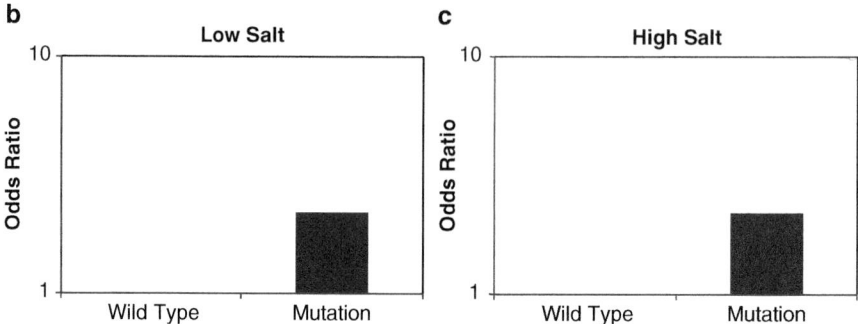

Fig. 17.3 Graphical display of the *logistic* model for hypertension without statistical interaction showing model coefficients: (**a**) combined; and separately for low (**b**) and high (**c**) salt intake

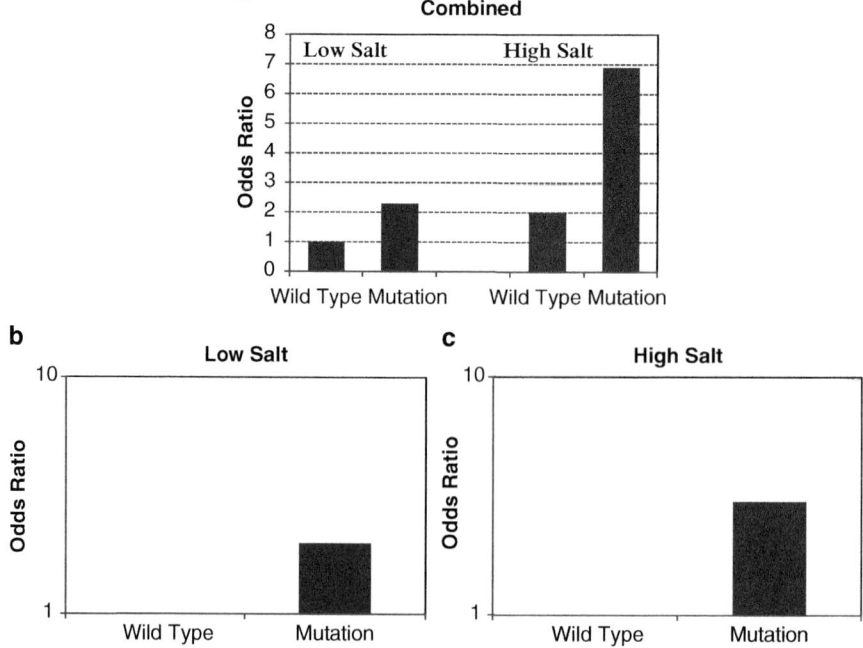

Fig. 17.4 Graphical display of the *logistic* model for hypertension with synergistic statistical interaction showing model coefficients: (**a**) combined; and separately for low (**b**) and high (**c**) salt intake

of the presence or absence of statistical interaction and the extent of the interaction; only the two-chart format is correct.

Such confusion arises because the scale upon which the odds ratio operates is *multiplicative* and charts reflect differences *additively*. The separate charts are more reliable because they contrast within exposure groups, separately for low and high salt intake, revealing accurately any differences as a true indication of statistical interaction. This reveals how much scale is important in our perception and hence interpretation of statistical interaction.

All regression models are scale dependent, but this matters greatly when seeking to interpret statistical interaction. There is nothing special about the scales adopted by models that use either the identity or *logit* link functions, as these links are used out of statistical convenience. The identity link may seem a natural choice for continuous outcomes, as it preserves the original scale of the outcome, and covariates operate additively on the original outcome scale. The *logit* link function has specific utility because model coefficients are interpretable as odds ratios (via exponentiation), and covariates therefore operate multiplicatively on the odds ratio scale. There are, however, an infinite number of possible scales upon which model covariates might relate to the outcome, depending upon the choice of link function. As there are only a handful of regularly used link functions, it is easy to overlook how arbitrary scale is, and how it always depends upon the choice of link function.

17.4 The Importance of Linearity in Statistical Interaction

Consider the following linear model:

$$y = \beta_0 + \beta_1 x + \beta_2 x^2 + \beta_3 z + \beta_4 xz + e \tag{17.6}$$

where y is a continuous outcome, β_0 is the intercept, x and z are two covariates that without loss of generality we assume to be continuous, β_i ($i = 1...4$) are covariate regression coefficients, and e is residual error, assumed to be normally distributed with mean zero and variance σ^2. This is a linear model that has a quadratic term in x and a product interaction term xz.

If we assume that x and z are correlated, i.e. collinear, then as the x-z correlation increases, collinearity increases between xz and x^2 (i.e. overlap between the 'explained' outcome variance increases). If we assume the relationship between y and x to be curvilinear, i.e. $\beta_2 \neq 0$, but assume there to be no xz interaction, i.e. $\beta_4 = 0$, the correct model we need to adopt is:

$$y = \beta_0 + \beta_1 x + \beta_2 x^2 + \beta_3 z + e. \tag{17.7}$$

Were we instead to adopt Eq. 17.6 but without the quadratic term (x^2):

$$y = \beta_0 + \beta_1 x + \beta_3 z + \beta_4 xz + e \tag{17.8}$$

a 'spurious' interaction (i.e. $\beta_4 \neq 0$) would be observed for the xz product interaction (Ganzach 1997). The collinearity between x and z effectively 'mops up' the unaccounted outcome variance that ideally should have been accommodated by the curvilinear relationship between y and x, and hence a non-zero statistical interaction is now observed. It is the assumption of linearity between the outcome y and covariate x that is not upheld which gives rise to the apparent statistical interaction.

It is therefore vitally important to verify model linearity assumptions, though this is rarely undertaken as rigorously as it should be. Whilst researchers may check model residuals, perhaps seeing if they are normally distributed and with constant variance, rarely do researchers verify implicit model assumptions of linearity. Statistical models that seek to emulate biological processes without due care regarding the issue of linearity amongst variable relationships are likely to observe statistical interactions that might be nothing more than artefact from a miss-specified model.

17.4.1 Example

Barrett's Oesophagus (often abbreviated by *BE* since the US spelling is Esophagus) is named after the doctor who first described the condition in 1957 (Barrett 1957) and is an abnormal lining of the oesophagus (gullet). The condition is found in about 10% of patients who seek medical care for heartburn and reflux (acid and bile moving into the gullet), and may progress in a minority of patients through a series of stages (such as dysplasia) to oesophageal cancer (Koppert et al. 2005). Adipose tissue (*AT*) is loose connective fatty tissue situated about the body. Its main role is to store energy in the form of fat. Obesity or being overweight depends upon the amount of body fat, especially adipose tissue. It is therefore adipose tissue that is crucial for some adverse outcomes of obesity, such as diabetes, since adipose tissue serves as an important endocrine organ. The formation of adipose tissue is controlled by the adipose gene. It is observed that there are sex differences in *BE* (Corley et al. 2009) and sex differences in the distribution of adipose tissue around the body (Ross et al. 1994). It has also been observed that *BE* is related to adipose tissue, though this might not be directly causal since the impact of adipose tissue on *BE* might operate via obesity inducing a greater risk of reflux (Moayyedi 2008). We therefore question if sex differences in *BE* might be explained by sex differences in adipose tissue, or if there is an 'interaction' between *sex* and *AT* in their joint association with *BE*. To do this we examine the following statistical model:

$$logit(BE) = \gamma_0 + \gamma_1 AT + \gamma_2 sex + \gamma_3 AT.sex + \xi \qquad (17.9)$$

where *BE* is binary (present or absent), *AT* is continuous, *sex* is binary (male or female), *AT.sex* is a product interaction, and ξ the binomial residual error. For some

17 Statistical Interactions and Gene-Environment Joint Effects

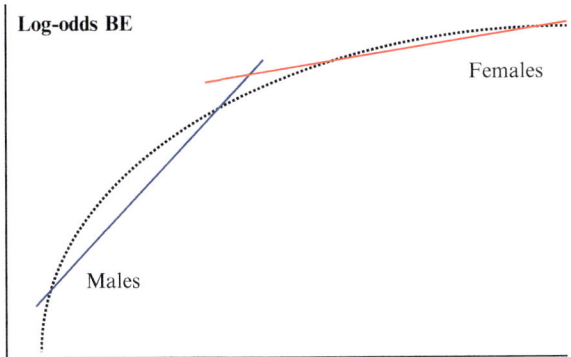

Fig. 17.5 The inter-relationships amongst Barrett's Oesophagus (*BE*), adipose tissue (*AT*) and sex: the underlying hypothesised relationship between the log odds of *BE* and *AT* is curvilinear; any linear relationship modelled using logistic regression might reveal different gradients for each sex, which manifests as an *AT.sex* statistical interaction within a regression model

researchers, evidence of a *biological* interaction between adipose tissue and sex is provided if a statistical interaction is observed, i.e. if $\gamma_3 \neq 0$. For such an interpretation to be correct, however, the assumption of linearity must be upheld between the log odds of *BE* and the continuous measure of *AT*.

We plot a hypothetical relationship between the log odds of *BE* and *AT* (Fig. 17.5), in which it is seen that the log odds of developing Barrett's Oesophagus increases with increasing levels of adipose tissue, though the rate of increase diminishes for larger adipose tissue levels; this yields an underlying relationship between the log odds of *BE* and *AT* that is curvilinear. This seems reasonable if obesity and increasing overweight lead to greater bouts of reflux, which in turn lead to an elevated risk of *BE*, and there becomes a point beyond which increasing obesity produces no further increases in reflux. In any event, one should anticipate curvilinear relationships as there is no natural biological reason to suppose that changes in the log odds of *BE* should be linearly related to changing *AT* levels (recall that the logistic scale is statistical convenience and has no biological basis). Further, if the association between *AT* and *BE* has no direct causal foundation, it is likely that common biological process would be sufficiently convoluted to yield a non-linear relationship.

Females have on average more adipose tissue for their weight than men. After accounting for overall weight differences one might anticipate that the distributions of *AT* levels for men and women would form a mixture, with the male mean *AT* value to the left of the female mean *AT* value along the adipose tissue axis in Fig. 17.5. Modelling men and women separately:

$$logit(BE^M) = \gamma_0^M + \gamma_1^M AT + \xi^M \ \& \ logit(BE^F) = \gamma_0^F + \gamma_1^F AT + \xi^F \qquad (17.10)$$

where superscripts denotes sex (M for males, F for females). Given different *AT* distributions for men and women, in conjunction with the overall curvilinear log odds *BE* ~ *AT* relationship, we would obtain different estimates for the log odds *BE* ~ *AT* slope for men and women, and we anticipate $\gamma_1^M > \gamma_1^F$. Differences in the two slopes is entirely due to the data for males and females lying on different parts of the curvilinear relationship between the log odds of *BE* and levels of *AT*.

The two separate models in Eq. 17.10 identically represent the combined model in Eq. 17.9, in which the product interaction term is non-zero. There is a statistical interaction between *sex* and *AT* in their jointly modelled association with *BE*, but this does not signify a joint biological process; it is consistent with *separate* biological processes, where sex affects *AT* levels and *AT* levels affect *BE* (via reflux, perhaps). The statistical interaction is a consequence of adopting the linear model approach when the underlying log odds *BE* ~ *AT* relationship is curvilinear (on the statistically convenient log odds scale for the binary outcome *BE*).

Where an underlying curvilinear relationship is overlooked within a linear model, statistical interaction is observed that might be referred to as 'spurious', yet the statistics are sound and the issue is one of interpretation. Statistical interaction is correctly estimated, though its cause (hence model interpretation) may be misguided. Statistical interaction need not be a reflection of joint biological action, as it is typically attributed, rather a consequence of an overlooked curvilinear relationship between outcome and (environmental) exposure. Without *a priori* knowledge of any underlying curvilinear relationships between the outcome and covariates, we would be too hasty in seeking to interpret statistical interaction without also evaluating the model assumption of linearity. Conversely, we might consider statistical interaction an indication of potential curvilinear relationships between outcome and model covariates, as we discuss later.

17.5 Effect Size of Joint Effects vs. Testing for Statistical Interaction

It might be argued that most diseases result from gene-environment joint effects and that the emphasis of research is to elucidate the magnitude of these effects. To describe the outcome contingent on a range of options, one is not compelled to assume any statistical model, i.e. to assume any particular model scale. Trying to compress the complexity of biology into the simplicity of a statistical model might be misguided and only mislead or misinform, as the information sought may not lend itself to the form of a statistical test, supporting or refuting a hypothesised mechanism; rather it should be more concerned with absolute effect size, which has clinical relevance. We therefore ask: *for what purpose do we test?* More insight might be gained by forgoing the questions 'if' and 'how' joint effects occur *biologically*, and instead ask 'to what extent' or 'by how much' are joint effects

Table 17.1 Summary of the case-control study investigating the joint association of both Factor V Leiden genetic mutation and the combined oral contraception pill (COCP) use with respect to deep vein thrombosis (DVT)

Factor V/COCP	Cases	Controls	OR
+/+	25	2	34.7
+/−	10	4	6.9
−/+	84	63	3.7
−/−	36	100	1.0
Totals	155	169	

observed in terms of their *effect size*, which can be derived irrespective of model scale.

For illustration consider the example of DVT, Factor V Leiden genetic mutation, and combined oral contraceptive pill (COCP) once more. We seek the joint association of genetic mutation and COCP with respect to DVT. At the outset we acknowledge that the environmental exposure (COCP) is not strictly categorical, since the COCP exposure varies according to dose and extent of use, though we return to this point later. For simplicity, therefore, we categorise this underlying continuous measure into present or absent, i.e. according to whether or not a woman uses the COCP. We then use a tabular method to examine statistical interaction, as suggested by Botto and Khoury (Botto and Khoury 2001). From a case-control study of DVT in relation to both Factor V Leiden genetic mutation and the COCP (Vandenbroucke et al. 1994), data are summarised in Table 17.1. Only point estimates are presented here, though attention should always additionally be given to confidence intervals.

As the analysis is undertaken using odds ratios, it is typical to consider the *multiplicative* scale. We might examine departure from a *multiplicative* model with no statistical interaction on the odds ratio scale by considering the observed (34.7) and expected ($3.7 \times 6.9 \times 1.0 = 25.7$) odds ratios. Departure is assessed as the ratio of observed to expected, i.e. $34.7/25.7 = 1.4$, which is a small deviation from 1.0 (perhaps statistically significant for large studies). Alternatively, we might examine departure from an *additive* model with no statistical interaction on the additive scale by considering the observed (34.7) and expected ($3.7 + 6.9 - 1.0 = 9.6$) odds ratios additively. Departure is assessed as the difference, i.e. $34.7 - 9.6 = 25.1$, which is substantively far from zero (most likely statistically significant, except for very small studies).

Is there any insight gained from formally *testing* either deviation if we do not know how to interpret the statistical interaction (whether present or absent) on either scale? It may be apparent that the multiplicative model fits the data better than the additive model, statistically speaking, suggesting that the joint effects of the genetic mutation and environmental exposure operate close to multiplicatively (on the odds ratio scale). From a public health perspective, however, what does the information in Table 17.1 really inform women considering the COCP?

Relative to not having Factor V Leiden genetic mutation and not using the COCP, taking the contraceptive increases a woman's relative risk (RR) for DVT by approximately 3.6 fold (since DVT is rare, OR $\approx$ RR). If there was no reason for the woman to suspect she had the genetic mutation, which has a prevalence of around 4.4% in Europe (Rees et al. 1995), these increased risks might not trouble her. On the other hand, if she was aware of a family history of DVT, she might suspect an elevated possibility of having the genetic mutation. Considering the relative risk of having both the mutation *and* using COCP (RR $\approx$ 34.7) compared to merely having the mutation (RR $\approx$ 6.9), she might instead seek to use an alternative contraception or explore being genetically tested.

There is no knowing how an individual woman would chose to use the information in Table 17.1. It is perhaps dubious to suppose that her interest would lie in the p-value of a formal test for a synergistic statistical interaction on the additive scale, or the indication that a multiplicative odds ratio scale fits the data better. The mental framework in which a woman's decisions are informed seems more likely to be based on the relative risk *effect sizes* (along with confidence intervals) than formal testing of statistical interaction on any scale. This begs the question why we focus on formal testing of statistical interaction. A related question is why are we so concerned about the statistical power of such tests? This is addressed later.

17.6 Non-causal Gene-Environment Attenuation

Gene-environment joint effects are often investigated via statistical interaction to evaluate if the environmental exposure *attenuates* the genetic effect, or vice versa. Despite seemingly to suggest a causal relationship that may not be appropriate, the pursuit of whether an environmental exposure operates differently according to genetic makeup is a legitimate question. Unless one knows *a priori* the exact relationship between outcome and continuous environmental exposure, however, it is not possible to model this explicitly and the environmental exposure (raw or transformed) may exhibit a curvilinear association with the outcome (via whichever link function is used for statistical convenience). Consequently, it becomes impossible to identify if the environmental effect on the outcome *differs* according to genotype unless the distribution of the environmental exposure is balanced across all levels of the genotype, which is typically ensured only if the genetic exposure is randomly assigned. Alternatively, the genetic effect must have no association with the environmental effect and there should be no intermediate variables linking the genetic and environmental factors. This is counterfactual to the notion of biological joint action of gene and environment.

Thus, where the underlying relationship between outcome and environmental exposure is too complex to be modelled explicitly, where random allocation of the genetic effect is ruled out, and the genetic and environmental effects are unrelated, one can legitimately seek to evaluate if the environmental exposure *attenuates* the genetic effect, or vice versa. But this would not be deemed *joint* action, in a biological mechanistic sense, and the effect of the environmental exposure on the outcome (if inferred to be causal) is noted only to differ by genotype; there is no inferred *direct* mechanistic relationship between environmental exposure and genotype. It should be noted that whilst epidemiologists cannot randomise genes, Mendelian randomisation (Davey and Ebrahim 2003) has been proposed to select individuals according to a genetic predisposition to succumb to, or evade, an environmental exposure. This may not always guarantee that the distribution of the environmental exposure is balanced across levels of the genotype if intermediate variables are involved jointly with both the genetic and environmental exposures.

17.7 Measurement Issues: Continuous vs. Categorical

Most concerns raised regarding the investigation of statistical interaction pertain to the use of at least one continuous exposure, as it is upon a continuous scale that interpretation becomes problematic. In the most part, simple genetic effects are categorical, though for complex traits, as with multiple gene-gene joint effects, categorical representation might be supplanted by an underlying *continuous* latent trait. Notwithstanding such instances, genetic effects are otherwise viewed as categorical. In contrast, environmental exposures are predominantly continuous, even if not always treated as such; there is typically an underlying continuum, even where the environmental exposure is quantified as present or absent, since there is often an underlying latent and continuous concept of *risk*.

Furthermore, environmental exposures may be measured correctly as continuous only to have measurement error introduced by categorisation, which is a common bad habit amongst epidemiologists, leading potentially to substantial biases in the estimates of statistical interaction (Greenwood et al. 2006; Tu et al. 2007). Worse still, when continuous measurement is possible, a study might choose to measure categorical exposures, thwarting any possibility of evaluating continuous data subsequently. So rarely are environmental exposures intrinsically categorical (i.e. not categorised continuous), and whenever an environmental exposure is treated as categorical, we must not fail to recognise its likely underlying continuous nature.

In the DVT example, the environmental exposure for oral contraception was categorical for simplicity, as this did not alter the relative importance of effect size over statistical interaction. In reality, women experience different doses of the COCP due to different periods of exposure and different pill formulations. In the hypothetical example where salt intake was categorised, interpretation of the statistical interaction for both the continuous and logistic outcome models is difficult, as there is no readily interpretable scale for the relationship between blood pressure and salt level that is not also dependent upon the threshold of the continuous environmental exposure. Were we to seek meaning from a model coefficient, its magnitude depends upon which model is adopted (*normal* or *logistic*), which thresholds were adopted for salt intake (and blood pressure in the logistic model), and whether or not the *BP-Salt* relationship is linear or not on either scale (it cannot be linear on more than one scale; it may not be linear on either conveniently adopted scale).

In the very limited circumstances that environmental exposures are intrinsically categorical, the interpretation of joint effects is straightforward, as with purely gene-gene interactions. For g genetic categories and e environmental categories, $g \times e$ joint effects are to be estimated. These could be evaluated as within Table 17.1, or within a regression model that could then consider, simultaneously, other potentially confounding factors (though interpretation of confounding needs careful consideration, as discussed in Chap. 4). The $g \times e$ joint effects of the gene-environment interaction are readily derived and their impact, hence interpretation, is observed directly via model coefficients along with confidence intervals. There is little more to interpret than the effect-size estimated.

17.8 To Test Linearity and Multivariate Normality

Focus thus far has been given to interpreting statistical interaction biologically, as this is the area of considerable misunderstanding and where most errors are reported in the literature. There is, however, *statistical* utility in understanding statistical interaction, which in some instances has biological utility also. It has been proposed in the statistical literature that testing the product term in a linear regression model is suitable for examining both *linearity* (between outcome and covariates via a suitable link function) and the *multivariate normality* of covariates (Cox and Small 1978; Cox and Wermuth 1994). Consider the statistical linear model with three continuous measures:

$$y = \beta_0 + \beta_1 x_1 + \beta_2 x_2 + \beta_3 x_1 x_2 + e \qquad (17.11)$$

where y is the outcome, x_i (i = 1...2) are covariates, β_i (i = 1...3) regression coefficients, and e is residual error, assumed to be normally distributed with mean zero and variance σ^2. If the variables y, x_1, and x_2 are multivariate normal, it can be shown mathematically that there is no statistical interaction (i.e. $\beta_3 = 0$), regardless of the bivariate correlation structure amongst all three variables (Tu et al. 2007). Were these variables to represent biological measures, this indicates that linearity and multivariate normality are upheld amongst all three measures. Conversely, any deviation from linearity or multivariate normality yields a statistical interaction. Biologically, interpretation is more about understanding outcome and covariate inter-relationships with respect to linearity and multivariate normality, and not joint biological action. Consider, for instance, the situation where the variables are multivariate normal (hence $\beta_3 = 0$) and x_2 is log-transformed:

$$y = \hat{\beta}_0 + \hat{\beta}_1 x_1 + \hat{\beta}_2 \ln(x_2) + \hat{\beta}_3 x_1 \ln(x_2) + \hat{e} \qquad (17.12)$$

where $\hat{\beta}_i$ (i = 1...3) are the revised regression coefficients, and $\hat{e}$ is the revised residual error. It is now highly implausible that the statistical interaction is zero (i.e. $\hat{\beta}_3 \neq 0$), though not as a consequence of anything that has biological meaning, since nothing has changed biologically between models Eq. 17.11 and Eq. 17.12; only the log-transformation of x_2 is different. Statistical interaction is generated where there was none before by transformation of the data. This would be true irrespective of which variable is transformed. If the outcome were transformed, this is analogous to using a non-identity link function, which is why the absence of statistical interaction on one scale (the *normal* scale) can become statistical interaction on a transformed scale (the *logit* scale).

Biological measures are often transformed for statistical convenience, e.g. positively skewed outcomes might be log-transformed to attain a more *normal* distribution (though it is model residuals and not variable values that must be normally distributed for *normal* models). Variable transformation is required amongst covariates only if the assumption of linearity is not upheld and this cannot be modelled via a curvilinear or some other parameterisation. Where model assumptions are not satisfied, the act of transformation to improve model performance will affect the statistical interaction. If biological measures are 'well behaved' and several such measures are multivariate normal (or multivariate log-normal if log-transformed), there will be few statistical interactions in a regression model. Alternatively, if biological measures are 'messy', or do not capture well the underlying processes under investigation (such that the data collected do not follow multivariate normality), then statistical interactions will be present, though these will have limited biological interpretation. If the modelling process indicates data transformation may be required to improve model performance, statistical interactions may come and go, even changing sign, merely due to data manipulation. Since nothing changes biologically, biological interpretation of statistical interaction in these instances is nonsensical.

The correct interpretation of statistical interaction is thus concerned with the outcome and covariates inter-relationships with respect to *linearity* and *multivariate normality*, and not joint biological action. Statistical interaction indicates that, as entered into the model, the outcome and covariates do not exhibit linearity and covariates do not exhibit multivariate normality. This can have utility if seeking to determine a scale upon which covariates exhibit multivariate normality, as with variables that are mechanistically closely linked. Where changes in one measure are thought to cause changes in others in a linear fashion, underlying multivariate normality might be anticipated. One could then seek the absence of statistical interaction to determine the correct *joint scale* of the variables.

17.9 Statistical Power to Test for Interaction

It is well documented that much larger sample sizes are required to test statistical interactions than for main effects (Greenland 1983), and it is a criticism directed at many studies for being too small to examine gene-environment interactions.

Notwithstanding the overzealous nature to test (and the associated undesirable dependency on p-values), the reasoning behind such sample-size criticisms is flawed, since the statistical power of an interaction is just as scale-dependent as the statistical interaction itself. Without a meaningful scale upon which the test is sought, there is no basis for power calculations; it is the confidence interval of the estimated effect size that is informative. Perversely, one might use existing data from pilot studies and transform away and test repeatedly until one finds a scale upon which the sample size needed is minimal. This strategy might save enormous amounts of money in epidemiology were it not pointless because interpretation of the interaction derived for a minimum sample size is meaningless if the scale adopted upon which the test is conducted has no interpretable utility.

Unfortunately, this issue is not just overlooked by researchers, since referees for journals and grants, as well as journal editors, can be quite over-enthusiastic, sometimes vigilant, in pursuit of power calculations for gene-environment interactions that have no interpretable utility. Were a meaningful scale found, upon which it is appropriate to interpret statistical interaction, and hence evaluate statistical power, it then becomes a matter of whether or not this scale lends itself to a viable model, where all model assumptions are met. Without due care and attention in considering model assumptions and model scale, most of what purports to be an investigation into statistical interaction is found wanting in both rigour and biological meaning.

17.10 Summary

Testing the effect of a risk factor on individuals may have a clear biological interpretation, but testing for statistical interaction between two factors has a mathematical interpretation, which is different. If the model has no biological analogue, hence no biological interpretation, then testing for statistical interaction might not contribute to biological understanding; indeed, it could confuse. Whilst the quantification of joint effects remains a legitimate aim, its utility does not lie in the elucidation of biological processes. There is an overreliance on the linear regression model, with too few checks and balances to verify model assumptions. There is also an overzealous interpretation of models invoking potential biological mechanisms.

Model scale and linearity assumptions are typically overlooked, potentially leading to confusion surrounding the interpretation of statistical interaction, particularly within the domain of gene-environment interaction. Such arguments have been made before, yet the previous literature that warned against these poor practices, continues to receive little acclaim, as pointed out two decades ago by Thompson when he reflected upon the even earlier debate on statistical interaction at the start of the 1980s: "A decade ago the concept of interaction among causes of disease was at the center of a lively debate. Since that time, controversy over the nature of interaction has largely subsided, although there seems never to have been an adequate resolution of the conceptual and pragmatic issues that had been raised" (Thompson 1991). He went on: "Unfortunately, choice among theories of pathogenesis is enhanced hardly at all by the epidemiological assessment of interaction ... What few causal systems can be rejected on the basis of observed results would provide decidedly limited etiological insight" (Thompson 1991).

Problems persist with the misinterpretation of statistical interaction and overzealous attempts to interpret statistical interaction with biological meaning. Researchers continue to pursue gene-environment interactions with no robust insight as to what they mean. There is now almost an obsession to include some form of formal testing for joint genetic and environmental effects wherever a study records both, without an adequate *a priori* statement of what it is that is being confirmed or refuted, either biologically or otherwise. This behaviour fuels attention to study sample size, pressuring researchers to seek statistical power sufficient for the elucidation of *significant* gene-environment statistical interactions. Consequently, there is a perceived and falsely legitimised demand for increasingly large epidemiological studies. Less attention is given to the estimated size of main effects and joint effects for clinical interpretation, or the evaluation of plausible underlying causal paths amongst the factors being considered. There is perhaps an unease to consider more sophisticated methods, such as structural equation modelling (SEM). This is why one author of this chapter and his colleague felt it necessary in 2001 to reaffirm the many points said throughout the previous decades and rehearsed here: "The prospects for epidemiology in the post-genomic era depend on understanding how to use genetic associations to test hypotheses about causal pathways, rather than modelling the joint effects of genotype and environment" (Clayton and McKeigue 2001).

It thus remains necessary to spell out repeatedly and vehemently the many issues associated with interpretation of statistical interaction in the hope to encourage better epidemiological practice and dispel persistent and inappropriate pursuit of the gene-environment statistical interaction. It is more appropriate to employ statistical models to understand causal pathways than pursue statistical interaction. Whilst statistical modelling (indeed statistical epidemiology) opens a window on the biological world for investigation of cause and effect, one has to know *how to investigate* what we go in search of, *how to see* what we find, and *how to interpret* what we see. Otherwise, we kid ourselves with nothing more than smoke and mirrors.

17.11 Further Reading

In addition to citations in this chapter, there are those provided in the papers commentating on the recurring debate surrounding statistical interaction within epidemiology by Thompson (1991) and by Clayton and McKeigue (2001).

Amongst the citations here, the more recent by Clayton (2009) is a good source for the genetics literature and a must for the more generic overview is the seminal review by Cox (1984).

References

Barrett, N. R. (1957). The lower esophagus lined by columnar epithelium. *Surgery, 41*(6), 881–894. available from: PM:13442856.

Botto, L. D., & Khoury, M. J. (2001). Commentary: Facing the challenge of gene-environment Interaction: the two-by-four table and beyond. *American Journal of Epidemiology, 153*(10), 1016–1020. available from: PM:11384958.

Clayton, D. G. (2009). Prediction and interaction in complex disease genetics: Experience in type 1 diabetes. *PLoS Genetics, 5*(7), e1000540. available from: PM:19584936.

Clayton, D., & McKeigue, P. M. (2001). Epidemiological methods for studying genes and environmental factors in complex diseases. *The Lancet, 358*(9290), 1356–1360. available from: PM:11684236.

Corley, D. A., Kubo, A., Levin, T. R., Block, G., Habel, L., Rumore, G., Quesenberry, C., & Buffler, P. (2009). Race, ethnicity, sex and temporal differences in Barrett's oesophagus diagnosis: A large community-based study, 1994–2006. *Gut, 58*(2), 182–188. available from: PM:18978173.

Cox, D. R. (1984). Interaction. *International Statistical Review, 52*(1), 1–24.

Cox, D.R., & Small, N. J. H. (1978). Testing multivariate normality. *Biometrika, 65*(2), 263–272. Available from: http://biomet.oxfordjournals.org/cgi/content/abstract/65/2/263.

Cox, D. R., & Wermuth, N. (1994). Tests of linearity, multivariate normality and the adequacy of linear scores. *Applied Statistics, 43*, 347–355.

Davey, S. G., & Ebrahim, S. (2003). 'Mendelian randomization': Can genetic epidemiology contribute to understanding environmental determinants of disease? *International Journal of Epidemiology, 32*(1), 1–22. available from: PM:12689998.

Ganzach, Y. (1997). Misleading interaction and curvilinear terms. *Psychological Methods, 2*(3), 235–247.

Greenland, S. (1983). Tests for interaction in epidemiologic studies: A review and a study of power. *Statistics in Medicine, 2*(2), 243–251. available from: PM:6359318.

Greenwood, D. C., Gilthorpe, M. S., & Cade, J. E. (2006). The impact of imprecisely measured covariates on estimating gene-environment interactions. *BMC Medical Research Methodology, 6*, 21. available from: PM:16674808.

Koppert, L. B., Wijnhoven, B. P. L., van Dekken, H., Tilanus, H. W., & Dinjens, W. N. (2005). The molecular biology of esophageal adenocarcinoma. *Journal of Surgical Oncology, 92*, 169–190. available from: PM:16299787.

Kupper, L. L., & Hogan, M. D. (1978). Interaction in epidemiologic studies. *American Journal of Epidemiology, 108*(6), 447–453. available from: PM:736024.

Moayyedi, P. (2008). Barrett's esophagus and obesity: The missing part of the puzzle. *American Journal of Gastroenterology, 103*(2), 301–303. available from: PM:18289199.

Rees, D. C., Cox, M., & Clegg, J. B. (1995). World distribution of factor V Leiden. *The Lancet, 346*(8983), 1133–1134. available from: PM:7475606.

Ross, R., Shaw, K. D., Rissanen, J., Martel, Y., de Guise, J., & Avruch, L. (1994). Sex differences in lean and adipose tissue distribution by magnetic resonance imaging: Anthropometric relationships. *American Journal of Clinical Nutrition, 59*(6). available from: PM:8198051.

Rothman, K. J., Greenland, S., & Walker, A. M. (1980). Concepts of interaction. *American Journal of Epidemiology, 112*(4), 467–470. available from: PM:7424895.

Rowntree, R. K., & Harris, A. (2003). The phenotypic consequences of CFTR mutations. *Annals of Human Genetics, 67*(Pt 5), 471–485. available from: PM:12940920.

Saracci, R. (1980). Interaction and synergism. *American Journal of Epidemiology, 112*(4), 465–466. available from: PM:7424894.

Thompson, W. D. (1991). Effect modification and the limits of biological inference from epidemiologic data. *Journal of Clinical Epidemiology, 44*(3), 221–232. available from: PM:1999681.

Tu, Y. K., Manda, S. O., Ellison, G. T., & Gilthorpe, M. S. (2007). Revisiting the interaction between birth weight and current body size in the foetal origins of adult disease. *European Journal of Epidemiology, 22*(9), 565–575. available from: PM:17641977.

Vandenbroucke, J. P., Koster, T., Briët, E., Reitsma, P. H., Bertina, R. M., & Rosendaal, F. R. (1994). Increased risk of venous thrombosis in oral-contraceptive users who are carriers of factor V Leiden mutation. *The Lancet, 344*, 1453–1457.

Vandenbroucke, J. P., van der Meer, F. J. M., Helmerhorst, F. M., & Rosendaal, F. R. (1996). Factor V Leiden: Should we screen oral contraceptive users and pregnant women? *British Medical Journal, 313*, 1127–1130.

Walter, S. D., & Holford, T. R. (1978). Additive, multiplicative, and other models for disease risks. *American Journal of Epidemiology, 108*(5), 341–346. available from: PM:727202.

Index

A
Additive measurement error, 34, 39

B
Backdoor principle, 197
Bayesian analysis, 23, 47, 138, 141
Berkson measurement error, 37
Best subset, 11, 12
Bias, 7, 11, 21, 34–36, 38, 40, 41, 47, 57–70, 100, 108, 125–128, 131, 132, 136, 173, 182, 183, 245, 256, 257, 264
Binomial distribution, 95, 96, 111, 293
Biomarkers, 33, 41, 49, 209, 210, 218

C
Casemix, 117, 119, 120, 123, 131–133, 136, 137
Classical measurement error, 36–37, 40, 42
Collider, 3, 4, 196–198
Confounding, 1–12, 34, 41, 58, 61, 65, 76, 119, 126, 132, 146, 174, 176, 178, 186, 196, 198, 243–250, 253, 255–257, 291, 306

D
Differential measurement error, 34, 38
Directed acyclic graphs, 1, 2, 5, 12, 47, 59, 60, 125, 126, 191–202
Direct effects, 196, 256

E
Errors-in-variables, 33, 46, 207, 213

G
Gene-environment interaction, 41, 291–293, 306–309
Generalised additive models, 128, 261–277, 279
G-estimation, 243–257
Growth mixtures models, 223–239

H
Hierarchical linear models, 75

I
Indirect effects, 195, 196, 256
Instrumental variables, 42, 43, 46, 48
Interaction, 25, 41, 79, 87, 126–128, 131, 192, 211, 224, 257, 261, 262, 271, 275, 279–284, 290–310

L
Latent class analysis, 117, 137
Latent classes, 46, 90, 97, 98, 106–109, 112, 117–138, 224, 225, 228–235, 237–239
Latent growth curve models, 205–220, 225
Latent variable methods, 46, 97, 124, 138, 185, 199–121, 206, 211
Logistic regression, 21, 35, 36, 43, 44, 48, 66, 88, 97, 138, 176, 192, 233, 246, 249, 251–253, 264, 271, 292, 293, 301

M
MAR. *See* Missing at random (MAR)
Markov chain Monte Carlo methods (MCMC), 24, 29, 47, 48, 73, 88–89, 144–145, 148, 163, 165

MCAR. *See* Missing completely at random (MCAR)
MCMC. *See* Markov chain Monte Carlo methods (MCMC)
Measurement error
  bias, 33–49, 126, 127, 131, 182, 183, 305
  loss of power, 33, 35, 40
  mechanisms, 37
Meta-analysis, 90, 173–187
Missing at random (MAR), 16–27, 30, 264, 284
Missing completely at random (MCAR), 16, 18–20
Missing data, 15–23, 25, 27–30, 46, 58, 133, 251
Missing Not At Random (MNAR), 17, 18, 20, 21, 30
MNAR. *See* Missing Not At Random (MNAR)
Mplus, 132, 206, 214, 216, 218, 219, 225, 230, 236–239
Multilevel modelling, 73–91, 121, 144, 205
Multilevel multiple imputation, 26–30
Multiple diseases, 81, 128, 292
Multiple imputation, 15–20, 23–30, 46
Multiplicative measurement error, 38, 41, 44
Multivariate disease mapping, 154
Multivariate random frailty effects model, 157–170

N
Non-differential measurement error, 34, 44
Nutrition epidemiology, 37, 41, 42

O
Over-dispersion, 96, 105, 108, 111, 147, 153

P
Performance evaluation, 111
Periodontal diseases, 73, 74, 77, 79, 209
Poisson distribution, 94–96, 100, 101, 104, 111, 112, 142, 143
Poisson spatial models, 142, 144, 147

Power, 33, 35, 40, 41, 46, 76, 138, 145, 182, 201, 216, 218, 230, 304, 308–309
Proportional hazards, 43, 45, 162, 252, 253, 257
Pseudo-randomisation, 117

Q
Quadrature, 46, 48

R
Random effects modelling, 77, 90, 123, 136, 143, 147, 150, 157, 159, 161, 163, 165, 170, 205, 211, 276
Random measurement error, 38, 42
Regression calibration, 38, 43–45, 47
Regression tree, 279–281, 284–286, 289, 290
Replicate samples, 42, 47

S
Selection bias, 57–70, 177, 245
SIMEX. *See* Simulation-extrapolation (SIMEX)
Simulation-extrapolation (SIMEX), 45–46
Spatial models, 114, 142–144, 147, 160, 162, 163, 165, 166, 170
Splines, 216, 224, 261, 269–273, 275, 276
Structural equation models, 47, 138, 154, 191–202, 205–208, 212–217, 219, 220, 224, 230, 309
Surrogate measures of exposure, 41
Survival analysis, 245, 251, 252, 254, 255
Systematic measurement error, 37, 42, 58

T
Time-varing covariate, 244, 246, 253

V
Validation samples, 41, 42, 44, 47

Z
Zero-inflated models, 93–114